Physical Activity and the Gastro-Intestinal Tract

The organs of the gastro-intestinal tract play an essential role in sustained physical activity, but their consideration in exercise-related literature has, to this point, been limited. *Physical Activity and the Gastro-Intestinal Tract* is the first book to explain the function and response to exercise of the gastro-intestinal system, in cases of both health and disease, and helps to shed light on the role they play in acute and chronic exercise.

Professor Roy Shephard synthesises previously disparate research to explain the physiology, function, pathology of disease and role of exercise in both health and chronic disease, covering topics including:

- physical activity and the oesophagus;
- gastro-duodenal function and physical activity;
- physical activity and peptic ulcers;
- physical activity and gastro-oesophageal cancers;
- physical activity and the function of the large bowel;
- physical activity and chronic intestinal inflammation.

With each chapter including a thorough bibliography and signposts to further reading, *Physical Activity and the Gastro-Intestinal Tract* provides a complete reference for understanding how exercise affects the function of the digestive organs. It is an important text for academics and upper-level students in sports medicine and exercise physiology, and for health professionals in preventative medicine.

Roy J. Shephard is Professor Emeritus of Applied Physiology in the Faculty of Kinesiology & Physical Education at the University of Toronto, Canada. He was Director of the School of Physical and Health Education (now the Faculty of Kinesiology & Physical Education) at the University of Toronto for 12 years (1979–1991), and he served as Director of the University of Toronto Graduate Programme in Exercise Sciences from 1964 to 1985.

Routledge Research in Physical Activity and Health

The *Routledge Research in Physical Activity and Health* series offers a multi-disciplinary forum for cutting-edge research in the broad area of physical activity, exercise and health. Showcasing the work of emerging and established scholars working in areas ranging from physiology and chronic disease, psychology and mental health to physical activity and health promotion and socio-economic and cultural aspects of physical activity participation, the series is an important channel for groundbreaking research in physical activity and health.

Physical Activity and the Gastro-Intestinal Tract
Responses in health and disease
Roy J. Shephard

Physical Activity and the Gastro-Intestinal Tract

Responses in health and disease

Roy J. Shephard

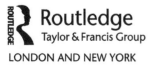

Routledge
Taylor & Francis Group

LONDON AND NEW YORK

First published 2017 by Routledge

2 Park Square, Milton Park, Abingdon, Oxon OX14 4RN

605 Third Avenue, New York, NY 10017

Routledge is an imprint of the Taylor & Francis Group, an informa business

First issued in paperback 2021

British Library Cataloguing in Publication Data
A catalogue record for this book is available from the British Library

Library of Congress Cataloging in Publication Data
Names: Shephard, Roy J., author.
Title: Physical activity and the gastro-intestinal tract : responses in health
and disease / Roy J. Shephard.
Description: Milton Park, Abingdon, Oxon ; New York, NY : Routledge,
2017. | Series: Routledge research in physical activity and health | Includes
bibliographical references and index.
Identifiers: LCCN 2016035809| ISBN 9781138244146 (hbk) | ISBN
9781315277103 (ebk)
Subjects: LCSH: Stomach–Diseases. | Physical fitness. | Exercise.
Classification: LCC RD540 .S484 2017 | DDC 617.4/3–dc23
LC record available at https://lccn.loc.gov/2016035809

ISBN: 978-1-138-24414-6 (hbk)
ISBN: 978-0-367-35452-7 (pbk)

Typeset in Times New Roman
by Wearset Ltd, Boldon, Tyne and Wear

Contents

Tables

x *Tables*

Preface

Since the burgeoning of sports science in the 1960s, a vast amount has been written concerning the acute and chronic exercise responses of the muscles and the cardio-respiratory system, but relatively little attention has been directed to the effects of physical activity upon the gastro-intestinal tract and other visceral organs. For instance, the index to the *Olympic Textbook of Science in Sport*[1] contains entries pointing to brief comments on liver glycogen and colon cancer, but there is no substantive mention of the oesophagus, the stomach, other aspects of hepatic or intestinal function, the kidneys and bladder, the gall bladder or the spleen. The muscles provide the immediate motive force for the athlete, and the cardiorespiratory system plays an essential immediate role in delivering oxygen and nutrients to the working muscles. However, sustained physical activity would not be possible without the contribution of the gastro-intestinal tract and the viscera. The fluid needed to dissipate heat, the energy provided by ingested fats and carbohydrates, and the essential amino acids needed for muscle hypertrophy are all delivered to the body via the gastro-intestinal tract. Critical steps in the provision of the prime energy source of glucose to the active muscles (glycolysis and gluconeogenesis) depend largely upon metabolic processes within the liver, and the regulation of fluid balance and the excretion of many unwanted by-products of metabolism depend upon the healthy functioning of the kidneys. Moreover, the function of the gut and many of the visceral organs is strongly influenced by a vigorous bout of physical activity, and a clear understanding of the impact of exercise upon the gastro-intestinal tract and the viscera is important to both the optimizing of athletic performance and enhancing the health of the general population.

Reasons why investigators have focussed upon the muscles and the cardiorespiratory system are not difficult to discern. Indices of gastro-intestinal and visceral function are less readily available, hampering evaluations of the response of these organs to physical activity. Further, the actions of the heart and lungs can be summarized by single and obvious primary measures of performance (the cardiac output and the respiratory minute volume, respectively), whereas the various segments of the gut and the viscera have multiple functions that cannot readily be represented by a single test measurement.

It is nevertheless important to bring together available information on the internal organs of the body, considering first their normal function and then examining how this is modified not only by various intensities and durations of acute physical activity, but also by repeated exercise sessions, whether the moderate training of the community fitness centre, the intensive preparation of the top athlete or the complex stresses of international competition itself. Both acute and chronic exercise can present not only benefits but also challenges to competitive performance and health status. Adverse consequences are particularly likely if intensive exercise is pushed to the point where most of the available cardiac output is directed to the claims of the muscles (for nutrients and oxygen) and the skin (for heat dissipation), leaving the gut and other viscera dangerously deprived of their normal blood supply.

As in most areas of physiology, much of the available information has been collected on men. However, where comparisons between the sexes have been drawn, few differences have so far been discovered. Studies range from small-scale experiments looking at physiological responses to the ingestion, metabolism and excretion of test substances to major epidemiological evaluations of large populations exploring changes in the risk of cancer and other chronic health conditions. The latter type of research has called for the careful selection of test groups, and not always completely successful attempts have been made to allow for the competing adverse health effects of such lifestyle factors as smoking history and alcohol consumption. Such studies have also required classification of an individual's habitual physical activity; until recently, this has involved using questionnaires with a limited reliability and validity, but there is now a growing tendency to replace questionnaires by objective monitors such as accelerometers.[2] Occasionally, there is recourse to evidence from animal experimentation, which facilitates biopsy and post-mortem examination of the internal organs, although caution is needed in applying such findings to humans, in part because of differences in body size and life span, and in part because the activity of the animals has often been enforced (for example by swimming to avoid drowning or running to escape and electrical shock).

The information that is presented in this text begins where possible with a brief sketch of early research, but the account is carried through to include the latest scientific articles, which are detailed in extensive bibliographies to each chapter. Conclusions are drawn using a minimum of technical jargon, so that the findings should be accessible not only to research investigators and students in sports medicine and kinesiology, but also to coaches, trainers and intelligent athletes.

The original plan was to summarize all of our current knowledge on responses to physical activity in both the gut and the other viscera in a single volume. However, as the writing of the book progressed, it became clear that the resulting text was becoming too large and cumbersome. In discussion with the publishers, I thus decided to focus a first volume on the reactions of the oesophagus, stomach, small and large intestines in health and disease, leaving to a later occasion discussion of similar issues for the liver, gall bladder, kidneys, urinary bladder, prostate and spleen.

I myself have learned much about a badly neglected area of sport and exercise science as the project has proceeded. I hope this will also be your experience.

Roy J. Shephard

Brackendale, BC, 2016

References

1 Maughan RJ. *The Olympic textbook of science in sport.* Oxford, UK, Wiley-Blackwell, 2009, pp. 1–426.
2 Shephard RJ, Tudor-Locke C. *The objective monitoring of physical activity: Contributions of accelerometry to epidemiology, exercise science and rehabilitation.* Dordrecht, Netherlands, Springer, 2016.

1   The classification of physical activity

This brief introductory chapter proposes a general categorization of physical activity that is appropriate to each of the topics discussed in this book. The impact of physical activity upon athletic performance, gastro-intestinal function and any related aspect of health depends upon the type of activity that is undertaken, and its pattern of intensity, frequency and duration.[1] We will thus define each of these key terms.

Types of physical activity

Physical activity implies any type of body movement produced by the skeletal muscles that results in a substantial increase in an individual's energy expenditure. The main potential components are the physical demands of occupational work, active physical leisure, exercise, sport and domestic chores, with occupational activity and leisure pursuits figuring largely in epidemiological studies.

Occupational work. The importance of occupational work to average daily energy expenditures has diminished greatly over the past 50 years, as workers have moved from agriculture to service and office jobs. Occupational activity is commonly assessed by job title, or by questioning employees on the time spent sitting, standing, lifting or engaging in heavy work. One problem with the use of job titles is that the physical demands of many occupations have diminished progressively through mechanization and automation.

The attraction of occupational activity for the epidemiologist is that an activity of relatively known intensity has been maintained for four to six hours per day, five days a week, for many years. However, there are often large socio-economic and cultural differences between "heavy" and "sedentary" workers, including the area of residence and features of lifestyle such as regular medical check-ups, smoking and alcohol consumption, and interest in and access to active leisure activities, and epidemiological analyses based on occupation must allow for these important covariates.

The standards of intensity also differ between occupational and leisure activity. Because heavy industrial work is sustained for 4–6 hours per day, and the pace is set by a supervisor, a machine or a conveyor belt, an energy expenditure of 31 kJ/min or more is judged as "very heavy" for a young or middle-aged worker. The situation may be further complicated by a task that involves only a small fraction of the body musculature, but requires maintenance of an awkward posture or involves exercise in a hot environment; such factors reduce the intensity of effort corresponding to a given intensity category.

Leisure activity. After work, a variable and growing period of commuting (usually passive, in a car, bus or train), completion of domestic chores and attention to personal hygiene, a typical person in developed societies now has three to four hours of "free" or discretionary time. This can be allocated between active and sedentary leisure pursuits and "do-it-yourself" tasks; automation of many domestic tasks is progressively increasing the discretionary component of daily life, but the growing cost of service industries is also increasing the need for many with smaller incomes to deal with household repairs. Although most epidemiologists have focussed on the active component of leisure time, some have also focussed on sedentary elements, such as the time spent watching television or working at a computer screen.

The volume of leisure activity is usually assessed by questionnaires that have a limited reliability and validity; in some instances, the absolute volume of activity may be exaggerated by a factor of three. There is growing interest in a more objective approach, using devices such as pedometers, accelerometers and GPS monitors. However, these instruments also have their problems, not recording such activities as swimming and cycling, and not taking account of energy spent in climbing hills. All data also suffer from the problem that leisure activity involves personal choice, and is highly seasonal; findings are thus likely to be invalid unless spread over the entire year.

Exercise. Exercise is a specific type of physical activity that is performed repeatedly with a specific purpose in mind, such as preparation for competition, or the improvement of health and fitness. In many with forms of chronic ill-health, the recommended mode of exercise, its intensity, frequency and duration, and speed of progression are regulated by a physician or a qualified health professional. Often, such exercise is undertaken in a fitness or rehabilitation class, and it is then possible to ascertain the energy expended with reasonable precision.

Sport. In North America, involvement in sport usually implies athletic competition or the use of a specially constructed facility such as a ski resort. However, in some European publications the term "sport" has been used to embrace many forms of leisure activity such as walking and jogging, as in UNESCO's "Sport for all" programme. The categorization of subjects by sport participation is controversial, because selection for many sports is based upon body build (which in itself influences vulnerability to many conditions). Moreover, high-level sport participation is generally a feature of adolescence and young adulthood, and by middle age many former athletes have become fatter and less active than their non-athletic counterparts.

Household and other chores. Household chores are often neglected in considering total weekly energy expenditures. The automation of much domestic equipment has certainly reduced energy expenditures around the home, but substantial physical effort is still demanded for the care of dependents, both young children and the elderly. This task still falls mainly to women, and is not captured adequately by many of the popular physical activity questionnaires. A growing number of workers are adding active commuting (cycling or walking) to their daily activity; this is a form of activity that is not easily neglected, and can be quantitated rather precisely.

Patterns of physical activity

Intensity. Often, the intensity of aerobic effort is described in semantic terms, such as a "moderate" or "heavy" effort", "brisk walking" or "vigorous getting about", and sometimes there is a perceptual anchor such as "sufficiently vigorous activity to work up a sweat", or "heavy enough exercise to make conversation difficult". But in order to compare studies, it is helpful to quantitate such descriptions. The level of effort needed to undertake a given task depends on a person's physical condition, and aerobic activity is thus conveniently categorized as a percentage of the individual's maximal oxygen intake ($\dot{V}O_{2max}$). Sweating and breathlessness typically imply a sustained bout of effort at 60–70% of an individual's maximal oxygen intake.

For a typical 30-minute bout of activity involving the large muscle groups of the body, intensities range from resting (<10% of $\dot{V}O_{2max}$) through light exercise (<35% of $\dot{V}O_{2max}$) to fairly light (<50% of $\dot{V}O_{2max}$), moderate (<70% of $\dot{V}O_{2max}$) and heavy (>70% of $\dot{V}O_{2max}$) to near maximal effort (100% $\dot{V}O_{2max}$, an intensity that can only be sustained for a few minutes). The oxygen intake can be measured directly when exercising maximally and when performing the activity of interest, but in epidemiological studies inferences are more usually drawn from the heart rate, expressed as a percentage of maximal heart rate.

Some authors have chosen to present their data in absolute rather than relative units (for instance, a measured or estimated energy expenditure, measured in kJ/min) or as metabolic equivalents (METs, ratios to resting metabolism), but then the categorization of intensity must take account of the fact that the maximal oxygen intake of a 65-year-old is only about a half of that found in a 20-year-old. Possible intensities for a young adult range from 1 to 13 METs, or 5.2 to 67.6 kJ/min, and in a 65-year-old the range is from 1 to 7 METs, or from 5.2 to 36.4 kJ/min. Furthermore, at any age the percentages corresponding to each descriptor diminish if the duration of exercise is extended for more than a few minutes, as for example when industrial activity is considered.

Frequency. The frequency of activity is commonly reported as the number of times a given form of activity is practised per week. However, this type of recording ignores the seasonal nature of many leisure pursuits. Preferably, the investigator should record the number of times the activity was performed in the past week or the past month, and overcome the problem of seasonal variations by questioning various members of the test sample at differing points during the year.

It is commonly assumed that to have an effect upon health, a bout of physical activity must have a minimum duration. At one time, note was only taken of periods longer than 15 or 30 minutes, but there is now growing recognition that some benefits can accrue from the accumulation of several short bouts as from a single 30-minute session at the same intensity of effort (for example, 3 activity periods of 10-minute durations) over the course of a day. This is particularly true of responses that are linked to a reduction of body fat. Inevitably, fat losses are linked to the cumulative increase of energy expenditure over the course of a day. Moreover, there is a continuing increase of energy expenditure for some minutes following a period of vigorous energy expenditure, and it is conceivable that this effect can be augmented if the day's physical activities are split into several segments.

Duration. The duration of exercise is usually recorded in minutes, but it is important to ensure that when this is reported a person includes only active time, omitting such factors as travelling to and from a gymnasium, changing and showering, discussions of exercise technique with a coach, and socializing with other exercisers.

Muscular versus aerobic activity. Muscular exercise is less often categorized than aerobic activity, although regular exercise for each of the main muscle groups of the body makes an important contribution to health. The intensity of a given isometric effort can be categorized as a percentage of the intensity of effort a person can make on a single occasion (the one-repetition maximum), and the cumulative stimulus can be expressed on this basis (for instance, 3 sets of 10 repetitions at 60% of 1 RM effort). Such information is sometimes available for participants in specific muscle-building programmes, but is rarely documented in population studies of physical activity.

Conclusions

Clarification of the effects of regular physical activity upon the normal functioning and health of the gastro-intestinal tract is dependent in part on a uniform and preferably objective categorization of activities between the studies performed in different laboratories. This chapter introduces methods of classifying the type of activity (occupational, leisure, exercise, sport, domestic and household chores) and its pattern (intensity, frequency and duration), noting also that muscular effort is often ignored in epidemiological assessments.

Reference

1 Bouchard C, Shephard RJ. Physical activity, fitness, and health: The model and key concepts. In: *Physical activity, fitness and health*. Bouchard C, Shephard RJ, Stephens T. (eds). Champaign, IL, Human Kinetics, 1992, pp. 77–88.

2 Physical activity and the oesophagus

Oesophageal motility and issues of gastro-oesophageal reflux

Introduction

When a person swallows, the ingested food or fluid passes through the oesophagus (gullet) and on into the stomach because of a sequential wave of motility, coordinated by the medulla oblongata and vagal innervation. At the upper end of the oesophagus, a muscular sphincter is normally kept closed, to prevent the swallowing of air during breathing. At the lower end, a second sphincter is also normally closed, restricting the reflux of acid and bile from the stomach into the oesophagus. During swallowing, a wave of contraction (peristalsis) passes along the length of the oesophageal wall at a speed of about 2 m/s, propelling the fluid or food forward, and the lower oesophageal sphincter relaxes briefly as food reaches the entrance to the stomach.[1] Disorders in this process lead to difficulties in swallowing (dysphagia) and chest pain as acid is regurgitated from the stomach and encounters the oesophageal wall.[2]

Physiology texts provide relatively little information as to how physical activity affects the behaviour of the oesophagus. Although many endurance athletes ingest nutritious fluids while they are actually competing, there are only a few studies concerning the effects of sport participation upon the mechanics of the healthy oesophagus.[3-8] Indeed, the classical and comprehensive review of Ingelfinger[1] made no reference to any changes in oesophageal function that might be brought about by exercise.

In this chapter, we look at available information on oesophageal function during exercise, including a possible increase in the risk of gastro-oesophageal reflux during vigorous physical activity, and the clinical problems caused by such reflux are considered in some detail. We next discuss the possible value of moderate exercise in preventing reflux, and the risks of increased reflux associated with vigorous physical activity and athletic participation. Recommendations are made for the treatment of this condition, and note is taken of the potentially serious complications, including oesophageal ulceration and haemorrhage, a permanent narrowing (stricture) of the oesophagus, a squamous cell metaplasia of the oesophageal lining and the development of an oesophageal adenocarcinoma.

Effects of physical activity upon oesophageal motility

Six studies detailed below have all pointed to a decrease of oesophageal motility in response to an acute bout of physical activity, with the greatest effects being seen at the highest intensities of effort (around 90% of maximal aerobic capacity).

Soffer *et al.*[9,10] evaluated the effects of graded exercise in a sample of 6 well-trained cyclists. Their protocol required 1 hour of exercise at 60% of maximal oxygen intake, followed by 45 minutes at 75% of maximal oxygen intake, and 10 minutes at 90% of maximum effort. The duration, frequency and amplitude of oesophageal contractions all declined as the intensity of exercise was increased, to become statistically significant when subjects were cycling at 90% of maximal aerobic effort. Episodes of gastro-oesophageal reflux, and the duration of acid exposure of the oesophagus were also increased when subjects were exercising at 90% of their maximal oxygen intake. Plasma concentrations of the hormones gastrin, motilin, glucagon, pancreatic polypeptide and vasoactive intestinal polypeptide were all monitored, but the decreases in oesophageal motility seemed to be independent of changes in the blood levels of these agents. Soffer *et al.* speculated that the cause of the observed changes might be an exercise-induced reduction in the volume of saliva swallowed, or a decrease of local blood flow to the oesophagus.

The same investigators made a parallel study of 9 untrained individuals who exercised on a cycle ergometer at intensities demanding 45%, 60%, 75% and 90% of their peak oxygen intakes.[11] Again, the amplitude, duration and frequency of oesophageal contractions decreased during physical activity, with the changes becoming statistically significant when the subjects were exercising at 90% of their peak heart rates (the equivalent of about 93% of maximal oxygen intake).

Van Nieuwenhoven *et al.*[12] had a group of 10 subjects cycle at a loading that was decreased gradually from 70% to 60% of their maximal short-term work rate over a period of 90 minutes. The peristaltic velocity in the oesophagus was increased by about a quarter while the subjects were cycling, However, the number of contractions over an unspecified interval (probably 90 minutes) was reduced from a resting average of 68 to only 24, and the duration of contractions and the peristaltic pressure were also somewhat decreased during this activity.

Choi *et al.*[13] exercised their subjects on a treadmill at 40% and 70% of their maximal heart rates. At the higher of the two intensities of effort, they found a decrease in both the frequency and the pressure of oesophageal contractions. Further, there were then significant increases in the number of reflux episodes and the duration of exposure of the oesophagus to acids.

Ravi *et al.*[14] examined changes in oesophageal motility with moderate treadmill exercise (walking at a speed of 5.2 km/h) in 135 individuals, including normal subjects, a group with high amplitude peristaltic waves (termed the "nutcracker" group), a group with diffuse oesophageal spasm and a group with frank gastro-oesophageal reflux disease (GERD). Standardized boluses of water were ingested while they were undertaking this activity. The normal, nutcracker and GERD groups all showed a decrease of peristaltic amplitude when walking, and those with oesophageal spasm showed a similar (but statistically non-significant) trend to less peristalsis. Gastro-oesophageal reflux was provoked in 13 of the 75 patients with GERD, despite the relatively mild intensity of effort.

Budzyński *et al.*[15] examined 63 patients with recurrent angina-like pain that was unresponsive to the reduction of gastric acid secretion by the administration of proton-pump inhibitor drugs. Performance of a Bruce treadmill test caused a decrease in the amplitude and effectiveness of oesophageal peristalsis in this group of individuals.

The distinction between gastro-oesophageal reflux (GER) and gastro-oesophageal reflux disease (GERD)

The disturbances of oesophageal motility induced by vigorous physical activity predispose to occasional regurgitation of some of the gastric contents into the oesophagus (gastro-oesophageal reflux, GER). GER is an almost universal phenomenon, particularly immediately after a person has eaten. The clinician only makes the more serious diagnosis of GERD if repeated gastro-oesophageal reflux is causing an excessive exposure of the oesophagus to gastric acids, with disturbing symptoms and the potential for mucosal injury and more serious long-term complications.

Uncertainties and disagreement around diagnostic criteria have hampered a clear distinction between GER and GERD, and thus consistent estimates of the prevalence of GER and GERD. In developed countries, the reported incidence of GER under resting conditions has ranged from 9% (in Italy) to 42% (in the USA).[16] Even more frequent GER has been reported during some forms of vigorous exercise.

Progression of GER to GERD adversely affects the individual's quality of life, with serious potential complications that include oesophageal ulceration (2 to 7% patients), oesophageal haemorrhage (<2%), oesophageal stricture (4 to 20%), metaplasia of the stratified squamous epithelium (Barrett's oesophagus, 10 to 15%), and the development of a very deadly oesophageal adenocarcinoma (0.5%).[17-21] However, with these important exceptions, GERD does not affect a person's survival prospects.[22]

Underlying anatomy and physiology

GER plainly results from a malfunction of the lower oesophageal sphincter. The action of this sphincter in preventing reflux of the stomach contents is normally reinforced by the restraints of the diaphragmatic crura and the phreno- oesophageal ligament.[23] Patients with GER show more frequent transient relaxations of the lower oesophageal sphincter than healthy individuals.[24] Oesophageal motility is ineffective, there is a loss of muscular tone in the lower oesophageal sphincter,[25] and a chronic malfunction of the normal gastro-oesophageal barrier.[26]

Reflux of the gastric contents into the proximal part of the oesophagus is important in increasing the severity of GER symptoms, and such reflux seems more likely to develop under ambulatory than under sedentary conditions.[27]

Factors predisposing to GER

Genetic and demographic factors may predispose an individual to GER. Links have also been suggested to obesity and other lifestyle variables, as well as to specific pathologies.

Genetic and demographic influences. A large Swedish twin study found heritability accounted for 31% of the liability to GERD.[28,29] Thus the common assertion of some paediatricians that a child will "grow out" of GER is not always warranted.[30,31] Several authors have noted that the prevalence of both GER and GERD is greater in women than in men,[32,33] increases with age[34,35] and is associated with a low educational level.[32,33] In one Swedish sample, the prevalence of GER in men peaked at an age of 50 to 70 years, but in women it continued to increase into old age.[36]

Lifestyle. Obesity and/or weight gain are usually considered as important risk factors for the GER that is seen under resting conditions,[25,32,37-52] and a measure of the central accumulation of body fat (a person's abdominal circumference) is closely linked to the severity of GERD.[53] In one report, severe obesity translated to a 3.3-fold increase in the risk of GER in men, and a 6.3-fold increase in women.[54] However, one questionnaire-based study of 820 Swedes, 135 with symptoms of GER, failed to find the generally accepted association with obesity; reasons for this anomaly remain unclear.[55]

In most studies, obesity has persisted as a risk factor after adjusting for the influence of multiple covariates.[32,56] Presumably because blood concentrations of the hormone ghrelin are inversely associated with obesity, there is also an inverse association between ghrelin levels, GER and GERD.[57]

Obesity seems to increase the prevalence of GER and GERD through a wide variety of mechanisms that include altered oesophageal and gastric motility, increased levels of sex hormones, increased intra-gastric[47,58] and intra-abdominal[39] pressures, and a deficit of the parasympathetic activity that normally keeps the tonus of the oesophagus higher than that of the stomach.[59] The action of regurgitated gastric acid can activate T-cells in the submucosal layers of the oesophagus, liberating cytokines that cause abnormalities of immune function.[60]

Some (but not all) investigators have found associations of GERD with other adverse lifestyle factors, including smoking,[33,38,43,48,61-64] a heavy consumption of alcohol,[48,61,63,65] and an excessive intake of salt.[62]

Association of reflux with other pathologies. GER and GERD have occasionally been linked with other pathologies, including psycho-social obesity and stress,[66] a poor quality of sleep and irregular dietary habits,[67] the irritable bowel syndrome,[68] non-alcoholic fatty liver disease,[69] and high serum levels of total cholesterol and triglycerides.[70]

Diagnosis and differential diagnosis of GERD

Diagnosis. Pathological gastro-oesophageal reflux may occur when a patient is erect, supine or both.[71] Diagnostic features differentiating GERD from GER include a drop in oesophageal pH below a value of 4.0 that is sustained for 10 seconds or longer and/or the presence of oesophageal spasm in more than 55% of spontaneous oesophageal contractions.[72] Observation during a one-hour period of dynamic changes in posture may be helpful in diagnosing ambiguous cases.[73] Often, GERD is unrelated to either meals or physical activity. It may occur at night, with two or more episodes of severe heartburn per week; such symptoms can adversely affect a person's well-being.

Any form of vigorous exertion can precipitate GER. Several reports examining the prevalence of GER during competitive events have unfortunately based their diagnosis upon the response to questionnaires such as the gastro-intestinal symptom-rating scale[74] which tally a range of epigastric complaints. Upper abdominal complaints are common in the endurance athlete, but they do not necessarily reflect the presence of GERD or even GER. One study of 25,640 triathlon participants noted reports of nausea, epigastric pain or vomiting in 8.9% of those who were questioned.[75] Often, such symptoms certainly reflect some degree of GER, but other possible causes include an excessive ingestion of "replacement" fluids, an exercise-induced slowing of gastric emptying, and a reduction of visceral blood flow with gastric or myocardial ischaemia.

About a third of GERD cases show an associated oesophagitis.[76] However, endoscopy and barium studies are not particularly helpful in looking for chronic inflammation of the oesophageal lining. Nor is diagnosis of GERD made easy by using oesophageal pressure manometers or barium ingestion to evaluate changes in local motility.[77-79] Better options include a decrease of symptoms in response to a decrease of gastric acid, brought about by the administration of high doses of a proton-pump inhibiting drug such as omeprazole for one week,[80] or the detection of gastric acid reflux by the continuous 24-hour monitoring of oesophageal pH.[81,82]

Differential diagnosis of GERD. GERD must be differentiated not only from the less serious condition of GER but also from other painful exercise-related conditions such as angina pectoris and visceral ischaemia, as well as the vague symptomatology associated with an overall dysfunction of visceral pain perception. One study concluded that less than a tenth of patients with a combination of chest pain and angiographically normal coronary arteries showed objective evidence of GERD.[83]

The differentiation of GERD from angina is not always an easy task, particularly when the epigastric pain is associated with periods of vigorous exercise.[7,15,80,84-88] The distal part of the oesophagus and the heart share a common afferent nerve pathway, and thus pain from either location is sensed over similar areas of the body surface. Moreover, acid stimulation of the oesophagus may precipitate a reflex spasm of the coronary arteries,[89,90] thus causing a combination of GERD and angina. The phenomenon of reflex spasm can be simulated by the deliberate instillation of 0.1 M hydrochloric acid into the oesophagus, but it is not seen in patients with denervated hearts (for instance, after cardiac transplantation). A study of 52 patients with angina pectoris found that 11 of the 52 individuals also had a high 24-h gastro-oesophageal reflux score; 10 of this group and 13 other patients all showed GER during performance of a Bruce treadmill test.[91]

Vigorous exercise induces a massive redistribution of blood flow from the viscera to the muscles and the skin. The resulting gastric ischaemia is one potential cause of severe epigastric pain,[92,93] although a reduction of local blood flow to the oesophagus may also be causing oesophageal dysfunction and thus GER.

Nevertheless, many acute episodes of atypical chest pain bear no apparent relationship to either a drop in oesophageal pH or to electrocardiographic abnormalities that would indicate a transient cardiac ischaemia. It has been suggested that a dysfunction of overall visceral perception leading to a low pain threshold may then be responsible.[100]

Acute effects of moderate and vigorous physical activity upon GER

Moderate physical activity and GER

There have been nine reports examining the acute effects of moderate physical activity upon the likelihood of developing gastro-oesophageal reflux[11,13,14,94–99] (see Table 2.1). With the exception of questionnaire observations on a post-dinner walk in 1825 Pakistanis,[95] all investigators have followed quite small groups of individuals, assessing the extent of gastro-oesophageal reflux objectively, by pH monitoring and/or manometry. Most authors have found little evidence of GER except with efforts at toe-touching,[98] and often moderate exercise (at an intensity of 70% of maximal oxygen intake or less) has even led to small improvements in gastro-oesophageal function.

Steady walking after a meal decreased the likelihood of GER by 17% during the first hour,[94] although the same subjects obtained a larger benefit simply from chewing gum. A multivariate analysis of the Pakistani data[95] showed that a post-dinner walk of unspecified length reduced the risk of GER by 34% relative to lying supine after a meal; in this study, benefit was also seen with a post-dinner interval of at least 3 hours before lying down to sleep.

Choi et al.[13] found that treadmill walking at 40% of maximal heart rate had no impact upon the likelihood of GER following a meal. Mendes-Filho et al.[96] used a pH meter and manometry to examine 29 patients with erosive and 10 patients with non-erosive GERD; light or brief exercise did not cause gastro-oesophageal reflux in this sample. Soffer et al.[11] had 9 untrained Americans perform cycle ergometry at 45%, 60% and 75% of their $\dot{V}O_{2peak}$, and again GER was not increased by exercise over this range of exercise intensities. Schoeman et al.[97] found that only 2 of 123 episodes of GER were associated with 10-minute bouts of either "*steady*" or "*rapid-as-possible*" treadmill walking. Another study

Table 2.1 Relationships between moderate physical activity and gastro-oesophageal reflux

Author	Population	Exercise	Diagnosis	Finding
Avidan et al.[94]	12 adults with GERD, 24 healthy	60 min of steady walking	pH monitoring	17% reduction in acid contact time in GERD group during 1st hr after meal
Choi et al.[13]	12 healthy males	Treadmill exercise at 40% and 70% of maximal heart rate after a meal	pH monitoring and manometry	Number and duration of reflux episodes, time when pH <4 all increased with exercise at >70% max heart rate
Karim et al.[95]	1875 Pakistanis (689 with GERD)	Post-dinner walk	Questionnaire	34% reduction of risk of reflux with post-dinner walk
Mendes-Filho et al.[96]	29 patients with erosive GERD, 10 with non-erosive GERD	Cycle ergometry	pH monitoring and manometry	Light or brief exercise did not cause reflux; reflux in erosive group with exercise at >70% $\dot{V}O_{2max}$
Ravi et al.[14]	135 untrained Irish adults	Treadmill walk, 1 km/h, then 5 min at 4.2 km/h	pH monitoring and manometry	Oesophageal pressures reduced during exercise; reflux in 13/75 patients with GERD
Schoeman et al.[97]	10 healthy Australians	10 min treadmill walking and 10 min rapid walking	pH monitoring and manometry	Relaxation of lower oesophageal sphincter not increased by walking or moderately vigorous exercise
Sodhi et al.[98]	25 patients with GERD	Toe touching from supine, sitting and standing positions	pH monitoring	Bending exercise provokes GER
Soffer et al.[11]	9 untrained Americans	Cycle ergometry at 45%, 60% and 75% of $\dot{V}O_{2peak}$	pH monitoring	GER not increased when exercising to 75% of $\dot{V}O_{2peak}$
Worobetz et al.[99]	6 healthy male athletes	120 min treadmill exercise at 50% of peak aerobic power	Manometry	Immediately post-exercise, increase in lower oesophageal sphincter pressure, no change of oesophageal motility

Abbreviations: GER = gastro-oesophageal reflux; GERD = gastro-oesophageal reflux disease; $\dot{V}O_{2peak}$ = peak oxygen intake; $\dot{V}O_{2max}$ = maximal oxygen intake.

found that walking at a pace of 4.2 km/h while engaging in wet swallows induced GER in only 13 of 75 subjects with known GERD.[14] Finally, Worobetz *et al.*[99] had 6 healthy male athletes perform 120 minutes of treadmill exercise at 50% of peak aerobic power; immediately post-exercise, they observed an increase in pressure at the lower oesophageal sphincter, while oesophageal motility remained unchanged.

Vigorous physical activity and GER

Vigorous physical activity generally provokes a decrease in the amplitude and effectiveness of oesophageal contractions and a decrease of oesophageal pressures.[15] Moreover, it is often associated with an increase of GER.[11,13,96,101–103] Both the prevalence and the duration of GER increase with the intensity of effort,[9,11,13,74,103,104] the threshold for the development of GER commonly being exercise that demands around 70% of the individual's $\dot{V}O_{2max}$.[101,104–107]

In one somewhat unlikely competitive scenario, exercise was performed at 70% of maximal heart rate only 30 minutes after a meal. In this situation, physical activity led to disorganized oesophageal contractions, increases in the number and duration of gastro-oesophageal reflux episodes, and the oesophageal pH remained below 4.0[13] for a longer time. Most reports have described decreases in oesophageal sphincter pressures as the intensity of cycle ergometer exercise was increased beyond 70% of the individual's peak aerobic power,[3,6,9,11,102,108,109] but one laboratory reported that 2 hours of treadmill running at 50% of maximal oxygen intake induced a modest increase of pressure at the lower oesophageal sphincter.[99,110] Van Nieuwenhoven *et al.*[12] also saw an increase of oesophageal peristaltic velocity when their subjects were operating a cycle ergometer at 70–90% of $\dot{V}O_{2max}$.

In addition to the mechanical factors predisposing to GER during vigorous exercise, other potential causes of abdominal symptoms include a reduced gastro-intestinal blood flow, a slowing of gastric emptying, air-swallowing,[102] an increase in intra-abdominal pressures,[87] and increases in the plasma concentration of hormones such as catecholamines.[99] However, *Soffer et al.* found no relationship between GER during exercise and the levels of hormones such as gastrin, motilin, glucagon, pancreatic polypeptide or vasoactive intestinal peptide.[9]

At least 15 reports have made laboratory evaluations of the effects of vigorous physical activity upon the incidence of GER[9,12,13,91,96,97,101–105,107,108,111,112] (see Table 2.2). All of these investigations have included an objective monitoring of oesophageal pH, and most have noted an increased risk of reflux.

Plainly, a substantial proportion of athletes who are symptom-free at rest develop GER during vigorous exercise, and sometimes the resulting symptoms can be sufficiently severe to cause a deterioration of performance or even an abandonment of competition. Thus, Peters *et al.*[113] found that some participants dropped out of a 4-day walking event due to various gastro-intestinal symptoms that likely included some cases of GER, and Rodriguez-Stanley *et al.*[114]

demonstrated that the experimental infusion of 0.1 N hydrochloric acid into the oesophagus caused a deterioration in the treadmill test performance of well-trained runners relative to controls who received a sham infusion. Nevertheless, not all changes of performance can be blamed on GER. Indeed, one reviewer concluded that the most common cause of abdominal discomfort in exercising athletes was a local ischaemia of the gut wall rather than a reflux of gastric acid into the oesophagus.[115]

Studies of sport participation and GER

Fifteen field studies have looked at the symptoms developed during vigorous exercise and participation in athletic events.[74,75,106,110,112,113,116–124] All except one of these investigations[112] relied upon symptom questionnaires that did not always differentiate clearly between GER and other upper and lower abdominal complaints (see Table 2.3).Upper abdominal symptoms were found more commonly in women than in men, and more commonly in young than in older runners.[122] Some 8.9% of a large sample of 25,640 French triathletes reported symptoms such as nausea, epigastric pain or vomiting during competition.[75] Other observers have noted various types of gastro-intestinal complaints in around 50% of athletes during an event,[4,125,126] for example 83% of marathon runners,[122] 50% of ultramarathon participants,[116] 83% of participants in a 3-peaks mountain biking event (58% of these contestants reporting upper abdominal symptoms),[110] and 24% of subjects who walked for 4 days (a total distance of 203 km for the men, and 164 km for the women).[113] Nevertheless, in most of these studies, lower abdominal symptoms such as diarrhoea were more common than upper abdominal complaints likely to have arisen from GER.

Factors predisposing to GER in athletes

At any given intensity of effort, GER as monitored by oesophageal pH monitoring seems to be less frequent during cycle ergometry (where body movement is relatively limited) than if the body is oscillating (as in treadmill running),[101] or if a Valsalva manoeuvre is undertaken (as in weight-lifters,[104]). Nevertheless, GER can occur even in cyclists,[107] particularly if a stooped position is adopted,[124] and it also is seen in 70%[112] of rowers, where a raised intra-abdominal pressure is suggested as a causal factor.[110,119,126,127]

Exercise in the prone position predisposes to GER, and complaints are very common in surf-boarders, particularly if they use short boards.[74] The odds ratio of GERD (defined as episodes of GER >2 times per week) was 4.6 times higher in surfers than in non-surfer athletes, and the likelihood of GERD also increased with the frequency and duration of surfing. Ingestion of a meal[101,106,112] or a sports drink rather than water shortly before exercising[119] predisposes to GER. The problem also seems to be exacerbated by gastric distension and air swallowing.[128] Dehydration can also lead to gastro-intestinal complaints (although not necessarily GER) during distance running.[120]

Table 2.2 Relationships between vigorous exercise and gastro-oesophageal reflux as seen in experimental studies

Author	Population	Exercise	Diagnosis	Finding
Choi et al.[13]	12 healthy males	Treadmill exercise at 70% of maximal heart rate after a meal	pH monitoring and manometry	Number and duration of reflux episodes, time when pH <4 all increased with exercise at 70% max heart rate
Clark et al.[101]	12 asymptomatic Americans (7 M, 5 F)	15 min cycling, 15 min rowing 15 min weight routine	pH monitoring	Association greatest for running, less for cycling, some effect from weight-lifting
Collings et al.[104]	American athletes (10 runners, 10 cyclists, 10 weight-lifters)	Standardized exercise (60 min at 65% max, 20 min at 85% of max)	pH monitoring and symptom evaluation	Association greatest in weight-lifters; mild reflux in cyclists, moderate in runners
Kraus et al.[102]	14 American runners	60 min running	pH monitoring	Reflux increased relative to baseline during running, reduced by 300 mg dose of ranitidine
Maddison et al.[108]	5 M, 2 F asymptomatic recreational cyclists	Four 5-min bouts of exercise at 90% of $\dot{V}O_{2max}$	Measurements of oesophageal, gastric and sphincter pressures	High intensity exercise reduces sphincter pressures, response unaffected by ingestion of sport drinks
Mendes-Filho et al.[96]	29 patients with erosive GERD, 10 with non-erosive GERD	Cycle ergometry	pH monitor and manometry	No reflux in erosive group with exercise at >70% of $\dot{V}O_{2max}$
Motil et al.[103]	One athletic girl, aged 11 yrs	Treadmill stress test	pH monitoring	No GER** over 24 h rest, but induced by treadmill test
Pandolfino et al.[111]	20 Americans (10 with GERD)	30 min running and 30 min resistance exercise (intensity not specified)	Endoscopy and manometry	Exercise caused 3-fold increase of acid exposure in controls and in those with GERD

Study	Subjects	Exercise protocol	Method	Findings
Peters et al. [105]	7 Dutch triathletes	50 min of running and cycling at 75% of $\dot{V}O_{2max}$ with intake of sports drinks	pH monitoring	Percent reflux time greater if running than cycling; GERD increased by drinking, sports drink > water, before exercise
Schoeman et al. [97]	10 healthy Australians	10 min vigorous cycle ergometry, 10 min treadmill walking and 10 min rapid walking	pH monitor and manometry	Relaxation of lower oesophageal sphincter not increased by walking or moderately vigorous exercise
Schofield et al. [91]	52 patients with angina pectoris	Bruce treadmill test	pH monitoring and manometry	10/11 patients with high 24-h reflux score, 13 other patients all showed reflux during exercise
Soffer et al. [9]	8 trained American cyclists	Cycle ergometry, 1 h at 60%+45min at 75% and 10 min at 90% of $\dot{V}O_{2peak}$	pH monitoring	Oesophageal acid exposure increased when exercising at 90% of $\dot{V}O_{2max}$
van Nieuwenhoven et al. [12]	10 healthy males	Cycle ergometry at 70% of $\dot{V}O_{2max}$	pH monitoring and pressure sensors	Peristaltic velocity increased while cycling, but no change in GERD
van Nieuwenhoven et al. [107]	10 symptomatic, 10 asymptomatic athletes	90 min cycling and running at 70% of aerobic power	pH monitoring	GERD running > cycling; Symptomatic subjects had more frequent and longer lasting reflux
Yazaki et al. [112]	17 healthy adults	Rowing, fasted running, running after a meal	pH monitoring	Gastro-oesophageal reflux in 70% of rowers, 45% of fasted runners, 90% of fed runners

Abbreviations: F = female; GER = gastro-oesophageal reflux; GERD = gastro-oesophageal reflux disease; M = male; $\dot{V}O_{2max}$ = maximal oxygen intake.

Table 2.3 Relationships between vigorous exercise and abdominal symptoms and/or gastro-oesophageal reflux as seen in field studies of athletes

Author	Population	Exercise	Diagnosis	Finding
Glace et al.[116]	19 volunteers	160-km ultramarathon	Questionnaire	Gastro-intestinal symptoms in 50%
Józków et al.[118]	100 patients with GERD	3 levels of habitual physical activity	IPAQ questionnaire	Neither self-reported symptoms nor GER differed between 3 activity groups
Keeffe et al.[117]	707 marathoners	A "hard run"	Questionnaire	Heartburn 9.5%, nausea 11.6%, vomiting 1.8%
Lopez et al.[75]	25,640 triathlon participants	French triathlon competition	Questionnaire	8.9% had upper gastric symptoms (nausea, epigastric pain or vomiting)
Norisue et al.[74]	185 surfers, 178 athletic non-surfers		Questionnaire	Odds ratio of GER >2/week 4.6 in surfers; prevalence is also related to frequency and duration of surfing
Peters et al.[119]	185 long-distance runners, 173 cyclists and 149 triathletes	Recent sport participation	Questionnaire	Runners – mainly lower GI symptoms cyclists upper and lower GI symptoms, frequently caused drop-out
Peters et al.[113]	Long-distance walkers, 79 M, 76 F	Walk 203 km (M), 164 km (F) over 4 days	Questionnaire	24% reported symptoms, commonly nausea, headache and flatulence

Reference	Subjects	Event	Method	Findings
Rehrer et al.[106]	55 male triathletes	Half Iron-man triathlon	Questionnaire	52% reported eructation, 48% flatulence, symptoms greatest when running
Rehrer et al.[121]	172 ultra-endurance runners	67-km run with 1900 m change of altitude to highest point	Questionnaire	43% complained of gastro-intestinal distress
Riddoch et al.[122]	471 marathoners	Marathon run	Questionnaire	Heartburn in 13%, nausea in 20%, vomiting in 4%
Sullivan[123]	110 triathletes	Triathlon	Questionnaire	Heartburn, nausea and vomiting in 24%
Verbeek et al.[124]	196 rowers, 439 other athletes	Rowing events	Questionnaire	GER symptoms in 51% of rowers
Worobetz and Gerrard[110]	70 endurance runners	Dunedin "Enduro" event	Questionnaire	58% developed upper gastro-intestinal symptoms
Yamake et al.[112]	17 healthy adults	Rowing, fasted and postprandial running	pH monitoring	GER in 70% of rowers, 45% of fasted runners, 90% of fed runners

Abbreviations: F = female; GER = gastro-oesophageal reflux; GERD = gastro-oesophageal reflux disease; GI = gastro-intestinal; M = male.

Another adverse factor is a large increase of the thoraco-abdominal pressure gradient. This is particularly likely to be seen when a person with asthma undertakes vigorous physical activity.[129,130] In such individuals, the reflux of gastric acid into the oesophagus is likely to trigger coughing and/or an asthma attack, and thus a vicious cycle of increasing respiratory effort and greater GER.[131] It has even been suggested that GER is one cause of exercise-induced asthma.[132] Some investigators have found no relationship between the severity of exercise-induced bronchial spasm and either GER or the administration of proton inhibitors,[133-135] but others have observed a reduction in the frequency of night-time asthma[130] and exercise-induced asthma[132] following treatment with omeprazole, one proton inhibitor.

Role of habitual physical activity in the management of GER

The effects of habitual physical activity upon oesophageal function and GER can be examined by relating prevalence of the disorder to questionnaire assessments of leisure activity, by making comparisons between occupational categories with differing levels of energy expenditure, or correlating the prevalence of GER with assessments of aerobic fitness (using the latter as a surrogate of habitual physical activity).

Any apparent benefit from regular physical activity[41,62] could reflect in part the impact of increased physical activity upon other components of personal lifestyle such as obesity, smoking and stress.[41,52] Physical activity is significantly associated with a lean body build, and with abstinence from cigarettes. Moderate physical activity also seems likely to encourage a reduction of stress, but on the other hand intensive athletic competition could augment stress levels. Many (but not all) studies of habitual physical activity have largely eliminated the influence of other aspects of personal lifestyle through extensive multivariate analyses.

Habitual recreational physical activity and GER

At least 13 reports have examined associations between habitual recreational physical activity and the risk of developing GER.[29,36,38,44-46,49,63,67,118,136-138] In general, a several-level classification of an individual's habitual leisure activity has been based upon questionnaire responses, and in all except two studies from the same laboratory,[118,138] the diagnosis of GER and/or GERD was also based upon questionnaire responses (see Table 2.4).

Eight of the 13 studies[29,36,38,44,49,63,67,137] found that participation in regular moderate physical activity was associated with a decrease in risk, although the extent of benefit varied widely between investigations. One multivariate analysis of 345 men and 500 women that included body mass index, smoking and the use of alcohol as covariates[38] found a 6.3 fold decrease in the odds of the Montreal definition of GERD when it compared individuals reporting high and low levels of habitual physical activity. Likewise, a multivariate analysis of data for 3153 cases and 40,210 controls in Norway[62] demonstrated that the risk of GER (here defined by severe or recurrent heartburn or regurgitation) was significantly diminished among those participating in vigorous exercise (jogging, cross-country skiing or swimming) for 30 minutes or more 1, 2 or 3 times per week (with respective odds ratios of 0.5, 0.6, and 0.7 for the active individuals after statistical adjustment of data for the effects of age, sex, body mass index, use of tobacco and coffee, table salt intake and dietary fibre in bread). Study of a Japanese population[44] suggested that even exercising as infrequently as once per month was associated with a 26% decrease in the risk of GERD as documented by the Carlsson-Dent questionnaire for the presence of this condition. One report also underlined that a moderate frequency of habitual physical activity reduced the risk of GERD in those who were obese, but not in those with a normal body mass.[136]

One report examined the effects of the intensity of habitual physical activity. Relative to those who engaged regularly in high intensity effort, frequent GER was 32% less common in those taking only light physical activity, and 54% less in those engaging in moderate physical activity.[49]

An 18-year follow-up investigation found that an increase of moderate habitual physical activity over the period of observation was associated with a substantially decreased risk of GER (odds ratio, 3.05), although apparently these data were not adjusted for covariates such as obesity.[137]

Two negative reports[118,138] were from the same laboratory. The most active members of their sample had a step count of 12,500 paces/day, equivalent to an hour of moderate activity or 30 minutes of vigorous activity per day. They found no relationship between habitual physical activity and either lower oesophageal pressures or GER (as assessed objectively by pH monitoring).[118,138] A third investigation with negative findings[46] was based upon a relatively small sample of 211 individuals. It found that an apparent association of GER with habitual physical activity disappeared if diet and body mass index were introduced into the analysis as covariates. Another negative report was based on a large sample (2035 men and 2350 women, including 472 people with GERD)[119]; a 3-level classification of habitual physical activity showed no relationship to GERD in those with a normal body mass, but a moderate frequency of physical activity did reduce the risk in those who were obese. The final report was based upon the reflux-prone exercise of surf-boarding; here, not surprisingly, frequent surfing led to a large increase in the incidence of GER.[74]

Occupational physical activity and GER

Two reports have studied the impact of heavy occupational activity upon the incidence of GERD.[29,139] The first of these surveys was based upon 3338 Chinese villagers; it found that relative to those with a "mild" burden of physical work, the odds ratio of manifesting GERD as assessed by a validated Chinese version of the reflux disease questionnaire was 1.29 for those with a "moderate" burden, and 3.43 for those with a "severe" burden of occupational activity.[139] The second investigation was based on twins living in Sweden, and it examined GER rather

Table 2.4 Habitual physical activity, occupational activity and aerobic fitness in relation to the risk of developing gastro-oesophageal reflux

Author	Population	Exercise	Diagnosis	Finding
Habitual physical activity				
Çela et al.[38]	345 men, 500 women	3-level activity classification	Symptom-reporting	6.3 fold increase in odds of GERD in low vs high activity individuals (adjusted for BMI, smoking and alcohol)
Djärv et al.[136]	4910 Swedish adults, 472 with GERD	3-level classification of frequency of physical activity	Questionnaire	Physical activity has no effect on GERD in normal weight individuals, but moderate frequency of exercise reduces risk in multivariate analysis for obese
Józków et al.[118]	100 patients with GERD	3 levels of physical activity defined by IPAQ	pH monitoring and questionnaire	Number of self-reported symptoms did not differ between 3 activity groups
Murao et al.[44]	2853 Japanese	Exercising less than once/month	Questionnaire	26% decrease in risk of GERD in exercisers with multivariate analysis
Nandurkar et al.[46]	211 Americans	Energy expenditure 7.3 MJ/d by questionnaire; 3-level PA classification	GERD questionnaire	Association of GER with exercise disappears if BMI and diet included as covariates
Nilsson et al.[62]	3153 cases, 40,210 controls	Habitual exercise bouts >30 min 1–3 times/wk	Severe or recurrent heartburn or regurgitation	Odds ratio of GERD 0.5–0.7 in exercisers vs control group
Nocon et al.[48,63]	7124 Germans	3-level questioning of sports participation	Questionnaire	Sports >2h/wk gives 25% protection against GERD
Norisue et al.[74]	185 Hawaiian surfers, 178 athletic non-surfers		Questionnaire	Odds ratio of GERD >2/week 4.6 in surfers; prevalence also related to frequency and duration of surfing

Study	Sample	Method	Findings
Pandeya et al.[49]	1580 Australian adults	3-level physical activity index	Questionnaire	Occasional reflux 11% higher with low physical activity; frequent reflux 32% lower with low than with high physical activity
Stake-Nilsson et al.[137]	18-year follow-up of 85 F, 52 M	Exercise questionnaire	Questionnaire	Odds ratio 3.05 for decrease of GERD with increase of exercise
Waśko-Cnopnik et al.[138]	100 patients with GERD symptoms	3 levels of habitual physical activity by IPAQ	pH monitor and manometry	No relationship of activity to reported habitual activity
Yamamichi et al.[67]	19,864 healthy Japanese	Exercising <30 min/day (questionnaire)	Questionnaire	GERD significantly related to low physical activity in multivariate analysis
Zheng et al.[29]	4083 twins with GERD, 21,383 controls	Physical activity at work, recreational physical activity	Questionnaire	"Much recreational physical activity" reduced risk of GER by 40%
Occupation				
Chen et al.[139]	1468 M, 1870 F in South China		Questionnaire	Odds ratio of 3.43 for those with strenuous work
Zheng et al.[29]	4083 twins with GERD, 21,383 controls	Physical activity at work, recreational physical activity	Questionnaire	Strenuous physical activity at work increased risk of GERD by 20%,
Fitness Level				
Hawrylkiewicz et al.[140]	6 F, 12 M with obstructive sleep apnoea	6-min walk test	12 of 18 patients had GERD, 14 had oesophagitis	Distance walked reduced 22% relative to normal controls

Abbreviations: F = female; GER = gastro-oesophageal reflux; GERD = gastro-oesophageal reflux disease; M = male.

than GERD. In a multivariate analysis, it found that "active" employment was associated with a reduced risk. However, the overall intensity of occupational work was probably lower in Sweden than in China, and individuals were classified in a different fashion; the odds ratios for manifesting GER relative to a corresponding twin involved in sedentary employment was 0.85 (for jobs that required standing and walking), 0.68 (for jobs that required standing, lifting and carrying) and 0.74 (for work that was classed as "physically strenuous").[29]

Aerobic fitness and GER

The study of Hawryłkiewicz *et al.* related a weak measure of aerobic fitness (the six-minute walking distance) to GERD.[140] Twelve individuals among a small sample of 6 women and 12 men with obstructive sleep apnoea had signs of GERD. In those who were affected by GERD, the six-minute walking distance tended to be shorter than in the remaining six individuals, although this difference was not statistically significant. Moreover, the group with GERD tended to be more obese, and this could account for any deficit in their walking performance.

Other potential treatments of gastro-oesophageal reflux

Although some studies have found benefit from regular, moderate physical activity, no treatment of gastro-oesophageal reflux has to date been entirely successful. The main focus has been upon prevention, sometimes also with recourse to specific drug treatment, and some authors have suggested that there is benefit in localized exercises designed to train the muscles of the diaphragm. It is particularly important to prevent progression of GER by clearing regurgitated stomach acid from the oesophagus. This can be done by encouraging salivation and resultant oesophageal peristalsis[141] following reflux.

General preventive measures

General recommendations designed to reduce the risk of GER may include sleeping with the head elevated (not always easy to arrange), and lifestyle changes that include alterations of diet and the timing of meals, together with attempts to reduce body mass in those who are obese[47,142–145]. A reduced frequency of GER often follows a reduction in body mass.[41,51,146–149] Other simple tactics to reduce reflux include a chewing of gum and a period of standing following a meal.[150]

One meta-analysis found no reduction of GER from a cessation of smoking, a reduction of alcohol consumption or modifications of diet.[148] A second report also noted little improvement of oesophageal function from the cessation of smoking.[151]

If a recreational exerciser is complaining of acute GER during bouts of physical activity, the problem can sometimes be corrected by changing the form of exercise (for instance, substituting cycling for running), reducing the intensity and/or the duration of effort,[21,104] or altering the timing and composition of meals relative to periods of exercise. Substantial meals should be taken at least three hours before exercising, while taking care to maintain fluid balance during a prolonged bout of physical activity.[21] One review concluded that GER was more likely if exercisers ingested hypertonic beverages containing carbohydrate or salt solutions rather than water.[41]

Pharmacological measures

If exercise-induced gastric pain is frequent, severe, and does not respond to modifications of diet and training, pharmacological measures may be proposed. These currently include the administration of antacids, histamine H_2-receptor blockers such as cimetidine or ranitidine (these are intended to inhibit stomach acid production and thus protect the oesophagus from further damage),[102] proton-pump inhibitors such as omeprazole or rabeprazole (these also limit the secretion of acid by the stomach)[7,102,119,145,152–156] and possibly drugs designed to inhibit lower oesophageal relaxation.[157]

Proton-pump inhibitors are at present the most popular choice of medication. In France, about 88% of cases of GERD are treated with proton-pump inhibitors, and 73% of these patients are also given lifestyle advice.[76] Unfortunately, proton-pump inhibiting drugs are costly,[158] and although they often reduce symptoms, it has yet to be demonstrated that they avert the long-term complications of GERD.[16] Moreover, although the gastric acid secretion is reduced by such drugs, they do not necessarily correct any impairment of athletic performance.[114]

Local diaphragmatic training

One further option is a course of diaphragmatic training. If the patient is willing to invest the effort, local exercises or osteopathic interventions designed to strengthen the diaphragm are said to help increase oesophageal sphincter pressures and thus reduce gastro-oesophageal reflux.[159–163]

Areas for further research

Much of the research to date has been based upon questionnaires that have looked both at gastro-intestinal symptoms and habitual physical activity. This is not a reliable way to determine either the prevalence of gastro-oesophageal reflux or factors modifying its incidence. There is thus a need for more objective research, based upon measurements of pH and pressures within the oesophagus, and personal monitors of habitual physical activity.

There has as yet been little examination of the possible contributions of diminished saliva production and decreased local blood flow to the slowing of oesophageal motility observed during vigorous exercise. There is also need for a closer control of covariates, particularly obesity, which some (but not all) investigators have found to be a significant factor modifying the exercise response.

There also remains scope for further attempts to find an effective remedy for those who suffer from gastro-oesophageal reflux, and have not benefitted from either moderate habitual activity or the other simple lifestyle changes suggested above. Given that the oesophagus penetrates the diaphragm, there seems logic in the suggestion that diaphragmatic training may be helpful, and the effectiveness of this form of treatment merits further investigation.

Practical implications

Although moderate intensities of physical activity usually improve oesophageal function and reduce the risk of gastro-oesophageal reflux, vigorous exercise commonly reduces motility and leads to an inappropriate relaxation of the sphincter at the lower end of the oesophagus, with an increased reflux of the acid contents of the stomach into the oesophagus. Occasional reflux of this type is a common enough phenomenon, and is reported by both athletes and sedentary individuals. In itself, it may be no more than a painful annoyance, but if it is frequent and left untreated it can progress to more serious clinical manifestations, including oesophageal ulceration, haemorrhage and stricture of the oesophagus, a cancerous change in the squamous cells of the oesophageal lining (Barrett's oesophagus), and a very deadly oesophageal adenocarcinoma.

The tendency to gastro-oesophageal reflux is exacerbated by both obesity and bouts of vigorous exercise (here defined as physical activity at intensities >70% of the individual's $\dot{V}O_{2max}$). The prevalence of GER is particularly marked during activities that involve rhythmic body movement (such as running), exercise in a prone position (for instance, surfing) and/or a sharp increase of intra-abdominal pressure (as in weight-lifting).

The main focus of prevention is upon regular moderate physical activity, coupled with simple changes of lifestyle – a decrease of body mass if a person is obese, sleeping with the head raised, and altering the timing of meals relative to bouts of exercise. The ability of regular moderate physical activity to reduce GER seems well established, and this should be a central component of any treatment plan, particularly for someone who currently has a sedentary lifestyle. If the symptoms of reflux are frequent during bouts of vigorous effort, a recreational exerciser may consider changing the type and/or intensity of physical activity that he or she practices. However, a change of sport is usually less feasible for the serious athlete.

Encouraging salivation may reduce the exposure of the oesophagus to acid during episodes of GER. The administration of proton-pump inhibitors can reduce symptoms, but it does not necessarily restore physical performance. Exercises to strengthen the diaphragm and thus increase oesophageal sphincter pressures may also be helpful, although their efficacy has yet to be established.

Conclusions

Moderate physical activity may enhance oesophageal motility, but if physical activity reaches an intensity greater than 70% of an individual's maximal oxygen intake it disrupts oesophageal mechanics, with inappropriate relaxation of the lower oesophageal sphincter and a reflux of gastric acid into the oesophagus. The immediate effect of such reflux is acute upper abdominal pain, but if the reflux is repeated many times, it can cause inflammation, ulceration, haemorrhage and cancerous change in the oesophageal wall.

Unfortunately, the prevalence of gastro-oesophageal reflux is uncertain, since in many investigations questionnaires have not distinguished such reflux from other causes of exercise-induced abdominal pain and discomfort. Simple measures to reduce oesophageal reflux include regular moderate physical activity, avoiding meals shortly before exercise, avoiding sudden increases of intra-abdominal pressure and the prone position when exercising, and changing one's sport or reducing the peak intensity of physical activity if severely affected. Commonly used drugs such as proton inhibitors, intended to reduce the acidity of the gastric contents, may alleviate symptoms, but do not seem to correct the impairments of athletic performance associated with gastro-oesophageal reflux.

References

1 Ingelfinger FJ. Esophageal motility. *Physiol Rev* 1958; 38(4): 533–584.
2 Peters L, Maas L, Petty D *et al*. Spontaneous noncardiac chest pain. Evaluation by 24-hour ambulatory esophageal motility and pH monitoring. *Gastroenterology* 1988; 84(4): 878–886.
3 Józków P, Waśko-Czopnik D, Medras M *et al*. Gastroesophageal reflux disease and physical activity. *Sports Med* 2006; 36: 385–391.
4 Moses FM. The effects of exercise on the gastrointestinal tract. *Sports Med* 1990; 9: 159–172.
5 Moses FM. Physical activity and the digestive processes. In: Bouchard C, Shephard RJ, Stephens T (eds). *Physical activity, fitness and health*. Champaign, IL: Human Kinetics; 1994, pp. 383–400.
6 Peters O, Peters P, Clarys JT *et al*. Esophageal motility and exercise. *Gastroenterology* 1988; 94: A351 (abstr.).
7 Shawdon A. Gastro-oesophageal reflux and exercise. Important pathology to consider in the athletic population. *Sports Med* 1995; 20: 109–116.
8 Shephard RJ. Physical activity and the visceral organs. In: Shephard RJ (ed.). *Year Book of Sports Medicine 2013*. Philadelphia, PA: Elsevier, 2013, pp. xv–xxviii.
9 Soffer EE, Merchant RK, Duethman G *et al*. The effect of graded exercise on esophageal motility and gastroesophageal reflux in trained athletes. *Gastroenterology* 1991; 100: A497 (abstr.).
10 Soffer EE, Merchant RK, Duethman G *et al*. Effect of graded exercise on esophageal motility and gastro-esophageal reflux in trained athletes. *Dig Dis Sci* 1993; 38(2): 220–224.
11 Soffer EE, Wilson J, Duethman G *et al*. Effect of graded exercise on esophageal motility and gastroesophageal reflux in nontrained subjects. *Dig Dis Sci* 1994; 39: 193–198.
12 van Nieuwenhoven MA, Brouns F, Brummer RJ. The effect of physical activity on parameters of gastrointestinal function. *Neurogastroenterol Motil* 1999; 11: 431–439.

13 Choi SC, Yoo KH, Kim TH *et al.* Effect of graded running on esophageal motility and gastro-oesophageal reflux in fed volunteers. *J Korean Med Sci* 2001; 16: 183–187.

14 Ravi N, Stuart RC, Byrne PJ *et al.* Effect of physical exercise on esophageal motility in patients with esophageal disease. *Dis Esophagus* 2005; 18: 374–377.

15 Budzyński J. Exercise-provoked esophageal motility disorder in patients with recurrent chest pain. *World J Gastroenterol* 2010; 16: 4428–4435.

16 Delaney BC. Review article: prevalence and epidemiology of gastro-oesophageal reflux disease. *Aliment Pharmacol Ther* 2004; 20(Suppl. 8): 2–4.

17 Koppert LB, Wijnhoven BP, van Dekken H *et al.* The molecular biology of esophageal adenocarcinoma. *Surg Oncol* 2005; 92(3): 169–190.

18 Modlin IM, Moss SF, Kidd M *et al.* Gastroesophageal reflux disease then and now. *J Clin Gastroenterol* 2004; 38: 390–402.

19 Rubenstein J, Taylor JB. Meta-analysis: the association of oesophageal adenocarcinoma with symptoms of gastro-oesophageal reflux. *Aliment Pharmacol Ther* 2010; 32(10): 1222–1227.

20 Shaheen NJ, Richter JE. Barrett oesophagus. *Lancet* 2009; 373 (9666): 850–861.

21 Parmalee-Peters K, Moeller JL. Gastroesophageal reflux in athletes. *Curr Sports Med Rep* 2004; 3: 107–111.

22 Ford AC, Forman D, Bailey AG *et al.* The natural history of gastro-oesophageal reflux symptoms in the community and its effects on survival: a longitudinal 10-year follow-up study. *Aliment Pharmacol Therap* 2013; 37: 323–331.

23 Mittal RK. Current concepts of the antireflux barrier. *Gastroenterol Clin North Am* 1990; 19(3): 501–516.

24 Schneider JH, Küper MA, Königstrainer A *et al.* Transient lower esophageal sphincter relaxation and esophageal motor response. *J Surg Res* 2010; 159: 714–719.

25 Gómez Escudero O, Herrera Hernández MF, Valdovinos Díaz MA. La obesidad y la enfermedad por reflujo gastroesofágico [Obesity and gastroesophageal reflux disease]. *Rev Invest Clin* 2002; 54(4): 320–327.

26 van Herwaarden MA, Samsom M, Smout AJ. Excess gastroesophageal reflux in patients with hiatus hernia is caused by mechanisms other than transient LES relaxations. *Gastroenterology* 2000; 119(6): 1439–1446.

27 Emerenziani S, Zhang X, Blondeau K *et al.* Gastric fullness, physical activity, and proximal extent of gastroesophageal reflux. *Am J Gastroenterol* 2005; 100: 1251–1256.

28 Cameron AJ, Lagergren J, Henriksson C *et al.* Gastroesophageal reflux disease in monozygotic and dizygotic twins. *Gastroenterology* 2002; 122: 55–59.

29 Zheng Z, Nordenstedt H, Pedersen NL *et al.* Lifestyle factors and risk for symptomatic gastroesophageal reflux in monozygotic twins. *Gastroenterology* 2007; 132(1): 87–95.

30 Gold BD. Gastroesophageal reflux disease: Could interventions in childhood reduce the risk of later complications? *Am J Med* 2004; 117(5A): 23S–29S.

31 Gold BD. Is gastroesophageal reflux disease really a life-long disease: Do babies who regurgitate grow up to be adults with GERD complications? *Am J Gastroenterol* 2006; 101: 641–644.

32 Dore MP, Maragkoudakis E, Fraley K *et al.* Diet, lifestyle and gender in gastroesophageal reflux disease. *Digest Dis Sci* 2008; 53: 2027–2032.

33 Hallan A, Bomme M, Hveem K *et al.* Risk factors for the development of new-onset gastroesophageal reflux symptoms. A population-based prospective cohort study: The HUNT study. *Am J Gastroenterol* 2015; 110: 393–400.

34 Fujiwara Y, Arakawa T. Epidemiology and clinical characteristics of GERD in the Japanese population. *J Gastroenterol* 2009; 44: 518–534.

35 Morozov SV, Stavraski ES, Isakov VA. Rasprostranennost' izzhogi u pozhilykh patsiy-entov v gorodskikh poliklinikakh v Rossii [The prevalence of heartburn in the elderly patients in urban outpatient clinics in Russia]. *Eksp Klin Gastroenterol* 2010; 12: 17–23.

36 Nilsson M, Johnsen R, Ye W *et al.* Prevalence of gastro-oesophageal reflux symptoms and the influence of age and sex. *Scand J Gastroenterol* 2004; 39: 1040–1045.

37 Anand G, Katz PO. Gastroesophageal reflux disease and obesity. *Rev Gastroenterol Disord* 2008; 8: 233–239.

38 Çela L, Kraja B, Hoti K *et al.* Lifestyle characteristics and gastroesophageal reflux disease: A population-based study in Albania. *Gastroenterol Res Pract* 2013: 936792, 1–7.

39 DeMarco D, Passaglia C. L'obesità e la malattia da reflusso gastroesofageo [Obesity and gastroesophageal reflux disease]. *Recenti Prog Med* 2010; 101(3): 106–111.

40 Eslick GD. Gastrointestinal symptoms and obesity: a meta-analysis. *Obesity Rev* 2012; 13: 469–479.

41 Festi D, Scaioli E, Baldi F *et al.* Body weight, lifestyle, dietary habits and gastro-esophageal reflux disease. *World J Gastroenterol* 2009; 15: 1690–1701.

42 Hampel H, Abraham NS, El-Serag HB. Meta-analysis: obesity and the risk for gastroesophageal reflux disease and its complications. *Ann Intern Med* 2005; 143: 199–211.

43 Islami F, Nassweri-Moghaddam S, Pourshams A *et al.* Determinants of gastro-esophageal reflux disease, including Hookah smoking and opium use. A cross-sectional analysis of 50,000 individuals. *PLoS ONE.* 2014; 9(2): e89256.

44 Murao T, Sakurai K, Mihara S *et al.* Lifestyle change influences on GERD in Japan: A study of participants in a health examination program. *Dig Dis Sci* 2011; 56: 2857–2864.

45 Murray L, Johnston B, Lane A *et al.* Relationship between body mass and gastro-oesophageal reflux symptoms: The Bristol Helicobacter project. *Int J Epidemiol* 2003; 32: 645–650.

46 Nandurkar S, Locke GR, Fett S *et al.* Relationship between body mass index, diet, exercise and gastro-oesophageal reflux symptoms in a community. *Aliment Pharmacol Ther* 2004; 20(5): 497–505.

47 Nilsson M, Lagergren J. The relation between body mass and gastro-oesophageal reflex. *Best Pract Res Clin Gastroenterol* 2004; 18(6): 1117–1123.

48 Nocon M, Labenz J, Willich N *et al.* Lifestyle factors and symptomatology of gastro-oesophageal reflux – a population-based study. *Aliment Pharmacol Ther* 2006; 23: 169–174.

49 Pandeya N, Green AC, Whiteman DC. Prevalence and determinants of frequent gastroesophageal reflux symptoms in the Australian community. *Dis Oesophagus.* 2012; 25: 573–583.

50 Rey E, Morenbo-Elola-Olaso C, Artalejo FR *et al.* Association between weight gain and symptoms of gastroesophageal reflux in the general population. *Am J Gastroenterol* 2006; 101: 229–233.

51 Singh AM, Lee J, Gupta N *et al.* Weight loss can lead to a resolution of gastro-esophageal reflux disease symptoms: A prospective intervention trial. *Obesity* (Silver Spring) 2013; 21(2): 284–290.

52 Vart P, Memon AR, Mirza SS *et al.* Does physical activity modify the gastro-esophageal reflux symptoms independent of obesity? Or obesity confounds the relationship between physical activity and gastroesophageal reflux symptoms? *J Pak Med Assoc.* 2011; 61(11): 1148–1149.

53 Corley DA, Kubo A, Levin TR *et al.* Abdominal obesity and body mass index as risk factors for Barrett's esophagus. *Gastroenterol* 2007; 133: 34–41.
54 Nilsson M, Johnsen R, Ye W *et al.* Obesity and estrogen as risk factors for gastro-esophageal reflux symptoms. *JAMA* 2003; 290: 66–72.
55 Lagergren J, Bergström R, Nyrén O. No relation between body mass and gastro-oesophageal reflux symptoms in a Swedish population based study. *Gut* 2000; 47: 26–29.
56 El Serag HB, Graham DY, Satia JA *et al.* Obesity is an independent risk factor for GERD symptoms and erosive esophagitis. *Am J Gastroenterol* 2005; 100: 1243–1250.
57 Rubenstein J, Morgenstern H, McConell D *et al.* Associations of diabetes mellitus, insulin, leptin, and ghrelin with gastroesophageal reflux and Barrett's esophagus. *Gastroenterol* 2013; 145(6): 1237–1244.
58 De Vries DR, van Herwaarden MA, Smout AJ *et al.* Gastroesophageal pressure gradients in gastroesophageal reflux disease: Relations with hiatal hernia, body mass index, and esophageal acid exposure. *Am J Gastroenterol* 2008; 103: 1349–1354.
59 Devendran N, Chauhan N, Armstrong D. GERD and obesity: is the autonomic nervous system the missing link? *Crit Rev Biomed Eng* 2014; 42(1): 17–24.
60 Falk GW, Jacobson BC, Riddell RH *et al.* Barrett's esophagus: prevalence-incidence and etiology-origins. *Ann NY Acad Sci* 2011; 1232: 1–17.
61 Friedenberg FK, Makipour K, Palit A *et al.* A population-based assessment of heartburn in urban black Americans. *Dis Esophagus* 2013; 26(6): 561–569.
62 Nilsson M, Johnsen R, Ye W *et al.* Lifestyle related risk factors in the aetiology of gastro-oesophageal reflux. *Gut* 2004; 53: 1730–1735.
63 Nocon M, Labenz J, Jaspersen D *et al.* Association of body mass index with heartburn, regurgitation and esophagitis: Results of the progression of gastroesophageal reflux disease study. *J Gastroenterol Hepatol* 2007; 22: 1728–1731.
64 Vossoughinia H, Salari M, Amirmajdi EM *et al.* An epidemiological study of gastro-esophageal reflux disease and related risk factors in urban population of Mashad, Iran. *Iran Red Crescent Med J* 2014; 16(12): e15832.
65 Veugelers PJ, Porter GA, Guernsey DL *et al.* Obesity and lifestyle risk factors for gastroesophageal reflux disease, Barrett esophagus and esophageal adenocarcinoma. *Dis Esophagus* 2006; 19(5): 321–328.
66 Stanghellini V. Relationship between upper gastrointestinal symptoms and lifestyle, psychosocial factors and comorbidity in the general population: results from the Domestic/International Gastroenterology Surveillance Study (DIGEST). *Scand J Gastroenterol Suppl* 1999; 231: 29–37.
67 Yamamichi N, Mochizuki S, Asada-Hirayama I. Lifestyle factors affecting gastro-esophageal reflux disease symptoms: a cross-sectional study of healthy 19864 adults using FSSG scores. *BMC Medicine* 2012; 10: 45.
68 Lovell R, Ford AC. Prevalence of gastro-esophageal reflux-type symptoms in individuals with irritable bowel syndrome in the community: A meta-analysis. *Am J Gastroenterol* 2015; 110: 393–400.
69 Miele L, Cammarota G, Vero V *et al.* Non-alcoholic fatty liver disease is associated with high prevalence of gastro-oesophageal reflux symptoms. *Digest Liver Dis* 2012; 44: 1032–1036.
70 Fujikawa Y, Tominaga K, Fujii H *et al.* High prevalence of gastroesophageal reflux symptoms in patients with non-alcoholic fatty liver disease associated with serum levels of triglyceride and cholesterol but not simple visceral obesity. *Digestion* 2012; 86: 228–237.

71 Demeester TR, Johnson LF, Joseph GJ *et al.* Patterns of gastroesophageal reflux in health and disease. *Ann Surg* 1976; 184: 459–469.

72 Budzyński J. Exertional esophageal pH-metry and manometry in recurrent chest pain. *World J Gastroenterol* 2010; 167(34): 4305–4312.

73 Schowengerdt CG. Dynamic position testing for the detection of esophageal acid reflux disease. *Digest Dis Sci* 2005; 50: 100–102.

74 Norisue Y, Onopa J, Kaneshiro M *et al.* Surfing as a risk factor for gastroesophageal reflux disease. *Clin J Sports Med* 2009; 19(5): 388–393.

75 Lopez A, Preziosi JP, Chateau P *et al.* Les troubles digestifs et l'automédication observés au cours d'une concurrence dans les athlètes d'endurance. Étude épidémiologique prospective au cours d'un championnat de triathlon [Digestive disorders and self medication observed during a competition in endurance athletes. Prospective epidemiological study during a triathlon championship]. *Gastroenterol Clin Biol* 1994; 18: 317–322.

76 Bretagne JF, Rey J-F, Caekaert A *et al.* Routine management of gastro-oesophageal reflux disease by gastroenterologists in France: A prospective observational study. *Digest Liver Dis* 2005; 37: 566–570.

77 Kahrilas PJ, Clouse RE, Hogan WJ. American Gastroenterological Association technical review on the clinical use of esophageal manometry. *Gastroenterol Clin Biol* 1994; 107: 1865–1884.

78 Lemire S. Assessment of clinical severity and investigation of uncomplicated gastroesophageal reflux disease and noncardiac angina-like chest pain. *Can J Gastroenterol* 1997; 11(Suppl. B): 37B–40B.

79 Pandolfino JE, Kahrilas PJ. Technical review on the clinical use of esophageal manometry. *Gastroenterology* 1995; 128: 209–224.

80 Botoman VA. Noncardiac chest pain. *J Clin Gastroenterol* 2002; 34: 6–14.

81 Kahrilas PJ, Quigley EMM. Clinical esophageal pH recording: a technical review for practice guideline development. *Gastroenterology* 1996; 110: 1982–1996.

82 Kouklakis G, Moschois J, Kountouras J *et al.* Relationship between obesity and gastroesophageal reflux disease as recorded by 3-hour esophageal pH recording. *Rom J Gastroeneterol* 2005; 14(2): 117–121.

83 Cooke RA, Anggiansah A, Smeeton NC *et al.* Gastroesophageal reflux in patients with angiographically normal coronary arteries: an uncommon cause of exertional chest pain. *Br Heart J* 1994; 72: 231–236.

84 Lenfant C. Chest pain of cardiac and noncardiac origin. *Metab Clin Exp* 2010; 59(Suppl. 1): S41–S6.

85 Liuzzo JP, Ambrose JA. Chest pain from gastroesophageal reflux disease in patients with coronary artery disease. *Cardiol Rev* 2005; 13: 167–173.

86 Ros E, Toledo-Pimentel V, Grande L *et al.* El dolor torácico de origen esofágico. La evaluación de 125 pacientes consecutivos con angina de reposo y coronarias angiográficamente normales. [Thoracic pain of esophageal origin. Assessment of 125 consecutive patients with resting angina and angiographically normal coronary arteries]. *Med Clin* (Barcelona) 1996; 106(3): 81–86.

87 Sik EC, Batt ME, Heslop LM. Atypical chest pain in athletes. *Curr Sports Med Rep* 2009; 8(2): 52–58.

88 Singh AM, McGregor RS. Differential diagnosis of chest symptoms in the athlete. *Clin Rev Allergy Immunol* 2005; 29: 87–96.

89 Budzyński J, Siatkowski M, Klopocka M *et al.* Związek pomiędzy wynikami elektrokardiograficznego próby wysiłkowej i intraesophageal pH u mężczyzn z

nietypowym bólem w klatce piersiowej. [Relationship between results of electrocardiographic exercise tests and intraesophageal pH in men with atypical chest pain]. *Pol Arch Med Wewn* 2000; 103(3–4): 133–138.

90 Chauhan A, Petch MC, Schofield PM. Cardio-oesophageal reflex in humans as a mechanism for "linked angina". *Eur Heart J* 1996; 17: 407–413.

91 Schofield PM, Bennett DH, Whorwell PJ *et al.* Exertional gastro-oesophageal reflux: a mechanism for symptoms in patients with angina pectoris and normal coronary angiograms. *BMJ (Clin Res Ed)* 1987; 294: 1459–1461.

92 Michel H, Larrey D, Blanc P. Troubles hépato-digestif dans la pratique medico-sportive. [Hepato-digestive disorders in athletic practice]. *Presse Méd* 1994; 23(10): 479–484.

93 ter Steege RW, Kolkman JJ, Huisman AB *et al.* Maagdarm-ischemie tijdens lichamelijke inspanning als een oorzaak van gastro-intestinale symptomen. [Gastrointestinal ischaemia during physical exertion as a cause of gastrointestinal symptoms]. *Ned Tijdschr Geneeskd* 2008; 152: 1805–1808.

94 Avidan B, Sonnenberg A, Schnell TG *et al.* Walking and chewing reduce postprandial acid reflux. *Aliment Pharmacol Ther* 2001; 15: 151–155.

95 Karim S, Jafri W, Faryal A *et al.* Regular post dinner walk can be a useful lifestyle modification for gastroesophageal reflux. *J Pak Med Assoc* 2011; 61(6): 526–530.

96 Mendes-Filho AM, Moraes-Filho JP, Nasi A *et al.* Influence of exercise testing in gastroesophageal reflux in patients with gastroesophageal reflux disease. *Arq Bras Cir Dig* 2014; 27(1): 3–8.

97 Schoeman MN, Tippett MD, Akkermans LMA *et al.* Mechanics of gastroesophageal reflux in ambulant healthy human subjects. *Gastroenterology* 1995; 108: 83–91.

98 Sodhi JS, Zargar SA, Javid G *et al.* Effect of bending exercise on gastroesophageal reflux in symptomatic patients. *Ind J Gastroenterol* 2008; 27: 227–231.

99 Worobetz LJ, Gerrard DF. Effect of moderate exercise on esophageal function in asymptomatic athletes. *Am J Gastroenterol* 1986; 81: 1048–1051.

100 Paterson WG, Abdollah H, Beck IT *et al.* Patients with atypical chest pain. *Digest Dis Sci* 1993; 38: 795–802.

101 Clark GS, Kraus BB, Sinclair J *et al.* Gastroesophageal reflux induced by exercise in healthy volunteers. *JAMA* 1989; 261: 3599–3601.

102 Kraus BB, Sinclair J, Castell DO. Gastroesophageal reflux in runners-characteristics and treatment. *Ann Intern Med* 1990; 112: 429–433.

103 Motil BB, Ostendorf J, Bricker JT *et al.* Case-report – exercise-induced gastro-esophageal reflux in an athletic child. *J Paediatr Gastroenterol Nutr* 1987 6: 989–991.

104 Collings KL, Pierce-Pratt F, Rodriguez-Stanley S *et al.* Esophageal reflux in conditioned runners, cyclists, and weightlifters. *Med Sci Sports Exerc* 2003; 35: 730–735.

105 Peters HP, Wiersma JWC, Koerselman J *et al.* The effect of a sports drink on gastroesophageal reflux during a run-bike-run test. *Int J Sports Med* 1999; 20: 65–70.

106 Rehrer NJ, van Kenemade M, Meester W *et al.* Gastrointestinal complaints in relation to dietary intake in triathletes. *Int J Sports Nutr* 1992; 2(1): 48–59.

107 van Nieuwenhoven MA, Brouns F, Brummer RJ. Gastrointestinal profile of symptomatic athletes at rest and during physical exercise. *Eur J Appl Physiol* 2004; 91: 429–434.

108 Maddison KJ, Shepherd KL, Hillman DR *et al.* Function of the lower esophageal sphincter during and after high intensity exercise. *Med Sci Sports Exerc* 2005; 37(10): 1728–1733.

109 Peters HP, de Vries WR, Vanberg-Henegouwen GP *et al.* Potential benefits and hazards of physical activity and exercise on the gastrointestinal tract. *Gut* 2001; 48: 435–449.

110 Worobetz LJ, Gerrard DF. Gastrointestinal symptoms during exercise in enduro athletes: prevalence and speculations on the aetiology. *N Z Med J* 1985; 98: 644–646.

111 Pandolfino JE, Bianchi LK, Lee TJ *et al.* Esophagogastric junction morphology predicts susceptibility to exercise-induced reflux. *Am J Gastroenterol* 2004; 99: 1430–1436.

112 Yazaki E, Shawdon A, Beasley I *et al.* The effect of different types of exercise on gastro-oesophageal reflux. *Austr J Sci Med Sport* 1996; 28: 93–96.

113 Peters HP, Zweers M, Backx FJ *et al.* Gastrointestinal symptoms during long-distance walking. *Med Sci Sports Exerc* 1999; 31: 767–773.

114 Rodriguez-Stanley S, Bemben D, Zubaidi S *et al.* Effect of esophageal acid and prophylactic rabeprazole on performance in runners. *Med Sci Exerc Sports* 2006; 38(9): 1659–1665.

115 de Oliveira EP, Burini RC. The impact of physical exercise on the gastrointestinal tract. *Curr Opin Clin Nutr Metab Care* 2009; 12: 533–538.

116 Glace B, Murphy C, McHugh M. Food and fluid intake and disturbances in gastrointestinal and mental function during an ultramarathon. *Int J Sport Nutr* 2002; 12(4): 414–427.

117 Keeffe E, Lowe D, Goss J *et al.* Gastro-intestinal symptoms of marathon runners. *West J Med* 1984; 141: 481–484.

118 Józków P, Waśko-Czopnik D, Dunajska K *et al.* The relationship between gastroesophageal reflux disease and the level of physical activity. *Swiss Med Weekly* 2007; 137: 465–470.

119 Peters HP, Bos M, Seebregts L *et al.* Gastrointestinal symptoms in long-distance runners, cyclists, and triathletes: prevalence, medication, and etiology. *Am J Gastroenterol* 1999; 94: 1570–1581.

120 Rehrer NJ, Janssen GME, Brouns F *et al.* Fluid intake and gastrointestinal problems in runners competing in a 25-km race and a marathon. *Int J Sports Med* 1989; 10(Suppl. 1): S22–S25.

121 Rehrer NJ, Brouns F, Beckers EJ *et al.* Physiological changes and gastro-intestinal symptoms as a result of ultra-endurance running. *Eur J Appl Physiol* 1992; 64: 1–8.

122 Riddoch C, Trinick T. Gastrointestinal disturbances in marathon runners. *Br J Sports Med* 1988; 22(2): 71–74.

123 Sullivan SN. Exercise-associated symptoms in triathletes. *Phys Sportsmed* 1987; 15(9): 105–110.

124 Verbeek RE, Kremer WCEM, van Baal JWPM *et al. Is rowing involved in the induction of esophageal adenocarcinoma: a literature review and questionnaire in active rowers?* Utrecht, Netherlands: Dept. of Gastroenterology, University Medical Centre, Utrecht, 2014.

125 Brouns F, Beckers E. Is the gut an athletic organ? Digestion, absorption and exercise. *Sports Med* 1993; 15: 242–257.

126 Waterman JJ, Kapur R. Upper gastro-intestinal issues in athletes. *Curr Sports Med Rep* 2012; 11(2): 99–104.

127 Bi L, Triadafilopoulos G. Exercise and gastrointestinal function and disease: An evidence-based review of risks and benefits. *Clin Gastroenterol Hepatol* 2003; 1: 345–355.

128 Dent J, Holloway RH, Toouli J *et al.* Mechanisms of lower oesophageal sphincter incompetence in patients with symptomatic gastro-oesophageal reflux. *Gut* 1988; 29: 1020–1028.

129 Ayazi S, Demeeter SR, Hsieh C-C *et al.* Thoraco-abdominal pressure gradients during the phases of respiration contribute to gastroesophageal reflux disease. *Dig Dis Sci* 2011; 56: 1718–1722.

130 Kiljander TO, Salomaa E-RM, Hietanen EK *et al.* Gastroesophageal reflux in asthmatics. A double-blind placebo-controlled crossover study with omeprazole. *Chest* 1999; 116: 1257–1264.

131 Kahrilas PJ, Smith JA, Dicpinigaitis PV. A causal relationship between cough and gastroesophageal reflux disease (GERD) has been established: a Pro/Con debate. *Lung* 2014; 192(1): 39–46.

132 Peterson KA, Samuelson WM, Ryujin DT *et al.* The role of gastresophageal reflux in exercise-triggered asthma: A randomized controlled trial. *Dig Dis Sci* 2009; 54: 564–571.

133 Ferrari M, Bonella F, Benini L *et al.* Acid reflux into the oesophagus does not influence exercise-induced airway narrowing in bronchial asthma. *Br J Sports Med* 2008; 42: 845–850.

134 Weiner P, Konson N, Sternberg A *et al.* Is gastro-oesophageal reflux a factor in exercise-induced asthma? *Resp Med* 1998; 92: 1071–1075.

135 Wright RA, Sagatellian MA, Simons ME *et al.* Exercise-induced asthma. Is gastroesophageal reflux a factor? *Dig Dis Sci* 1996; 41(5): 921–925.

136 Djärv T, Wikman A, Nordenstedt H *et al.* Physical activity, obesity and gastroesophageal reflux disease in the general population. *World J Gastroenterol* 2012; 18(28): 3710–3714.

137 Stake-Nilsson K, Hultcrantz R, Unge P *et al.* Changes in symptoms and lifestyle factors in patients seeking healthcare for gastrointestinal symptoms: an 18-year follow-up study. *Eur J Gastroenterol Hepatol* 2013; 25: 1470–1477.

138 Waśko-Cnopnik D, Józkow P, Dunaiska K *et al.* Associations between the lower esophageal sphincter function and the level of physical activity. *Ann Clin Exp Med* 2013; 22(2): 185–191.

139 Chen M, Xiong L, Chen H *et al.* Prevalence, risk factors and impact of gastroesophageal reflux disease symptoms: a population-based study in South China. *Scand J Gastroenterol* 2005; 40(7): 759–767.

140 Hawryłkiewicz I, Dziedzic D, Plywaczeski R *et al.* Współistnienie obniżonej wydolności wysiłkowej chorych na obturacyjny bezdech senny z występowaniem refluksu żołądkowo-przełykowego. [The coexistence of impaired exercise tolerance in patients with obstructive sleep apnea with gastroesophageal reflux]. *Pneumonol Alergol Pol* 2008; 76: 83–87.

141 Kahrilas PJ, Lee TJ. Pathophysiology of gastroesophageal reflux disease. *Thorac Surg Clin* 2005; 15(3): 323–333.

142 Kendrick ML, Houghton SG. Gastroesophageal reflux disease in obese patients: the role of obesity in management. *Dis Esophagus* 2006; 19: 57–63.

143 Reavis KM. Management of the obese patient with gastroesophageal reflux disease. *Thorac Surg Clin* 2011; 21(4): 489–498.

144 Csendes A, Burdiles P. Fundamentos científicos para el tratamiento médico a base de dieta modificación, hábitos de vida y las actitudes del paciente en la enfermedad por reflujo gastroesofágico crónico. [Scientific foundations for medical treatment based on modifying diet, lifestyle habits, and patient attitudes in chronic gastroesophageal reflux disease]. *Cir Esp* 2007; 81(2): 64–69.

145 Peters HPF, DeKort AF, Van Krevelen H *et al.* The effect of omeprazole on gastro-oesphageal reflux and symptoms during strenuous exercise. *Aliment Pharmacol Ther* 1999; 13: 1015–1022.

146 Anand G, Katz P. Gastroesophageal reflux disease and obesity. *Gastroenterol Clin North Am* 2010; 39(1): 39–46.

147 Friedenberg FK, Xanthopoulos M, Foster GD *et al.* The association between gastro-esophageal reflux disease and obesity. *Am J Gastroenterol* 2008; 103: 2111–2122.

148 Kaltenbach T, Crockett S, Gerson LB. Are lifestyle measures effective in patients with gastroesophageal reflux disease? An evidence-based approach. *Arch Intern Med* 2006; 166: 965–971.

149 Ness-Jensen E, Lindam A, Lagergren J *et al.* Weight loss and reduction in gastro-esophageal reflux: A population-based cohort study: the HUNT study. *Am J Gastroenterol* 2013; 103: 376–382.

150 Bujanda L, Cosme A, Muro N *et al.* Influencia del estilo de vida en la enfermedad por reflujo gastroesofági. [Influence of lifestyle in patients with gastroesophageal reflux disease]. *Med Clin* (Barcelona) 2007; 128(14): 550–554.

151 Ness-Jensen E, Lindam A, Lagergren J *et al.* Tobacco smoking and improved gastro-esophageal reflux: A prospective population-based cohort study: The HUNT study. *Am J Gastroenterol* 2014; 109: 171–177.

152 Holtmann G, Adam B, Liebregt T. Review article: the patient with gastro-oesophageal reflux disease – lifestyle advice and medication. *Aliment Pharmacol Ther* 2004; 20(Suppl. 8): 24–27.

153 Jian R, Hassani Z, Kebir S *et al.* Management of gastro-esophageal reflux disease in primary care. Results from an observational study of 2,474 patients (AO). *Gastroenterol Clin Biol* 2007; 31(1): 72–77.

154 Kinoshita Y. Review article: treatment for gastro-oesophageal reflux disease-lifestyle advice and medication. *Aliment Pharmacol Ther* 2004; 20(Suppl. 8): 19–23.

155 Simons SM, Kennedy RG. Gastrointestinal problems in runners. *Curr Sports Med Rep* 2004; 3: 112–116.

156 Tytgat GN. Review article: treatment of mild and severe cases of GERD. *Aliment Pharmacol Ther* 2002; 16(Suppl. 4): 73–78.

157 Coron E, Hatlebakk JG, Galmiche JP. Medical therapy of gastroesophageal reflux disease. *Curr Opin Gastroenterol* 2007; 23(4): 434–439.

158 Rubenstein J, Chen JW. Epidemiology of gastroesophageal reflux disease. *Gastroenterol Clin North Am* 2014; 43(1): 1–14.

159 Eherer A. Management of gastroesophageal reflux disease: lifestyle modification and alternative approaches. *Dig Dis Sci* 2014; 32(1–2): 149–151.

160 Chaves RC, Suesada M, Polisel F *et al.* Respiratory physiotherapy can increase lower esophageal sphincter pressure in GERD patients. *Resp Med* 2012; 106: 1794–1799.

161 da Silva RCV, de Sá CC, Pascual-Vaca ÁO *et al.* Increase of lower esophageal sphincter pressure after osteopathic intervention on the diaphragm in patients with gastroesophageal reflux. *Dis Esophagus* 2013; 26: 451–456.

162 Nobre e Souza MA, Lima MJV, Martins GB *et al.* Inspiratory muscle training improves antireflux barrier in GERD patients. *Am J Physiol* 2013; 305: G862–G867.

163 Ding Z, Wang ZF, Sun XH *et al.* Gémó xùnliàn zài huànzhě bùtóng shíqí wèi shíguǎn fǎn liú bìng de zhìliáo jīlǐ. [Therapeutic mechanism of diaphragm training at different periods in patients with gastroesophageal reflux disease]. *Zhonghua Yi Xue Za Zhi* 2013; 93(40): 3215–3219.

3 Optimizing gastro-duodenal function during physical activity

Introduction

An athlete can sustain brief periods of physical activity without ingestion of any additional fluid or metabolites. However, the loss of fluid equivalent to 3–4% of body mass is enough to impair human performance, and after 60–90 minutes of vigorous endurance activity, depletion of glycogen reserves in the muscles and liver also limits muscle and brain function. During prolonged periods of physical activity, the primary roles of the stomach and duodenum are thus to allow the absorption of sufficient fluid and minerals to replace sweat losses and to augment depleted muscular and hepatic glycogen reserves. If the stomach and duodenum fail to fulfil these functions, not only is physical performance impaired,[1,2] but dehydration can ultimately progress to death from heat stroke,[3,4] a catastrophe well recognized among both athletes and workers in deep underground mines. If a prolonged bout of heavy exercise is contemplated, it is thus important to know how to optimize the delivery of fluid and carbohydrate to the circulation of the exerciser. This implies an understanding of how to maximize rates of gastric emptying for various nutrients, factors influencing their subsequent uptake by the circulation, and how these processes are modified when people are engaged in various types and intensities of physical activity.

This chapter thus considers the influence of physical activity upon various aspects of gastric and duodenal function, using this background to make some practical recommendations for meeting the nutritional needs of those who engage in prolonged and vigorous endurance activity. We begin with some comments on methodology, and then consider the impact of various patterns of physical activity upon gastric and duodenal function, relating these findings to the optimal choice of beverage for fluid replenishment in various types of sport. Detailed examination of the influence of habitual physical activity upon common gastro-duodenal pathologies, including peptic ulcers and gastro-oesophageal cancers is deferred to the following two chapters.

Methods of studying gastric function

The approaches both to study gastro-duodenal function and to express gastric motility have an important influence upon the conclusions that are drawn. Many measuring techniques can only be used at rest or during the recovery period immediately following a bout of physical activity, and the erroneous assumption is sometimes made that the functional patterns observed at rest and during recovery are the same as those found during a bout of vigorous physical activity.

Rate of gastric emptying

Early qualitative data on the rate of gastric emptying were obtained either by direct observation of gastric contractions in individuals with gastric fistulae,[5,6] or by radiographic visualization of the rate of emptying of a barium sulphate suspension from the stomach. The average speed of emptying of the barium sulphate suspension was found to match that of water, at least under resting conditions,[7] although sometimes the suspension tended to separate from solid food, thus providing misleading information on the emptying of a normal meal. More recent approaches to measuring the rate of gastric emptying include sequential aspiration of the stomach contents, ultra-sonography, scintigraphy, and determinations of abdominal impedance.

Gastric aspiration. One of my former mentors at Guy's Hospital in London (Maurice Campbell) and his colleagues introduced the concept of assessing gastric emptying rate by using an oral or naso-pharyngeal tube to aspirate from the stomach the remnants of a porridge test meal one hour after it had been ingested.[8] The added contribution of gastric secretions was estimated by assuming that these secretions had a known and constant chlorine ion content.[9] Details of the emptying process were explored by retaining differing volumes of fluid in the stomach for differing times on different days.

Multiple observations were made over periods as long as four weeks. However, considerable subject cooperation was required, as at each visit subjects had to travel into central London without breakfast, undergo a rather unpleasant intubation and then retain a large volume of an unpleasant tasting test-meal in the stomach for an hour or more. A further important limitation to this approach was a considerable intra-individual day-to-day variation in the emptying rate for any given volume of fluid.[10,11]

The difficulty of day-to-day variation in gastric motility is now circumvented by multiple sampling on a single day, using double-lumen catheters and a non-absorbable marker.[12] By repeated instillation of the marker dye, it is possible to determine residual gastric volumes at various times after commencing a bout of physical activity.[13] Further, the contribution of gastric secretions to the total stomach contents can now be examined in terms of the dilution of a second non-absorbable marker, introduced into the stomach at the beginning of the experiment.[12]

Nevertheless, the prolonged presence of an oral or naso-pharyngeal catheter is not particularly pleasant for a subject, and may in itself modify gastric emptying rates.[14] Possibly, this issue can be overcome by the use of very thin catheters,[15] but the complexity of double- and triple-lumen intubation still limits observations to small studies carried out in a research setting, usually with the subjects who are resting rather than exercising.

Ultrasonography. Rather than tracking changes in the volume of the entire stomach, ultrasonography usually assesses changes of cross-sectional area in one predetermined region of the stomach (the antrum) following ingestion of a test meal.[16,17] Most ultrasonographic data have been collected under resting conditions, although a few studies have also been completed immediately following a bout of physical activity.[18,19]

Scintigraphy. Quantitative studies of gastric emptying in resting subjects can be obtained by radio-nuclide imaging. Indium or [99m]technetium-labelled diethylene triamine penta-acetic acid (DTPA) markers are added to the nutrient solutions that are ingested.[20,21] It is not always easy to persuade volunteers to ingest radioactive materials. Technetium has the advantage of a relatively short radioactive half-life, allowing repeated measurements on the same subject without excessive exposure to radiation. The technetium is neither absorbed nor adsorbed by the gut mucosa. However, if a solid meal is ingested, the radioactive marker may dissociate from the other nutrients, giving an unreliable measure of the rate of emptying for the meal itself.[21] Scintigraphy often suggests slower gastric emptying rates than direct aspiration of the stomach contents, perhaps in part because emissions continue to be counted from radioactive fluid that has already passed through the pylorus and into the duodenum or other parts of the body.[22]

A comparison of data between ultrasonography and scintigraphy also shows some systematic differences.[23,24] Ultrasonography is currently considered as the reference methodology.

Impedance techniques. Other potential options for measuring the rate of gastric emptying are impedance epigastrophagy[25] and applied potential tomography.[26] Both of these techniques are based upon the greater electrical conductivity of fluids relative to solid tissues. Epigastrophagy measures the electrical impedance between a single pair of electrodes placed anterior to and posterior to the stomach, whereas applied potential tomography employs a bank of 16 electrodes to determine changes in the resistivity of a thick cross-section of the upper abdomen. Both of these techniques have the advantage of being non-invasive, but as with most impedance technology, a number of interfering factors preclude any close relationship between abdominal impedance and the fluid content of the stomach. Thus, these approaches have not replaced ultrasonography or scintigraphy for most studies of gastric emptying.[25]

Data handling. Gastric emptying rates have often been expressed simply as a volume transfer, expressed in mL/min. However, this is an unsatisfactory approach, since the emptying of the stomach is an exponential process that depends in part upon the remaining volume of the gastric contents.[27,28] One immediate manifestation of this problem is an apparent diminution in the inhibitory effects of ingested glucose upon gastric emptying as observations continue.[29] This finding reflects the common practice of drinking the glucose solution and any comparison beverage as a single bolus. The glucose solution is emptied more slowly than, for example, a comparable amount of water. Larger relative volumes of glucose drinks thus persist in the stomach as observations continue, and the greater remaining volume of fluid in the stomach maintains a higher rate of emptying than that for water.

A few investigators have opted to express data as half-emptying times, although these also vary, depending upon the initial volume of the gastric contents.

In order to interpret emptying rates appropriately, it is necessary to standardize the volume of fluid that is initially ingested, the period of observation, and any additional fluid that is drunk over the course of the study.

Evaluating duodenal motility and nutrient absorption

Motility. Local movement within the intestines can be visualized from the displacement of radio-opaque markers.[30,31] Pressure-sensitive radio-telemetry capsules can also monitor the movement of pressure waves created by slowly migrating motor complexes within the wall of the intestine.[32]

The combined motility of the stomach and small intestine can be examined by ingesting a solution of lactulose. The lactulose is not absorbed by either the stomach or the small intestine, but it undergoes fermentation to hydrogen within five minutes of entering the large intestine.[33] The hydrogen can be readily detected in samples of expired air, thus providing an estimate of the time that has been taken for the lactulose marker to be carried from the mouth to the large intestine.

Absorption of nutrients. Triple-lumen tubes allow the direct collection of intestinal contents from regions of specific interest,[34] although problems of interpretation can arise if samples are drawn from an unrepresentative film of unstirred fluid that lies in immediate contact with the intestinal endothelium.[35] Other limitations of the triple-lumen approach are that it only measures the flux of metabolites in one small segment of the intestines, and that it does not allow for possible changes in gut contents due to secretions from the stomach or more proximal regions of the small intestine. Moreover, local intestinal motility tends to be modified by the inflatable balloons that are used to isolate the gut segment under investigation, and this may in turn affect the rate of absorption of nutrients. Finally, if a person has engaged in very heavy and prolonged exercise, ischaemic damage to the integrity of the intestinal endothelium may allow the absorption of what are supposedly "unabsorbed" marker substances such as polyethylene glycol.

By examining the movement of radioactive markers into the circulation, data can be collected on the speed of a combination of gastric emptying and intestinal absorption. In a typical protocol,[36] solutions containing a water isotope (D_2O) and a non-absorbed marker (polyethylene glycol) are infused into the small intestine via the first of the three tube lumens, usually at a speed that is representative of the anticipated rate of gastric emptying.[37] One alternative approach is to ingest small volumes of fluid repeatedly, so that gastric emptying rather than an external infusion of fluid supplies an appropriate volume of fluid to the small intestine.[38] Aspiration of samples through the second lumen of the catheter, some

10–20 cm distal, provides a measure of admixture with endogenous secretions, and samples collected through the third lumen 20–60 cm beyond that examine the absorption of water and solutes into the blood stream. The net movement of water into or out of the gut can be assessed in terms of changes in concentration of the polyethylene glycol, which (in the absence of visceral ischaemia) is presumed to be unabsorbed.[34]

Other investigators have based their research upon the uptake of ^{13}C acetate. This radioactive marker is absorbed in the small intestine, but not in the stomach. If ^{13}C acetate is added to the ingested fluid, a qualitative comparison of the speed of gastric emptying for various carbohydrate solutions can be deduced from the respective times to a peaking of $^{13}CO_2$ concentrations in expired gas.[39–41]

Physical activity and other factors modifying gastro-duodenal function

A multitude of biological factors acting within both the stomach and the duodenum can modify the rate of gastric emptying,[21,42] and the influence of many of these factors is likely to be modified during a bout of vigorous physical activity.

Intra-gastric influences

Within the stomach, the most potent factor influencing the rate of emptying is the initial volume of the gastric contents. Mechano-receptors in the stomach wall are stimulated as this volume is increased. The response of a resting individual was described by Naylor Hunt[28] as early as 1951. Unfortunately, this classical and careful research was ignored by some subsequent investigators. Rehrer et al.[43] also inferred a volume effect from the faster gastric emptying that was seen during the first 20 minutes following fluid ingestion. Because of a diminishing gastric volume, emptying usually proceeds much more slowly once 60–70% of a drink has reached the small intestines. Reflex effects upon the stomach arising from the accumulation of metabolites in the duodenum can sometimes cause hypertonic solutions to empty in a quasi-linear rather than an exponential fashion.[44]

Costill and Saltin[27] found that gastric emptying peaked at a rate of around 25 mL/min following the ingestion of 600 mL of fluid. Incidentally, they chose a larger volume of ingested fluid than that used in many of the other published studies. One immediate corollary of the volume effect is that the average rate of gastric emptying is increased if filling of the stomach is maintained by drinking small volumes of fluid throughout an experiment. Duchman et al.[45] found that emptying rates reached values as high as 41.5 mL/min when their subjects ingested an initial 750 mL of water, followed by a further 180 mL every subsequent 10 minutes.

Food composition also has an important influence on the rate of gastric emptying. Solutions containing carbohydrate polymers have been used to test the influence of the caloric density of a drink (the energy content per unit volume) versus its osmolality. Such studies suggest that caloric density is the more important determinant of emptying rates,[46–48] although it remains possible that because polymers are rapidly hydrolysed to simple carbohydrates once they reach the duodenum, a reflex feedback to the stomach from a build-up of osmotic pressure in the duodenum is the real limiting factor.[49] Other possible modifying influences are the bulk/weight of any solids, the food particle size, liquidity, and the temperature of the ingested material.

Duodenal influences

There are many potential factors within the duodenum that can modify the rate of gastric emptying. These feedback influences include acid receptors in the proximal part of the duodenum,[50] and duodenal osmotic receptors that are sensitive to local concentrations of electrolytes and carbohydrates.[51]

Studies in the rat have shown that the delayed gastric emptying provoked by vigorous physical activity (15 minutes of swimming against an added load equal to 5% of body mass) can be countered by administering a sodium bicarbonate solution 40 minutes prior to exercise; this intervention acts by reducing the normal inhibitory effects of the duodenal acidosis that develops during vigorous physical activity.[52]

The duodenal accumulation of metabolites that can slow gastric emptying is modified by enzyme availability and by the absorption of nutrients and fluids from the small intestine. The rate of absorption depends in turn upon interactions between sodium and glucose concentrations, and effects from a decrease in splanchnic blood flow, possibly including an ischaemic inhibition of active mineral uptake by the energy-dependent sodium pumps in the gut wall.[42]

The entry of fats into the jejunum stimulates a production of the hormone enterogastrone, and this causes a reflex inhibition of gastric motility, as does the local breakdown of protein and the liberation of amino acids.[53] A variety of other hormones (including catecholamines, gastrin, motilin, secretin, glucagon, gastric inhibitory polypeptide, somatostatin and endorphins) can also modify small intestinal function.[21,54]

Physical activity and gastric emptying

Popular literature has long maintained that an exercise-induced retention of fluid and food in the stomach can hamper athletic performance, not only by limiting the uptake of carbohydrates and fluids, but also by causing disabling symptoms during and after an event.[55,56] However, objective data do not support such contentions; physical activity does not seem to modify the rate of gastric emptying, at least at intensities of effort below 70% of an individual's $\dot{V}O_{2max}$.

Historical background

William Beaumont[5] had the opportunity to make extensive studies on a man with a gastric fistula due to a gunshot wound. Beaumont concluded (p. 85) that "moderate exercise conduces considerably to healthy and rapid digestion", whereas (p. 86) "severe and fatiguing exercise ... retards digestion". Some 80 years later, Carlson[6] made further observations on dogs, on another human subject with a gastric fistula and on four healthy laboratory workers. He observed (p. 210) "Standing or walking in situ has no effect on the gastric tonus or the hunger contractions ... but running in situ promptly inhibits the gastric contractions".

Maurice Campbell and his associates[8] made semi-quantitative observations on gastric emptying, measuring the remnants of a porridge test meal aspirated from the stomach one hour after it had been ingested. Mild exercise increased the proportion of the meal emptied from the stomach over the hour, but running a total distance of one to four miles caused abdominal discomfort and increased the gastric residue, particularly in those subjects who were unfit. Hellebrandt and his colleagues[57] followed the gastric emptying of a mixture of porridge, water and barium sulphate, using the techniques of fluoroscopy and manometry in addition to gastric aspiration. Again, they found that mild exercise enhanced gastric emptying, but that "violent and exhaustive" exercise caused an initial inhibition of both gastric emptying and acid secretion. This article cited other early reports suggesting that mild exercise either had little influence upon the motor power of the stomach[58] or speeded emptying,[59,60] whereas violent running inhibited gastric peristalsis.[58]

Influence of ingested fluid volume upon gastric emptying

Early studies at Guy's Hospital had addressed the important issue of the initial volume of gastric contents.[28] Emptying of a relatively inert citrus pectin meal with a "neutral" osmotic pressure varied linearly with gastric volume, from 5 mL/min at an initial volume of 200 mL to 20 mL/min at an initial volume of 600 mL.

Mitchell and Voss[61] extended these observations to individuals who were engaged in physical activity. They had subjects ingest 200, 300 or 400 mL of a 7.5% carbohydrate solution every 15 minutes during 2 hours of cycling at an intensity of effort that induced an oxygen consumption 70% of the individual's $\dot{V}O_{2max}$. The rate of gastric emptying showed a progressive increment over this range of fluid intakes, although the authors cautioned that an excessive rate of ingestion of fluid could cause the gastric volume to exceed its optimal value of 600 mL, with a resultant risk of abdominal discomfort and a deterioration in exercise performance. Mudambo *et al.*[62] noted that the rate of gastric emptying stimulated by ingestion of fluid (400 mL every 20 minutes) was about a third greater during moderate sustained exercise (an alternation of 15-minute runs at 50% of $\dot{V}O_{2max}$ and 10-minute walks for a total of 3 hours) than when subjects were resting.

Influence of exercise intensity

Although large inter-individual differences in gastric emptying rates have been seen under resting conditions,[63] investigators have generally assumed that the effects of exercise upon gastric motility are similar in "slow" and "fast" emptiers. Quantitative studies have generally confirmed the findings of early qualitative reports (see Table 3.1). Among 9 small-scale studies of moderate exercise at intensities up to 70% of $\dot{V}O_{2max}$, 4 investigations (1 with measurements made post-exercise) showed no change in gastric emptying,[27,64–66] and in the remaining 5 studies (1 based on post-exercise data) a small speeding of emptying was seen.[18,67–70] Animal experiments have suggested that any exercise-related stimulation of gastric emptying is dependent upon intact vagal innervation.[71]

At higher intensities of effort, six of seven studies found that exercise slowed the rate of gastric emptying.[18,19,27,68,72,73] However, recovery of normal function was rapid post-exercise, and even intensive sprinting had no effects on gastric emptying 30 minutes later.[66]

The effects of moderate exercise seem similar for liquids and for solid food such as a typical evening meal of entrée and dessert,[67] a comprehensive meal,[70] or radioactively labelled stewed beef.[69] Likewise, 10 minutes of vigorous cycle ergometer exercise at 85% of maximal heart rate delayed the emptying of a semi-solid meal of chicken broth and beans.[19]

Maughan *et al.*[73] used heavy water (^2H_2O) to study the overall gastro-duodenal absorption of water, finding a slowing of its uptake as the intensity of effort was increased from 40 to 62 and then to 80% of the individual's $\dot{V}O_{2max}$.

Influence of the type of physical activity

Despite substantial differences in abdominal mechanics between walking and running,[74] the two types of activity generally have comparable effects upon the rate of gastric emptying at any given intensity of effort.[68] Houmard *et al.*[75] saw no difference of gastric emptying between cycle ergometry and running when subjects were exercising at an intensity of effort demanding 75% of their $\dot{V}O_{2max}$, and Rehrer *et al.*[76] also reported that gastric emptying was initially similar for treadmill running and cycle ergometry when exercising at 70% of $\dot{V}O_{2max}$. The similarity of emptying continued for hypertonic drinks, but if a hypotonic drink was ingested, emptying became slightly faster for cycling than for running after the activity had continued for 40 minutes. Rehrer *et al.*[76] concluded that any differences relating to the mode of physical activity were small, and could not account for the greater prevalence of abdominal symptoms when running relative to cycling.

There seem to be some differences of gastro-duodenal response between continuous and intermittent exercise. Leiper *et al.*[77] compared steady-state cycle ergometer exercise at 66% of $\dot{V}O_{2max}$ with intermittent exercise at intensities averaging either 66% or 75% of $\dot{V}O_{2max}$. Over the first 20 minutes of effort, gastric emptying rates were essentially unchanged by constant exercise, but in contrast emptying dropped to 60% and 31% of resting values for the 2 intensities of intermittent exercise. Likewise, gastric emptying during the intermittent exercise of a five-a-side soccer game was much slower than when walking (period 1 of the game, 34%, period 2, 60% of the walking value[78]). Again, data collected during an intermittent shuttle run showed an emptying rate that was 73% of the walking value following the ingestion of placebo solutions, and 60% of the walking value for the emptying of a carbohydrate/electrolyte solution.[79]

Table 3.1 Effects of moderate and vigorous physical activity upon the rate of gastric emptying

Author	Subjects	Exercise modality	Gastric methodology	Findings
Moderate exercise				
Beaumont[5]	Man with gastric fistula	Unspecified type and duration	Direct visualization	"Conduces considerably to healthy and rapid digestion"
Cammack *et al.*[67]	7 healthy volunteers	Cycle ergometry at heart rate of 120 beats/min 5 in every 10 min for 6 hours	Technetium sulphur colloid	Rate of gastric emptying faster than at rest in 6/7 subjects
Campbell *et al.*[8]	Laboratory workers	Mild exercise	Aspiration of a porridge test meal at 1 hour	Gastric emptying increased
Carlson[6]	Man with gastric fistula, 4 healthy lab workers, dogs	Standing, walking *in situ*	Direct visualization	No effect on gastric tonus or hunger contractions
Costill and Saltin[27]	15 men	Cycle ergometry at 40–70% of $\dot{V}O_{2max}$	Aspiration after 15 minutes	No effect on gastric emptying
Evans *et al.*[66]	5 men, 3 women	Cycling at 33% of peak power		No effect on emptying 30 min post-exercise
Fordtran and Saltin[64]	4 men, 1 woman	Treadmill exercise at average 71% of $\dot{V}O_{2max}$	Aspiration after 1 hour	Exercise had no effect on emptying of either water or 13.3% glucose/ 0.3% saline
Franke *et al.*[70]	10 healthy men	Moderate walking, 4 km/h on treadmill		Half-time of emptying of solid meal decreased from 123 to 107 min. Gastric emptying unaffected by associated alcohol intake

Study	Subjects	Exercise	Method	Result
Hellebrandt and Tepper[57]		Mild exercise	Fluoroscopy, manometry and gastric aspiration	Gastric emptying enhanced
Marzio et al.[18]	Ultrasonography (11 normal subjects), scintigraphy (6 normal subjects)	Treadmill exercise (30 min at 50% of maximal heart rate)	Measurements immediately post-exercise	Gastric emptying of water accelerated after exercise
Moore et al.[69]	10 healthy men	Treadmill walking at 3.2 and 6.4 km/h	Radioactively labelled stewed beef	Gastric half-emptying time decreased from rest (72.6 min) to 44.5 min (3.2 km/h) and 32.9 min (6.4 km/h)
Neufer et al.[68]	10 healthy men	Treadmill walking (at 28, 41 or 56%) or running (57% or 65%) of $\dot{V}O_{2max}$	Aspiration after 15 minutes	Small increase of emptying, similar for walking and running
van Nieuwenhoven et al.[65]	10 well-trained men	90 min of cycle ergometry at 70% of maximal power output		No change of gastric emptying
Heavy exercise				
Beaumont[5]	Man with gastric fistula	Severe and fatiguing exercise, unspecified type and duration	Direct visualization	"Retards digestion"
Brown et al.[19]	Ultrasonography	10 min of cycle ergometry at 85% of maximal heart rate		Gastric emptying of semi-solid chicken broth and beans delayed by exercise
Campbell et al.[8]	Laboratory workers	Running 1–4 miles	Aspiration of a porridge test meal at 1 hour	Abdominal discomfort, slowed gastric emptying, particularly if subjects unfit

continued

Table 3.1 Continued

Author	Subjects	Exercise modality	Gastric methodology	Findings
Carlson[6]	Man with gastric fistula, 4 healthy lab workers, dogs	Running *in situ*	Direct visualization	Inhibits gastric contractions
Costill and Saltin[27]	15 men	Cycle ergometry at 80–90% of $\dot{V}O_{2max}$	Aspiration after 15 minutes	Slowing of gastric emptying
Evans et al.[66]	5 men, 3 women	Ten 1-min sprints at peak power	Measurements 30 minutes post-exercise	No effect on gastric emptying
Hellebrandt and Tepper[57]		Violent and exhaustive exercise	Fluoroscopy, manometry and gastric aspiration	Gastric secretion reduced, emptying slowed
Marzio et al.[18]	Ultrasonography (11 normal subjects), scintigraphy (6 normal subjects)	Treadmill exercise (30 min at 70% of maximal heart rate)	Measurements immediately post-exercise	Gastric emptying of water slowed after exercise
Maughan et al.[73]	6 healthy men	Cycle ergometry at 42, 61 or 80% of $\dot{V}O_{2max}$	Plasma accumulation of ^2H	Overall absorption slowed progressively as intensity of exercise increased
Neufer et al.[68]	10 healthy men	Treadmill running at 75% of $\dot{V}O_{2max}$	Aspiration after 15 minutes	Gastric emptying slower than for lower intensities of effort
Ramsbottom and Hunt[72]	6 young men	20 minutes of cycle ergometry at 125 watts	Aspiration	30% increase of gastric residual volume with exercise in 4/6 subjects

Abbreviations: $\dot{V}O_{2max}$ = maximal oxygen intake.

Influence of training status

Anecdotal evidence has suggested that aerobic training may facilitate gastric emptying during physical activity.[80] However, experimental data show that any effect of such training upon the rate of gastric emptying is quite small, and it may arise because when a person is exercising at a fixed absolute intensity of effort, the relative loading is higher for sedentary than for well-conditioned individuals.

Carrió *et al.*[81] compared gastric emptying between marathon runners and sedentary controls. Under resting conditions, respective half-times for the emptying of an egg omelette sandwich plus 200 mL of orange juice were 67.7 and 85.3 minutes. Moreover, running 20–22.5 km over 90 minutes had no effect upon gastric emptying in the well-trained runners. Rehrer *et al.*[43] compared responses to cycle ergometry at 50% and 70% of peak working capacity between 8 trained and 8 untrained subjects. Exercise did not affect the gastric emptying of water, but it did slow the emptying of some isotonic and hypertonic drinks, especially at 70% of maximal working capacity. Nevertheless, this study found no differences of gastric emptying between trained and untrained subjects.

Strid *et al.*[31] compared the gastric emptying rates of orienteers between their rest week and a week when they were undertaking heavy training (running one to two h/day). The training regimen induced an acceleration of colonic transit, but had no effect upon gastric emptying. A high habitual level of physical activity apparently speeds overall oro-caecal transit,[82] but there seems to be a compensatory adaptation of intestinal carbohydrate transport, since the d-xylose uptake as measured by urinary xylose excretion or breath hydrogen production is not compromised by the faster movement of food through the gut in well-trained individuals.

Influences of temperature, osmolality and hypohydration upon the rate of gastric emptying

Gastric emptying proceeds more slowly with the ingestion of warm (35°C) than with cold (5°C) solutions.[83,84] A slowing of emptying also occurs with drinks that have a glucose concentration >139 mM.[27] Owen *et al.*[85] and Ryan *et al.*[86] found that under hot environmental conditions, the presence even of hypotonic concentrations of glucose slowed gastric emptying relative to water.

The environmental temperature is an important determinant of gastric responses. Owen *et al.*[85] compared 2-hour treadmill runs at 65% of $\dot{V}O_{2max}$, finding that residual volumes in the stomach varied positively with both the osmolality of the drink and environmental temperature (35° vs 25°C). Neufer *et al.*[87] had subjects carry out 15-minute bouts of treadmill exercise at 50% of $\dot{V}O_{2max}$ in neutral (18°C), warm (35°C), and hot (49°C) conditions, on one occasion when also substantially dehydrated (a 5% decrease in body mass). Gastric emptying was significantly slowed at 49°C, and a slowing was also seen at 35°C if the subject was dehydrated.[87]

Subjects can normally ingest 150–600 mL of fluid periodically while they are running or cycling, with minimal resulting gastro-intestinal complaints.[43,76] However, a 4% reduction of body mass by either sauna exposure or running in the heat slowed gastric emptying more than would be normally anticipated when running on the treadmill at 60% of the individual's maximal speed, and 6 of 16 dehydrated runners also reported gastric discomfort when drinking under these conditions.[88] Other investigators have also found that dehydration has an adverse effect upon gastric emptying.[27,64]

Van Nieuwenhoven *et al.*[89] examined changes in the overall absorption of nutrients by the ^{13}C method. They induced a 3% loss of body mass by sauna exposure, and assessed the rate of gastric emptying from the subsequent ^{13}C enrichment of breath samples. During cycle ergometry at 70% of the individual's maximal working capacity, the average time to reach a peak enrichment of ^{13}C in expired air was 23.6 minutes when the subject was dehydrated, compared with 17.1 minutes when he or she was euhydrated. Ryan *et al.*[90] induced a slightly lesser degree of dehydration (a 2.7% reduction of body mass) and opted for a slightly lower intensity of exercise (cycle ergometry at 65% of $\dot{V}O_{2max}$). Under these conditions, they saw no impairment of either gastric emptying or absorption of a water placebo.

Influences of stress and habituation upon gastric emptying

There is limited evidence that emotional stress may delay gastric emptying,[4] and this could be a further factor modifying gastro-duodenal function when athletes are engaged in competition. Many manifestations of emotional stress are alleviated by habituation, but it is unclear whether this is true of its effects upon gastric emptying. Lambert *et al.*[91] examined the habituation of a small group of runners to drinking sufficient fluid to match sweat losses over 6 successive 90-minute treadmill runs at 65% of $\dot{V}O_{2max}$. Although gastric discomfort had lessened by run 6, the rate of gastric emptying remained unchanged over the six trials.

Possible mechanisms modifying the rate of gastric emptying during vigorous physical activity

The mechanisms that slow gastric emptying during vigorous physical activity remain unclear, but they may include an exercise-induced increase of sympathetic nerve tone, and the release of catecholamines and opiates.[92–95] Effects may also arise from an altered duodenal absorption of metabolites, for instance due to a reduction of visceral blood flow and the resulting development of visceral ischaemia.

Physical activity and gastric secretions

Gastric secretions increase with the ingestion of hypertonic fluids.[96] A substantial number of reports have examined interactions between physical activity and the secretion of acid, but much less attention has been paid to the effects of physical activity upon the other constituents of gastric secretion.

Gastric acid secretion and physical activity

Campbell *et al.*[8] surmised that vigorous physical activity reduced gastric acid secretion, although they recognized that the aspiration of stomach contents one hour after a meal reflected overall acidity rather than the amount of acid that had been secreted during their experiment. Hammar *et al.*[97] concluded from a review of the literature and experiments on dogs that strenuous physical activity decreased both basal acid output and the additional acid that was secreted by the stomach in response to the stimuli of food and histamine; the inhibitory effects of vigorous physical activity were independent of local vagal innervation, and cross-transfusion experiments suggested that some hormone was involved.

Sullivan[98] concluded from a literature review that although mild exercise had little effect upon gastric secretions, moderate to vigorous physical activity inhibited the basal, meal and histamine-simulated acid production of the stomach, although not the maximal acid secretion that could be induced by administration of pentagastrin. Others showed that the inhibition of acid secretion continued for some period following a bout of exercise,[99,100] was inversely related to the fitness of the individual, and was exacerbated by the emotional excitement of competition.[101]

The findings from some more recent studies support these findings (see Table 3.2). Although 3 reports found no change of acid secretion with exercise at intensities demanding up to 75% of maximal power output, whether subjects had ingested water, a hypertonic glucose/electrolyte solution, or a liquid or a solid meal,[64,65,102] in 4 other reports there was some reduction in both basic acid secretion and the secretory response to the ingestion of 5% glucose during or following exercise, despite somewhat lower intensities and shorter durations of effort.[72,99,100,103]

Two authors compared the exercise responses of healthy individuals and those with peptic ulcers. Zach *et al.*[100] found that an hour of cycle ergometer exercise at 50% of an individual's maximal heart rate reduced acid secretion during and following exercise in both healthy individuals and in those with gastric ulcers, but in those with duodenal ulcers the same dose of exercise increased acid secretion. Likewise, Canalles *et al.*[103] reported that one hour of exercise in the training zone decreased the basal secretion of acid relative to resting conditions in healthy individuals; however, in those with peptic ulcers, acid secretion was further increased during the test exercise.

Physical activity and other gastric secretions

Physical activity can induce a decrease in some other gastric secretions. Zach *et al.*[100] found that an hour of cycle ergometer exercise at 50% of the individual's maximal heart rate reduced both the volume of gastric secretion and its

Table 3.2 Effects of physical activity upon gastric secretions

Author	Sample	Exercise modality	Findings	Comments
Campbell et al.[8]	Laboratory workers	Running 1–4 miles	Gastric acid secretion presumed reduced	Conclusions based on acidity of gastric contents
Canalles et al.[103]	10 healthy individuals, 16 patients with duodenal ulcer	60 min of exercise in training zone	Basal secretion of acid decreased relative to rest	Acid secretion increased in patients with peptic ulcers
Feldman and Nixon[102]	Healthy adults	Cycle ergometer exercise at 50% or 75% of maximal power output 45 min after steak meal	No change of gastric secretory response relative to resting conditions 45 min after eating a steak meal	
Fordtran and Saltin[64]	4 men, 1 woman	Treadmill exercise for 1 hour at average 71% of $\dot{V}O_{2max}$	No change in acid retrieved from stomach relative to resting conditions following ingestion of water or 13.3% glucose/electrolyte	
Hammar and Öbrink[97]	Dogs	Treadmill running, 30–60 min at 6.2 km/h	Inhibition of food or histamine-stimulated secretion in Heidenhain pouch animals	Inhibitory effect of exercise could be transmitted to another dog via blood
Hellebrandt and Tepper,[57] Hellebrandt and Miles[101]	Young female physical education student	Comparison of mild and exhaustive exercise	Mild exercise did not affect peak acidity; violent and exhaustive exercise reduced it	Gastric aspiration. Effects of exercise exacerbated by competition

Study	Subjects	Protocol	Findings	
Hoelzel[104]			Acidity of gastric contents reduced, mucin increased during quiescence	Increased lactate secretion in gastric juice during exercise
Markiewicz et al.[99]	14 healthy men	20 minutes of cycle ergometry at 125 watts	Basic gastric secretion unchanged during exercise, but declined during 20 min of recovery	
Ramsbottom and Hunt[72]	6 young men	20 minutes of cycle ergometry at 125 watts	20% decrease in acid secretion with exercise following ingestion of 5% glucose	
van Nieuwenhoven et al.[65]	10 well-trained men	90 min of cycle ergometry at 70% of maximal power output	No change of intra-gastric pH relative to rest following standard liquid breakfast (4 mL/kg)	
Zach et al.[100]	25 healthy individuals, 15 gastric and 54 duodenal ulcer patients	60 minutes of cycle ergometry at 50% of maximal heart rate	In healthy individuals, decreased basic secretion of gastric fluid and acid content during exercise and recovery	Gastric ulcer patients respond similarly to healthy individuals; in duodenal ulcer patients, exercise increases acid secretion

Abbreviation: $\dot{V}O_{2max}$ = maximal oxygen intake.

electrolyte content. Oektedalen *et al.*[105] noted a decrease in meal-stimulated gastrin secretion in army cadets during the course of participation in an arduous four-day field-training exercise. However, the secretion of other gastro-intestinal hormones (gastrin, motilin, glucagon, pancreatic polypeptide and vasoactive intestinal peptide) was unaffected by exercise at intensities up to 90% of $\dot{V}O_{2max}$.[106,107]

Physical activity and other aspects of gastro-duodenal function

Vigorous physical activity may modify the rate of transit of materials through the small intestine, as well as changing the rate of absorption of various nutrients. Very heavy and prolonged physical activity may also compromise the normal mucosal barrier to the absorption of intestinal endotoxins.

Influence of physical activity upon small intestinal transit

Physical activity seems to have only minor effects upon small intestinal motility. Harrison *et al.*[108] saw no change in the displacement of radio-opaque intestinal markers with 25–45 minutes of jogging, and Ollerenshaw *et al.*[109] also found no significant change in the rate of displacement of radioactive markers with exercise at intensities inducing heart rates of up to160 beats/min. However, cycle ergometry for 90 minutes at 70% of maximal working capacity increased peristaltic velocity slightly, from an average of 4.0 to 4.9 cm/sec.[65]

The use of radio-telemetry capsules demonstrated a slowing of migrating motor complexes in the intestinal wall of young and healthy volunteers following a 19-km walk,[32] and this prolonged bout of physical activity delayed the transit of radio-opaque capsules through the intestines.[30] Soffer *et al.*[110] noted that very vigorous exercise tended to increase phase 3 postprandial intestinal motor activity. No effect was seen when exercising at 60% of $\dot{V}O_{2max}$ but intestinal activity was augmented at 80% of $\dot{V}O_{2max}$, and this response became even more marked at 90% of $\dot{V}O_{2max}$. Peters *et al.*[111] had subjects run and cycle at about 70% of $\dot{V}O_{2peak}$ for a total of 170 minutes. This shortened the time to the onset of phase 3 intestinal contractions, from a resting value of 183 minutes to 152 minutes following the ingestion of water, and to 63 minutes after ingestion of a carbohydrate solution.

Walking at 5.6 km/h up a 2% grade shortened the oro-caecal transit time substantially,[112] but this could reflect a speeding of gastric emptying rather than an increase of small intestinal motility. More vigorous physical activity has usually had little effect upon motility of the small intestine. For instance, a 6-hour cycle ergometer ride at an average heart rate of 117 beats/min had no effect upon the overall transit time for a solid meal, as measured by the breath hydrogen technique.[67] Likewise, one hour of cross-country running at an intensity of 70% of $\dot{V}O_{2max}$ did not alter the overall transit time of female athletes as assessed by pH telemetry,[113] and 90 minutes of cycle ergometry at 70% of $\dot{V}O_{2max}$ did not change the oro-caecal transit time in 10 well-trained men.[65] However, Meshkinpour *et al.*[114] found a slowing of lactulose transit from mouth to caecum when sedentary individuals undertook 60 minutes of treadmill walking at 4.5 km/hour, and others have reported a slowing of overall transit at high intensities of effort (treadmill running at 60% and 90% of $\dot{V}O_{2max}$ and interval running).[115,116]

A week of heavy training (running one to two h/day) speeded the passage of radio-opaque markers through the small intestine of orienteers;[31] however, this seems an immediate effect of the increased physical activity rather than a cumulative response to training.

Physical activity and other factors influencing duodenal and jejunal absorption

The body quickly normalizes the characteristics of fluids in the small intestine. Hypertonic solutions are rapidly brought to isotonicity by a secretion of water into the gut[117] and the absorption of nutrients.[118] In contrast, if the intestinal contents initially contain little or no electrolytes, sodium is rapidly secreted into the gut to restore normal electrolyte concentrations,[34,119] with an associated flux of water into the intestinal lumen.

In terms of maximizing an individual's overall carbohydrate uptake, the rate of transfer of nutrients across the intestinal endothelium is more critical than the rate at which a drink empties from the stomach.[120] Intestinal glucose uptake is an energy-dependent process, linked to active sodium transport across the gut wall, and the rate of transfer is generally thought to depend on luminal concentrations of both glucose and sodium, as well as energy supply to the sodium pump. In contrast, fructose is absorbed passively, so that the ingestion of a solution containing a mixture of glucose and fructose could theoretically increase the movement of water into the blood stream relative to glucose alone.[121]

Water is absorbed mainly in the first 25 cm of the intestines (the duodenum), and in this sector the movement of water is essentially a passive process, driven by local gradients of osmotic pressures. There is a large osmotic gradient between the gut and the blood, favouring the absorption of water relative to an isotonic 6% glucose solution.

In the second and third 25 cm segments of the intestines (the jejunum) the resistance to transfer of nutrients at the gut wall is greater, but here glucose transport is an active process.[122] Water is absorbed along with solutes, giving carbohydrate/electrolyte solutions some advantage over water alone as a means of rehydration.[123] However, the concentration of carbohydrate needed to optimize the speed of water absorption is relatively low (an isotonic, rather than a hypertonic, solution).

The differing patterns of intestinal absorption described by various investigators[37,124–126] depend in part on the intestinal segments where measurements have been made. If data are averaged over the entire first 75 cm of the small intestine, there seems to be little difference of fluid absorption from water and carbohydrate/electrolyte solutions. There are other effects related to methodology.

Gisolfi et al.[127] determined water absorption from differences in polythene glycol concentrations along the intestinal segment, and Fordtran and Saltin[64] based their estimates on the constant infusion of a non-absorbable marker, whereas other investigators have examined the urinary excretion of non-metabolized carbohydrates, both actively absorbed compounds such as 3-O-methyl-d-glucose and passively absorbed d-xylose.[65,128]

It is conceivable that intensive exercise (particularly if combined with heat exposure) could impair the absorption of nutrients, either directly (by reducing local visceral blood flow) or less directly (by causing ischaemic damage to the active transport mechanisms that pump sodium ions and carbohydrates through the endothelial membrane of the intestines). In dogs, the intestinal absorption of glucose and xylose was significantly reduced when visceral blood flow had decreased by 50%,[129] and in humans, the absorption and excretion of 3-methyl glucose was decreased with 3 hours of walking at 4.8km/h in 38°C heat.[129] However, hypohydration alone (a 12.7% reduction of body mass) did not reduce the intestinal absorption of water during 85 minutes of cycling at 65% of $\dot{V}O_{2max}$.[90]

Under temperate conditions, some authors have found that even prolonged exercise (60–90 minutes) at intensities <70% of $\dot{V}O_{2max}$ has little effect upon intestinal fluid absorption.[34] Studies with a steady perfusion of fluids through the first orifice of a triple-lumen tube indicated that treadmill running at 64–78% of $\dot{V}O_{2max}$ did not alter the absorption of water, glucose or sodium ions in the proximal jejunum and ileum.[64] Gisolfi et al.[127] compared 1 hour of cycle ergometer exercise at 30, 50, or 70% of $\dot{V}O_{2max}$ with resting responses; again, the duodeno-jejunal absorption of either water or solute was unaffected by physical activity over this range of intensities. However, van Nieuwenhoven et al.[65] found that cycle ergometry at 70% of an individual's maximal working capacity decreased the active jejunal absorption of glucose as assessed by changing lactulose/rhamnose concentrations, possibly reflecting an adverse effect of local ischaemia on ATPase activity in the jejunal wall. Likewise, Lang et al.[128] observed decreases in both the active jejunal absorption of 3-O-methyl glucose and the passive absorption of d-xylose with exercise at 70% of $\dot{V}O_{2max}$, relative to rates seen when exercising at 30% and 50% of $\dot{V}O_{2max}$. Maughan et al.[73] also reported a decrease in the uptake of deuterated water with cycle ergometry at either 40%, 62% or 80% of $\dot{V}O_{2max}$, although their data left unclear whether there had been a reduction in gastric emptying or a slowing in the intestinal absorption of the deuterated water. Barclay and Turnberg,[130] using the triple-lumen perfusion technique, found a substantial reduction in the intake of both water and sodium ions with cycle ergometer exercise evoking a 40–50% increase of heart rate. One important difference between this and the other studies cited was that the perfusate used by Barclay and Turnberg contained electrolytes but no glucose, thus eliminating the normal effects of the active transport of glucose upon water intake.

There are a number of active transporters of amino acids in the intestinal wall,[131] and these mechanisms could be adversely affected if visceral ischaemia were to develop during vigorous and prolonged physical activity. Existing studies suggest no increase and sometimes a decrease of water absorption if amino acids are added to carbohydrate solutions; possibly, the amino acids compete with the carbohydrates for available sodium ions.[132]

Physical activity and intestinal barrier function

The gut mucosa normally offers a very effective barrier to the penetration of intestinal toxins into the circulation. However, one final effect of the visceral ischaemia induced by heavy and prolonged physical activity is to reduce the efficacy of the mucosal barrier, potentially allowing endotoxins to enter the blood stream.[133,134] Training may be helpful in avoiding this problem, because it reduces the extent of visceral ischaemia that develops at any given absolute intensity of effort.[135]

Practical implications for nutrition of the athlete

What are the practical implications of the above findings? One important application seems to provide data for optimizing nutrition of the athlete during prolonged physical activity. It appears that activity at intensities <70% of $\dot{V}O_{2max}$ can be sustained for quite long periods (60–90 minutes) with little effect upon either gastric emptying or the intestinal absorption of replacement fluids and nutrients.[34,64] Thus, investigators often compare the merits of various athletic drinks in terms of their respective gastric emptying rates as measured under resting conditions (see Table 3.3). In contrast, at higher intensities of exercise, there are negative effects upon all stages of nutrient intake: gastric emptying, gastric secretions, intestinal motility and fluid absorption.

The main nutritional concerns of the endurance athlete are to minimize the depletion of fluid and carbohydrate reserves during a competitive event. Although there can be small losses of fluid in expired gas, urine and faeces, the main reason for water depletion in the athlete is sweating, with cumulative losses ranging from 3 to 10 L in long-distance running events.[136–140] Moreover, there are significant decrements of performance if dehydration is sufficient to cause a weight loss >3–4%. In a hot environment, the primary need is for fluid replacement, and the optimal fluid to ingest is then probably water, but under cooler conditions, the main concern may be to maintain waning carbohydrate reserves,[141–145] and then there is benefit in adding carbohydrate to the ingested fluid.

Nevertheless, many high intensity activities are not pursued for long enough to deplete either carbohydrate or fluid reserves, and the focus should then be upon a choice of fluid that the runner finds agreeable and does not cause gastric discomfort.

Coyle and Montain[146] argued that there were no trade-offs between fluid and carbohydrate needs if an athlete was sweating at a rate of less than 1 L/h. In contrast, when subjects exercised in a warm environment (31°C) for 1 hour at 80% of $\dot{V}O_{2max}$, additive gains of performance were obtained by providing both water and carbohydrate.[147] Our early experience was with post-coronary marathon

Table 3.3 Influence of the composition of drinks upon the rate of gastric emptying

Author	Subjects and exercise type	Exercise intensity	Fluid composition	Gastric emptying
Dickinson et al.[148]	5 endurance athletes, running	Treadmill, 75% of $\dot{V}O_{2max}$ for 90 min	Isotonic drink (<2% carbohydrate) vs 7% carbohydrate, vs 4 mg/kg caffeine vs 7% carbohydrate + caffeine	Gastric emptying slowed by 7% carbohydrate, but speeded by caffeine
Duchman et al.[45]	8 males, resting	No exercise	Water, vs 2% glucose/4% sucrose vs 10% glucose	Emptying 41.4 vs 30.1 vs 25.7 mL/min
Gant et al.[149]	9 male soccer players, running	60 min shuttle running	Water vs carbohydrate/electrolyte	No difference water (18.2 mL/min) vs carbohydrate/electrolyte (16.3 mL/min)
Gonzálvez et al.[150]	26 well-trained cyclists, cycle ergometry	60 min of exercise at 70% $\dot{V}O_{2max}$	10.3% carbohydrates with protein and fruit juice vs 15.2% carbohydrates	Faster gastric emptying with 10.3% carbohydrates
Houmard et al.[75]	10 well-trained male bi- and triathletes, treadmill and cycle ergometry	75% of $\dot{V}O_{2max}$	Water vs 7% glucose	Emptying 8.8 (rest) vs 8.2 (running) vs 8.5 (cycling) mL/min, no difference water or 7% glucose
Kavanagh et al.[151]	9 middle-aged men (5 post-coronary) in marathon run	Running 11.8 km/h for 212 min	Water vs Erg (53 g/L glucose, 354 mOsmol/L) vs Special solution 41 g/L glucose, 278 mOsmol/L	Water intake 547 mL/h, Erg 428 mL/h, Special solution 281 mL/h
Leese et al.[39]	6 healthy subjects (5 male, 1 female), treadmill	Inclined treadmill, 70% of $\dot{V}O_{2max}$	Water vs 18.5% sucrose vs 18.5% glucose vs 18.5% glucose polymer	Peak appearance of $^{13}CO_2$ water 30 min, sucrose 54 min, glucose-polymer 59 min, glucose 62 min

Study	Subjects	Exercise protocol	Treatment	Findings
Leiper et al.[79]	8 healthy trained males, walking and performing intermittent shuttle run	15-min bouts of exercise	Water vs 6.4% carbohydrate/electrolyte	Emptying, first 15 min for walking and shuttle run 17.3, 10.7 mL/min (water), 10.7, 6 mL/min for carbohydrate
MacLaren et al.[20]	5 males, cycle ergometry	cycle ergometry at 70% of $\dot{V}O_{2peak}$, for 45 min	5% glucose vs isosmotic maltodextrin	No difference of gastric emptying
Maughan et al.[13]	6 healthy males, resting		2.3%, 7% glucose vs iso-energetic 6% soy protein hydrolysate vs 12% soy	Half-emptying times 2% glucose 13 min, 7% glucose 25 min, 6% soy 36 min, 12 and soy 80 min
Mitchell et al.[152]	8 trained male cyclists, intermittent cycle ergometry	12 min at 70% of $\dot{V}O_{2max}$, 3 min rest for 2 hours	Water vs 5% vs 6% vs 7.5% carbohydrate	653 mL/h water; only 5% carbohydrate slightly slower emptying (632 mL/h)
Mitchell et al.[153]	10 trained male cyclists, cycle ergometry	Cycling 105 min at 70% of $\dot{V}O_{2max}$, with final 15 min sprint	Water vs 6%, 12% or 18% glucose	12 or 18% glucose slow relative to water (445 mL/h vs 605 mL/h).
Murray et al.[154]	5 healthy men, 1 woman at rest		Water vs 6% sucrose vs 4% sucrose/2% glucose, vs 6% maltodextrin vs 6% glucose as 400 mL bolus	Emptying rate 0–20 min: water 18.8 mL/min, sucrose 18.4 mL/min, sucrose/glucose 16.9 mL/min, maltodextrin 16.6 mL/min, glucose 16.1 mL/min
Murray et al.[155]	8 males, 2 females, cycle ergometry	7 0 min cycle ergometry at 60% of $\dot{V}O_{2max}$	Water vs 6% vs 20% carbohydrate	[13]C gastric emptying and absorption similar for water and 6% carbohydrate, slower for 20% carbohydrate
Näveri et al.[156]	5 resting male subjects		3% glucose vs 3% glucose polymer vs 5% glucose polymer vs 10% glucose polymer	Emptying 3%, 5%, 10% when tested as exponential functions

continued

Table 3.3 Continued

Author	Subjects and exercise type	Exercise intensity	Fluid composition	Gastric emptying
Neufer et al.[157]	21 male, 4 female runners on treadmill	Slower than normal running speed (50–70% of $\dot{V}O_{2max}$) for 15 min	Water vs 5% maltodextrin vs 3% maltodextrin 2% glucose vs 4.5% maltodextrin 2.5% fructose	Emptying of water faster with exercise (331 mL in 15 min) than at rest (258 mL in 15 min); significantly slower if glucose in mixture (218 mL in 15 min), but effect of fructose minimal
Owen et al.[85]	5 fit males, treadmill exercise in heat	Running at 65% of $\dot{V}O_{2max}$ for 2 hours	Water vs 10% glucose polymer, 194 mOsmol/kg, vs 10% glucose 586 mOsmol/kg	Emptying: sweetened water, 354 mL/h, 10% glucose, 246 mL/h, 10% glucose polymer 306 mL/h. Effects of osmolality and environmental temperature
Ramsbottom and Hunt[72]	6 male undergraduates, cycle ergometry	Intensities to 100 W	750 mL of 5% glucose	Exercise at 100 W slowed emptying in 4/6 subjects
Rehrer et al.[43]	8 trained, 8 untrained males, cycle ergometry	50%, 70% W_{max}	Sweetened water vs 15% glucose, vs 15% maltodextrin/3% fructose vs 7% sucrose	Emptying of water (600 mL in 20 min) unaffected by exercise
Rehrer et al.[76]	9 male triathletes, treadmill and cycle ergometer	70% W_{max}	Flavoured water vs isotonic disaccharide vs hypertonic maltodextrin	Isotonic emptying at 60 min cycling ~ 830 mL/h, running ~ 760 mL/h at 60 min; hypertonic ~ 650 mL/h t 60 min for both cycling and running
Rehrer et al.[158]	8 males, cycle ergometer	70% of $\dot{V}O_{2max}$ for 80 min	Water vs 4.5% glucose vs 17% glucose vs 17% maltodextrin	Average over 80 min water 15.7 mL/min, 4.5% glucose 15.3 mL/min, 17% maltodextrin 10.8 mL/min, 17% glucose 9.8 mL/min

Reference	Subjects	Exercise protocol	Treatments	Results
Ryan et al.[90]	Healthy volunteers (5 M, 2 F), cycle ergometry	cycle ergometry, 85 min at 65% of $\dot{V}O_{2max}$	Water vs 6% vs 8% vs 9% carbohydrate	Dehydration (2.7% body mass) does not impair gastric emptying or fluid uptake of water, but water flux less with 8% and 9% carbohydrate
Ryan et al.[86]	8 trained males, cycle ergometer exercise in heat	Cycle ergometry at 60% of $\dot{V}O_{2peak}$ for 3 hours	Water vs 5% glucose, 300 mOsmol/kg, vs 5% glucose polymer, 82 mOsmol/kg, vs 3.2% glucose/1.8% fructose, 156 mOsmol/kg	Emptying: water 1032 mL/h, glucose, 974 ml/h glucose/fructose, 983 mL/h, glucose polymer, 1025 mL/h. Exercise slowed emptying of 2 commercial isotonic drinks and of 15% glucose, effects >at 70% than at 50% W_{max}
Seiple et al.[48]	6 resting male subjects		400 mL bolus, water vs 3% glucose polymer/2% fructose vs 5% glucose polymer/2% fructose	Data corrected for gastric secretion. No difference for 3 solutions (12.0–12.6 mL/min for first 30 min)
Sole and Noakes[159]	7 endurance-trained athletes, treadmill exercise	Running at 75% of $\dot{V}O_{2peak}$	Water vs 15% glucose/polymer	Emptying at rest faster for 15% glucose polymer than 15% glucose (20 mL/min vs 13.5 mL/min); during exercise 12.5 mL/min vs 10 mL/min
Vist and Maughan[160]	6 healthy males	Resting	Water vs 2, 4 and 6% glucose	600 mL bolus, emptying over first 20 min 27–28 mL/min (water, 2% glucose), 17.7 mL/min (4% glucose) and 16.4 mL/min (6% glucose)
Zachwieja et al.[161]	8 male cyclists	105 min at 75% of $\dot{V}O_{2max}$, 15 min self-paced	Water vs carbonated drink vs 10% carbohydrate vs 10% carbohydrate carbonated	13% slowing of gastric emptying with 10% carbohydrate, no difference in either gastric emptying or exercise performance with carbonation

Abbreviations: $\dot{V}O_{2max}$ = maximal oxygen intake; $\dot{V}O_{2peak}$ = peak oxygen intake; W = watts; W_{max} = maximal working capacity.

runners; they were preloaded with 200 mL of fluid immediately before their event, and were offered an additional 200 mL of fluid every 2.6 km of their run. This data suggested that the overall fluid balance and plasma mineral ion composition of the participants was maintained slightly better by drinking water than by the ingestion of other beverages containing minerals and carbohydrates.[151] Such a choice would not of course be appropriate during the recovery period, when water without the inclusion of some salt would become unpalatable and would stimulate urine production.[162]

With very prolonged activity in a hot environment, the ingested fluid can also usefully contain some electrolytes. Consensus recommendations are for 20–30 mE/L of Na^+, and 2–5 mE/L of K^{+140}; in addition to replacing sweat losses of mineral ions, the sodium stimulates thirst, and facilitates the absorption of glucose.

We will now look in more detail at methods of optimizing the absorption of water, carbohydrate and sodium ions during physical activity; we will consider the value of amino acids and other potential additives; and will discuss tactics for minimizing abdominal symptoms.

Optimizing water absorption

In some segments of the gut, water is absorbed in parallel with the active transport of carbohydrates, so that intestinal fluid absorption generally occurs more quickly from an isotonic carbohydrate/electrolyte solution than from water alone.[125,163,164] Indeed, Gisolfi *et al.*[127] found that intestinal fluid absorption was increased as much as six-fold by adding carbohydrate (2% glucose and 6% sucrose) to a simple electrolyte solution (20 mE Na^+, 2.6 mE K^+).

However, not all studies have seen increases of water absorption from the addition of carbohydrates to the ingested fluid. Wheeler and Banwell[165] reported that the jejunal absorption of fluid was similar for water and for 5% glucose polymer/2% fructose, and that the replacement of a part of the glucose polymer by sucrose actually decreased water absorption. Gisolfi *et al.*[166] also found no difference in the total fluid absorption from the duodenum and jejunum when they compared a water placebo with a 6% glucose solution over a wide range of osmolalities (197–414 mOsmol/kg of water).

Optimizing carbohydrate absorption

Initial differences in the osmolality of carbohydrate drinks are quickly attenuated by the secretion or absorption of water in the proximal duodenum, and for this reason the rate of uptake of a 6% glucose solution does not vary over osmolalities ranging from 186 to 403 mOsmol/kg.[126]

Although high concentrations of carbohydrate slow the delivery of fluid from the stomach into the duodenum, they usually increase the net delivery of carbohydrate into the circulation.[47,167,168] ^{13}C tests have shown that when riding a cycle ergometer to exhaustion at 80% of $\dot{V}O_{2max}$, the percentage of exogenous carbohydrate oxidized is much greater with ingestion of a 17% glucose solution than with a drink containing 4.5% glucose.[169] Moodley *et al.*[170] compared the oxidation of 7.5%, 10% or 15% glucose, sucrose and glucose-polymers during 90 minutes of cycle ergometry at 70% of $\dot{V}O_{2max}$. In keeping with subsequent observations,[169] although the percentage of ingested fluid delivered to the intestines decreased as carbohydrate concentrations increased, the total oxidation of ingested nutrient was greatest for a 15% carbohydrate solution.[170] The rate of oxidation was also greater for a mixture containing carbohydrate polymers than for glucose or sucrose, this benefit increasing with polymer chain length. Such findings negate an earlier hypothesis that the rate of gastric emptying is regulated to achieve a constant delivery of metabolic energy.

Solutions containing two or more carbohydrates can stimulate differing active absorption mechanisms, thus potentially increasing the intake of both carbohydrate and water.[121,171,172] However, for an active athlete sucrose and fructose are less desirable metabolites than glucose. Sucrose is hydrolyzed to fructose, and because this is absorbed slowly, it tends to draw fluid from the blood stream into the intestines.[165] Fructose is also a less desirable nutrient, since it must be converted to glucose in the liver before it can be metabolized by the skeletal muscles.

Because of limitations in intestinal transport mechanisms and/or hepatic metabolism, the usage of exogenous carbohydrate appears to peak at a rate of about 1.0–1.5 g/min.[173–175]

Optimizing sodium ion absorption

The inclusion of sodium ions in a drink generally facilitates the jejunal uptake of glucose and associated water,[167,176–178] although one dissenting report found no differences in intestinal absorption of 6% carbohydrate between solutions containing 0, 25 or 50 mE/L of Na+.[119,179]

The value of including amino acids in athletic drinks

There has been recent interest in adding amino acids to athletic drinks, with a view to maximizing anabolism during and immediately following a bout of physical activity.[180] When exercising at 65% of $\dot{V}O_{2max}$, the rate of gastric emptying does not differ between a 6% solution of carbohydrate alone, and that same solution reinforced by the addition of 1.5% protein.[181] Some[182,183] but not all[184,185] investigators have claimed enhanced endurance, as well as reduced muscle damage[183,186] with the addition of 1.8–2.0% protein to 6–7% glucose beverages. However, any gain of physical performance may reflect the increased energy content of the drink rather than a specific benefit from its protein content.[187]

Other potential additives to nutrient drinks

Athletes are sometimes given fixed schedules, indicating the points during an event when they should drink specified volumes of fluid. But if fluid intake is on a voluntary basis, the volume ingested can be increased substantially by the addition of certain flavourings.[188] Despite the potential negative effect of duodenal acidity upon gastric emptying, several studies have shown that for any given carbohydrate content, the rate of gastric emptying is largely unaffected by carbonation of a beverage.[161,189,190] If a drink contains a high content of either acid or electrolytes, this can slow the rate of gastric emptying, but little effect is seen at the concentrations of acids and electrolytes found in most athletic beverages.[167] The addition of caffeine speeds the gastric emptying of 7% glucose when a person is exercising at 75% of $\dot{V}O_{2max}$.[148] However, if a drink contains even low concentrations of caffeine, diuresis is increased, with negative consequences for hydration of the exerciser.

If a very hot or very cold drink is provided, gastric emptying is slowed until the fluid has remained in the stomach long enough to reach a "neutral" temperature.[29,191]

The emptying of solid meals is influenced by particle size. Thus, large cubes of chicken liver were emptied more slowly than homogenized food or solutions where particles were smaller than 1 mm.[192–195]

Minimizing abdominal symptoms

Depending on age, state of training, type, duration and particularly the intensity of effort, 20–50% of endurance competitors develop various gastro-intestinal symptoms when they are exercising.[135,196–200] How far does the choice of drink influence the prevalence of such symptoms? Factors contributing to such complaints include an overloading of the stomach and duodenum from an inappropriate diet, mechanical stimulation of the colon, exercise-induced hormonal changes, pre-race stress and anxiety, the development of visceral ischaemia, and possibly the absorption of endotoxins. Probably for mechanical reasons, complaints are more frequent with running than with cycling.[201] Mechanical stimulation of the gut increases the release of vasoactive intestinal peptide, which probably contributes to the symptoms experienced during vigorous physical activity.[202] Oektedalen *et al.*[105] found that high polypeptide levels persisted for up to two hours following completion of a strenuous five-day military exercise.

Symptoms are increased by the ingestion of high concentrations of carbohydrate,[203] for instance 6.9% saccharose/maltodextrin,[204] or 8% rather than 6% carbohydrate/electrolyte solutions,[205] presumably because the high osmolality reduces the rate of gastric emptying and/or the intestinal absorption of fluid. Symptoms are also increased by dehydration. Reasons for this need to be clarified, but one explanation could be that the resulting decrease in blood volume increases the extent of visceral ischaemia and thus slows the absorption of nutrients from the intestines.[88] Individuals with marked abdominal symptoms show a longer oro-caecal transit time, but a higher intestinal permeability; possibly, this allows the absorption of endotoxins, contributing to the abdominal discomfort.[201]

Areas for further research

Future investigations will need to reassess much of the published information on the choice of nutrient fluids for those who are exercising hard in an adverse environment, looking at the circulatory absorption of water, minerals and nutrients rather than just simply studying their rate of gastric emptying. Moreover, information should be collected during prolonged and vigorous exercise, rather than simply applying data collected under resting conditions. There is also a need to adjust the initial volumes of ingested fluids to realistic levels that athletes are likely to find acceptable during competition. A further gap in current knowledge concerns the impact of the emotional and mental stress of athletic competition[42,167] upon gastro-duodenal function, and practical methods of attenuating any adverse effects that arise from such stressors.

There remains scope to explore what factors cause the sudden transition from a neutral or weak positive effect of exercise to an inhibition of gastric emptying and nutrient uptake at an exercise intensity between 70% and 75% of the individual's maximal oxygen intake, and to determine how far the altered gastro-duodenal function impedes athletic performance in terms of nutrition and abdominal symptoms. If adverse effects prove to be substantial, there will be a need to seek possible countermeasures. Further, why are such problems exacerbated by hypohydration? Is this an expression of greater visceral ischaemia when the blood volume is also reduced, or are other factors involved?

Finally, there is a need to resolve the controversy concerning the usefulness of adding amino acids to carbohydrate containing beverages.

Conclusions

For the exerciser, the primary roles of the stomach and duodenum are to maintain optimal fluid and carbohydrate reserves during sustained exercise. Gastric emptying can be studied by serial aspiration of a test meal, ultrasonography, scintigraphy and impedance techniques, with ultrasonography being the current reference standard. Uptake of nutrients into the blood stream can be followed by noting the rate of appearance of radio-isotopes of carbon and hydrogen in expired air. The rate of gastric emptying is critically dependent upon gastric volume, both at rest and during exercise. Although moderate physical activity may cause a small speeding of gastric emptying, at the intensities of effort likely during sustained endurance competition (>70% of $\dot{V}O_{2max}$), there is some decrease of gastric motility, with associated decreases in the gastric secretion of acid, a decrease of jejunal motility, and a reduced absorption of nutrients. The effects of physical activity upon gastric function are not affected by the mode of exercise, but are increased by intermittent activity, heat exposure, dehydration and emotional stress, and if the ingested fluid contains a high concentration of carbohydrates; on the other hand, they are probably diminished by training and habituation.

Much of the focus of gastric physiological research to date has been upon determining the rate of gastric emptying for various athletic drinks under resting conditions; however, these findings are not necessarily applicable during vigorous exercise. Moreover, gastric emptying is but one step in the process of fluid and carbohydrate absorption. The focus of future research must shift to optimizing the intestinal absorption of nutrients during vigorous exercise. In a hot environment, the emphasis should be upon providing hypotonic or isotonic drinks that maximize the throughput of water, whereas in cooler environments, the focus can be upon hypertonic solutions that increase the intake and metabolism of carbohydrate at the expense of a smaller fluid intake. Training responses may also be enhanced if fluids contain amino acid supplements.

References

1 Gordon B, Cohn LA, Levine SA *et al.* Sugar content of the blood in runners following a marathon. *JAMA* 1925; 185: 508–509.
2 Pitts GL, Johnson RE, Consolazio CF. Work in the heat as affected by intake of water, salt and glucose. *Am J Physiol* 1944; 142: 253–259.
3 Knochel JP. Dog days and psoriasis. How to kill a football player. *JAMA* 1975; 233: 513–515.
4 Maughan RJ and Leiper JB. Limitations to fluid replacement during exercise. *Can J Appl Physiol* 1999; 24(2): 173–187.
5 Beaumont W. *Experiments and observations on the gastric juice and the physiology of digestion.* Edinburgh, Scotland: MacLachlan & Stewart, 1838.
6 Carlson AJ. *The control of hunger in health and disease.* Chicago, IL: University of Chicago Press, 1916.
7 Ramsbottom N, Knox MT, Hunt JB. Gastric emptying of barium sulphate suspension compared with that of water. *Gut* 1977; 18(7): 541–542.
8 Campbell JMH, Mitchell G, Powell ATW. The influence of exercise on digestion. *Guy's Hosp Rep* 1928; 78: 279–283.
9 Hunt JN. A modification to the method of George for studying gastric emptying. *Gut* 1974; 17: 812–813.
10 Beckers E, Rehrer NJ, Saris WH *et al.* Daily variation in gastric emptying when using the double sampling technique. *Med Sci Sports Exerc* 1991; 23(10): 1210–1212.
11 Irvine EJ, Tougas G, Lappaleinen R *et al.* Reliability and inter-observer variability of ultrasonographic measurement of gastric emptying rate. *Dig Dis Sci* 1993; 38(5): 803–810.
12 Beckers E, Rehrer NJ, Brouns F *et al.* Determination of total gastric volume, gastric secretin and residual meal using the double sampling technique of George. *Gut* 1988; 29: 1725–1729.
13 Maughan RJ, Leiper JB, Vist GE. Gastric emptying and fluid availability after ingestion of glucose and soy protein hydrolysate solutions in man. *Exp Physiol* 2003; 89: 101–108.
14 Read NW, Al Janabi MN, Bates TE *et al.* Effect of gastrointestinal intubation on the passage of a solid meal through the stomach and small intestine in humans. *Gastroenterology* 1983; 84(6): 1568–1572.
15 Müller-Lissner SA, Pimmel C, Will N *et al.* Effect of gastric and transpyloric tubes on gastric emptying and duodenogastric reflux. *Gastroenterology* 1982; 83: 1276–1279.
16 Bolondi L, Bortolotti M, Santi V *et al.* Measurement of gastric emptying time by real-time ultrasonography. *Gastroenterology* 1985; 89(4): 752–759.

17 Darwiche G, Almér LO, Björgell O *et al.* Standardized real-time ultrasonography in healthy subjects and diabetic patients. *J Ultrasound Med* 1999; 18: 673–682.

18 Marzio L, Formica P, Fabiani F *et al.* Influence of physical activity on gastric emptying of liquids in normal human subjects. *Am J Gastroenterol* 1991; 86(10): 1433–1436.

19 Brown BP, Ketelaar MA, Schulze-Delrieu K *et al.* Strenuous exercise decreases motility and cross-sectional area of human gastric antrum. A study using ultrasound. *Dig Dis Sci* 1994; 39(5): 940–945.

20 MacLaren D, Miles A, O'Neill I *et al.* Use of radionuclide imaging to determine gastric emptying of carbohydrate solutions during exercise. *Br J Sports Med* 1996; 30: 20–23.

21 Minami H, McCallum RW. The physiology and pathology of gastric emptying in humans. *Gastroenterology* 1984; 86: 1592–1610.

22 Beckers E, Leiper JB, Davidson J. Comparison of aspiration and scintigraphic techniques for the measurement of gastric emptying rates of liquids in humans. *Gut* 1992; 31: 115–117.

23 Darwiche G, Björgell O, Thorsson O *et al.* Correlation between simultaneous scintigraphic and ultrasonographic measurement of gastric emptying in patients with type 1 diabetes mellitus. *J Ultrasound Med* 2003; 22(5): 459–466.

24 Franke A, Harder H, Singer MV. Reliability of the [^{13}C]-acetate breath test in the measurement of gastric emptying of ethanol solutions: a methodological study. *Scand J Gastroenterol* 2004; 39(8): 722–726.

25 Mangnall YF, Barnich C, Brown BH *et al.* Comparison of applied potential tomography and impedance epigastrography as methods of measuring gastric emptying. *Clin Phys Physiol Meas* 1988; 9(3): 249–254.

26 Avill R, Mangnall YF, Bird NC *et al.* Applied potential tomography. A non-invasive technique for measuring gastric emptying. *Gastroenterology* 1987; 92(4): 1019–1028.

27 Costill DL, Saltin B. Factors limiting gastric emptying during rest and exercise. *J Appl Physiol* 1974; 37: 679–683.

28 Hunt JN, Spurrel WR. The pattern of emptying of the human stomach. *J Physiol* 1951; 113: 157–168.

29 Noakes TD, Rehrer NJ, Maughan RJ. The importance of volume in regulating gastric emptying. *Med Sci Sports Exerc* 1991; 23(3): 307–313.

30 Evans DF, Foster GE, Hardcastle JD. Does exercise affect small bowel motility in man? *Gut* 1989; 24: A1012.

31 Strid H, Simrén M, Störsrud S *et al.* Effect of heavy exercise on gastrointestinal transit in endurance athletes. *Scand J Gastroenterol* 2011; 46: 673–677.

32 Evans DF, Foster GE, Hardcastle JD. Does exercise affect the migrating motor complex in man? In: Roman C, (ed.). *Gastrointestinal motility*. Lancaster, MA: MTP Press, 1984, pp. 277–284.

33 Van Wyk M, Sommers DK, Steyn AGW. Evaluation of gastrointestinal motility using the hydrogen breath test. *Br J Clin Pharmacol* 1985; 20: 479–481.

34 Schedl HP, Maughan RJ, Gisolfi C. Intestinal absorption during rest and exercise: Implications for formulating oral rehydration beverages. *Med Sci Sports Exerc* 1994; 26: 267–280.

35 Strocchi A, Levitt MD. A reappraisal of the magnitude and implications of the intestinal unstirred layer. *Gastroenterology* 1991; 101: 843–847.

36 Davis JM, Amb DR, Burgess WA *et al.* Accumulation of deuterium oxide (D2O) in body fluids following ingestion of D2O-labelled beverages. *J Appl Physiol* 1987; 63: 2060–2066.

37 Gisolfi CV, Summers RW, Schedl HP *et al.* Human intestinal water absorption: Direct vs indirect measurements. *Am J Physiol* 1990; 258: G216–G222.

38 Lambert GP, Chang RT, Joensen D *et al.* Simultaneous determination of gastric emptying and intestinal absorption during cycle exercise in humans. *Int J Sports Med* 1996; 17: 48–55.

39 Leese GP, Bowtell J, Mudambo S *et al.* Post-exercise gastric emptying of carbohydrate solutions determined using the ^{13}C acetate breath test. *Eur J Appl Physiol* 1995; 71: 306–310.

40 Meyer-Wyss B, Mossi S, Beglinger C *et al.* Gastric emptying measured non-invasively in humans with a ^{13}C acetate breath test. *Gastroenterology* 1991; 100: A469.

41 van Nieuwenhoven MA, Wagenmakers AJM, Senden JMG *et al.* Performance of the [^{13}C] acetate gastric emptying test during physical exercise. *Eur J Clin Invest* 1999; 29: 922–928.

42 Brouns F, Saris WHM, Rehrer NJ. Abdominal complaints and gastrointestinal function during long-lasting exercise. *Int J Sports Med* 1987; 8: 175–189.

43 Rehrer NJ, Beckers E, Brouns F *et al.* Exercise and training effects on gastric emptying of carbohydrate beverages. *Med Sci Sports Exerc* 1989; 21(5): 540–549.

44 Brouns F. Gastric emptying as a regulatory factor in fluid uptake. *Int J Sports Med* 1998; 19 (Suppl.): S125–S128.

45 Duchman SM, Bleiler TL, Schedl HP *et al.* Effects of gastric function on intestinal composition of oral rehydration solutions. *Med Sci Sports Exerc* 1990; 22 (Suppl.): S89.

46 Coyle EF, Costill DL, Fink WJ *et al.* Gastric emptying rates for selected drinks. *Res Quart Ex Sport* 1978; 49(2): 119–124.

47 Hunt JN, Smith JL, Jiang CL. Effect of meal volume and energy density on the gastric emptying rate of carbohydrates. *Gastroenterology* 1985; 89: 1326–1330.

48 Seiple RS, Vivian VM, Fox EL *et al.* Gastric emptying characteristics of two polymer-electrolyte solutions. *Med Sci Sports Exerc* 1983; 15(5): 366–369.

49 Gisolfi CV, Duchman SM. Guidelines for optimal replacement beverages for different athletic events. *Med Sci Sports Exerc* 1992; 24(6): 679–687.

50 Hunt JN, Knox MT. The slowing of gastric emptying by nine acids. *J Physiol* 1969; 201(1): 161–179.

51 Barker GR, Coichrane GM, Corbett GA *et al.* Actions of glucose and potassium chloride on osmoreceptors slowing gastric emptying. *J Physiol* 1974; 237(1): 183–186.

52 Silva MTB, Palheta-Junior RC, Sousa DF *et al.* bicarbonate treatment prevents gastric emptying delay caused by acute exercise in awake rats. *J Appl Physiol* 2014; 116: 1133–1141.

53 Shapiro H, Woodward ER. Inhibition of gastric motility by acid in the duodenum. *J Appl Physiol* 1955; 8: 121–127.

54 Galbo H. Gastro-entero-pancreatic hormones. In: Galbo H, (ed.). *Hormonal and metabolic adaptations to exercise.* New York, NY: Thieme, 1983.

55 Olivares CJ. Toughest ironman ever. *Triathlete.* 1988; 52: 33–42.

56 Zieve FJ. Correspondence. *Mil Med* 1986; 151: 131–132.

57 Hellebrandt FA, Tepper RH. Studies on the influence of exercise on the digestive work of the stomach. II. Its effects on emptying time. *Am J Phsiol* 1934; 107: 355–363.

58 Dickson and Wilson. Cited by Hellebrandt & Tepper.[57]

59 Nielsen. Cited by Hellebrandt & Tepper.[57]

60 Kasabach. Cited by Hellebrandt & Tepper.[57]

61 Mitchell G, Voss KW. The influence of volume on gastric emptying and fluid balance during prolonged exercise. *Med Sci Sports Exerc* 1991; 23(3): 314–319.

62 Mudambo S, Leese GP, Rennie MJ. Gastric emptying in soldiers during and after field exercise in the heat measured with the [^{13}C]acetate breath test method. *Eur J Appl Physiol* 1997; 75: 109–114.

63 Foster C, Thompson NN. Serial gastric emptying studies: effect of preceding drinks. *Med Sci Sports Exerc* 1990; 22(4): 484–487.

64 Fordtran JS, Saltin B. Gastric emptying and intestinal absorption during prolonged severe exercise. *J Appl Physiol* 1967; 23: 331–335.

65 van Nieuwenhoven MA, Brouns F, Brummer RJ. The effect of physical exercise on parameters of gastrointestinal function. *Neurogastroenterol Motil* 1999; 11: 431–439.

66 Evans GH, Shirreffs SM, Watson P *et al.* Gastric emptying rate and perceived hunger after rest and exercise in man. *Br J Sports Med* 2010; 44: i20–i1.

67 Cammack J, Read NW, Cann PA *et al.* Effect of prolonged exercise on the passage of a solid meal through the stomach and small intestine. *Gut* 1982; 23: 957–961.

68 Neufer PD, Young AJ, Sawka MN. Gastric emptying during walking and running. *Eur J Appl Physiol* 1989; 58: 433–439.

69 Moore JG, Datz FL, Christian PE. Exercise increases solid meal gastric emptying rates in men. *Dig Dis Sci* 1990; 35(4): 428–432.

70 Franke A, Harder H, Orth AK *et al.* Post-prandial walking but not the consumption of alcoholic digestifs or espresso accelerates gastric emptying in healthy volunteers. *J Gastrointest Liv Dis* 2008; 17: 27–31.

71 Wang Y, Kondo T, Suzukamo Y *et al.* Vagal nerve regulation is essential for the increase in motility in response to mild exercise. *Tohuku J Exp Med* 2010; 222(2): 155–163.

72 Ramsbottom N, Hunt JN. Effect of exercise on gastric emptying and gastric secretion. *Digestion* 1974; 10: 1–8.

73 Maughan RJ, Leiper JB, McGaw BA. Effects of exercise intensity on absorption of ingested fluids in man. *Exp Physiol* 1990; 75: 419–421.

74 Rehrer NJ, Meijer GA. Biomechanical vibration of the abdominal region during running and bicycling. *J Sports Med Phys Fitness* 1991; 31(2): 231–234.

75 Houmard JA, Egan PC, Johns RA *et al.* Gastric emptying during 1 h of cycling and running at 75% VO2max. *Med Sci Sports Exerc* 1991; 23: 320–325.

76 Rehrer NJ, Brouns F, Beckers E *et al.* Gastric emptying with repeated drinking during running and bicycling. *Int J Sports Med* 1990; 11: 238–243.

77 Leiper JB, Broad NP, Maughan RJ. Effect of intermittent high-intensity exercise on gastric emptying in man. *Med Sci Sports Exerc* 2001; 33(8): 1270–1278.

78 Leiper JB, Prentice AS, Wrightson C *et al.* Gastric emptying of a carbohydrate-electrolyte drink during a soccer match. *Med Sci Sports Exerc* 2001; 33(11): 1932–1938.

79 Leiper JB, Nicholas CW, Ali A *et al.* The effect of intermittent high-intensity running on gastric emptying of fluids in man. *Med Sci Sports Exerc* 2005; 37(2): 240–247.

80 Rehrer NJ. Fluid and electrolyte balance during ultra-endurance sport. *Sports Med* 2001; 31(10): 701–715.

81 Carrió I, Estorch M, Serra-Grima R *et al.* Gastric emptying in marathon runners. *Gut* 1989; 30: 152–155.

82 Harris A, Lindeman AK, Martin BJ. Rapid orocecal transit in chronically active persons with high energy intake. *J Appl Physiol* 1991; 70(4): 1550–1553.

83 Gershon-Cohen J, Shay H, Fels S. The relation of meal temperature to gastric motility and secretion. *Am J Roentgenol Rad Therap Nucl Med* 1940; 43: 237–242.

84   Webber DE, Nouri M, Bell FR. A study of the effects of meal temperature on gastric function. *Pflüg Archiv* 1980; 384(1): 65–68.

85   Owen MD, Kregel KC, Wall PT *et al*. Effects of ingesting carbohydrate beverages during exercise in the heat. *Med Sci Sports Exerc* 1986; 18: 568–575.

86   Ryan AJ, Bleiler TL, Carter JE *et al*. Gastric emptying during prolonged cycling in the heat. *Med Sci Sports Exerc* 1989; 21: 51–58.

87   Neufer PD, Young AJ, Sawka MN. Gastric emptying during exercise: Effects of heat stress and hypohydration. *Eur J Appl Physiol* 1989; 58: 433–439.

88   Rehrer NJ, Beckers EJ, Brouns F *et al*. Effects of dehydration on gastric emptying and gastrointestinal distress while running. *Med Sci Sports Exerc* 1990; 22(6): 790–795.

89   van Nieuwenhoven MA, Vriens BEPJ, Brummer RJ *et al*. Effect of dehydration on gastrointestinal function at rest and during exercise in humans. *Eur J Appl Physiol* 2000; 83: 578–584.

90   Ryan AJ, Lambert GP, Shi X *et al*. Effect of hypohydration on gastric emptying and intestinal absorption during exercise. *J Appl Physiol* 1998; 84(5): 1581–1588.

91   Lambert GP, Lang J, Bull A *et al*. Fluid tolerance while running: Effect of repeated trials. *Int J Sports Med* 2008; 29: 878–882.

92   Bortz WM, Angwin P, Mefford I *et al*. Catecholamines, dopamine, and endorphin levels during extreme exercise. *N Engl J Med* 1980; 305: 466–467.

93   Rees MR, Clark RA, Holdsworth CD. The effect of beta-adrenoreceptor agonists and antagonists on gastric emptying in man. *Br J Clin Pharmacol* 1980; 10: 551–554.

94   Allen M. Activity generated endorphins: a review of their role in sports science. *Can J Appl Sports Sci* 1983; 8: 115–133.

95   Bi L, Triadafilopoulos G. Exercise and gastrointestinal function and disease: An evidence-based review of risks and benefits. *Clin Gastroenterol Hepatol* 2003; 1: 345–355.

96   Brener W, Hendrix F, McHugh PR. Regulation of gastric emptying of glucose. *Gastroenterology* 1983; 85: 76–82.

97   Hammar S, Öbrink KJ. The inhibitory effect of muscular exercise on gastric secretion. *Acta Physiol Scand* 1953; 28(2–3): 151–162.

98   Sullivan SN. The effect of running on the gastrointestinal tract. *J Clin Gastroenterol* 1984; 6: 461–465.

99   Markiewicz K, Cholewa M, Gorski L *et al*. Effect of physical exercise on gastric basal secretion of healthy men. *Acta Hepatogastroenterol* 1977; 24: 377–380.

100 Zach E, Markiewicz K, Lukin M *et al*. Das Verhalten der basalen Magensäure-S ekretion während des Trainings und Restitution in chronischen Magen- und Zwölffingerdarmgeschwür Patienten [The behaviour of basal gastric secretion during exercise and restitution in chronic gastric and duodenal ulcer patients]. *Dtsch Z Verdaungs Stoffwechselkr* 1982; 42(2–3): 53–63.

101 Hellebrandt FA, Miles MM. The effect of muscular work and competition on gastric acidity. *Am J Physiol* 1932; 102: 258–266.

102 Feldman M, Nixon JV. Effect of exercise on postprandial gastric secretion and emptying in humans. *J Appl Physiol* 1982; 53(4): 851–854.

103 Canalles P, Diago M, Tomé A *et al*. El ejercicio físico y la secreción de ácido gástrico [Physical exercise and gastric acid secretion]. *Rev Espan Enferm Dig* 1990; 77(3): 179–184.

104 Hoelzel F. The relation between the secretory and motor activity in the fasting stomach (man). *Am J Physiol* 1925; 73: 463–469.

105 Oektedalen O, Flaten P, Opstad PK. LPP and gastric response to a liquid meal and oral glucose during prolonged severe exercise, caloric deficit and sleep deprivation. *Scand J Gastroenterol* 1982; 19: 619–624.

106 Soffer EE, Merchant RK, Duethman G *et al.* The effect of graded exercise on esophageal motility and gastroesophageal reflux in trained athletes. *Gastroenterology*. 1991; 100: A497.

107 Soffer EE, Wilson J, Duethman G *et al.* Effect of graded exercise on esophageal motility and gastroesophageal reflux in nontrained subjects. *Dig Dis Sci* 1994; 39: 193–198.

108 Harrison RJ, Leeds AR, Bolster NR *et al.* Exercise and wheat bran: effect on whole-gut transit. *Proc Nutr Soc* 1980; 39: 22A.

109 Ollerenshaw KJ, Norman S, Wilson CG *et al.* Exercise and small intestinal transit. *Nucl Med Comm* 1987; 8: 105–110.

110 Soffer EE, Summers RW, Gisolfi C. Effect of exercise on intestinal motility and transit in trained athletes. *Am J Physiol* 1991; 260: G698–G702.

111 Peters HP, De Vries DR, Akkermans LM *et al.* Duodenal motility during a run-bike-run protocol: the effect of a sports drink. *Eur J Gastroenterol Hepatol* 2002; 14(10): 1125–1132.

112 Keeling WF, Martin BJ. Gastrointestinal transit during mild exercise. *J Appl Physiol* 1987; 63: 978–981.

113 Rao KA, Yazaki E, Evans DF *et al.* Objective evaluation of small bowel and colonic transit time using pH telemetry in athletes with gastrointestinal symptoms. *Br J Sports Med* 2004; 38: 482–487.

114 Meshkinpour H, Kemp C Fairster R. Effect of aerobic exercise on mouth to cecum transit time. *Gastroenterology* 1989; 96: 938–941.

115 Moses FM, Ryan C, DeBolt J *et al.* Oral-cecal transit time during a 2hr run with ingestion of water or glucose polymer. *Am J Gastroenterol* 1988; 83: 1055.

116 Moses F, Singh A, Villanueva V *et al.* Lactose absorption and transit during prolonged high intensity running. *Am J Gastroenterol* 1989; 84: 1192.

117 Sessions RF, Reynolds VH, Ferguson JL. Correlation between intraduodenal osmotic pressure changes and Cr51-blood volumes during induced dumping in men with normal stomachs. *Surgery* 1982; 52: 266–279.

118 Case GL, Philips RW, Lewis LD *et al.* Effects of osmolarity of liquid nutrient diets on plasma equilibration of water and carbohydrate in yucatan miniature swine. *Am J Clin Nutr* 1981; 34: 1861–1867.

119 Gisolfi C, Summers RW, Schedl HP *et al.* Effect of sodium concentration in a carbohydrate-electrolyte solution on intestinal absorption. *Med Sci Sports Exerc* 1995; 27(10): 1414–1420.

120 Hawley JA, Dennis SC, Nowitz A *et al.* Exogenous carbohydrate oxidation from maltose and glucose ingested during prolonged exercise. *Eur J Appl Physiol* 1992; 64: 523–527.

121 Shi X, Summers RW, Schedl HP *et al.* Effects of carbohydrate type and concentration and solution osmolality on water absorption. *Med Sci Sports Exerc* 1995; 27(12): 1607–1615.

122 Harig JM, Soergel KH, Barry J *et al.* Brush border membrane vesicles formed from human duodenal biopsies exhibit Na^+-dependent concentrative L-leucine and D-glucose uptake. *Biochem Biophys Res* 1988; 156: 164–170.

123 Lambert GP, Chang RT, Xia T *et al.* Absorption from different intestinal segments during exercise. *J Appl Physiol* 1997; 83(1): 204–212.

124 Hunt JN, Elliott EJ, Fairclough PD *et al.* Water and solute absorption from hypotonic glucose electrolyte solutions in human jejunum. *Gut* 1992; 33(4): 479–483.
125 Leiper JB, Maughan RJ. Absorption of water and electrolytes from hypotonic, isotonic and hypertonic solutions. *J Physiol* 1986; 373: 90P.
126 Shi X, Summers RW, Schedl HP *et al.* Effects of solution osmolality on absorption of select fluid replacement solutions in human duodenojejunum. *J Appl Physiol* 1994; 77(3): 1178–1184.
127 Gisolfi C, Spranger KJ, Summers RW *et al.* Effects of cycle exercise on intestinal absorption in humans. *J Appl Physiol* 1991; 71(6): 2518–2527.
128 Lang J, Gisolfi C, Lambert GP. Effect of exercise intensity on active and passive glucose absorption. *Int J Nutr Exerc Metab* 2006; 16(5): 485–493.
129 Williams JH, Mager M, Jacobson ED. Relationship of mesenteric blood flow to intestinal absorption of carbohydrates. *J Lab Clin Med* 1964; 63: 853–862.
130 Barclay GR, Turnberg LA. Effect of moderate exercise on salt and water transport in the human jejunum. *Gut* 1988; 29: 816–820.
131 Stevens BR. Vertebrate intestine apical membrane mechanisms of organic nutrient transport. *Am J Physiol* 1992; 263(3 Pt. 2): R456–R463.
132 Leiper JB. Intestinal water absorption – implications for the formulation of rehydration solutions. *Int J Sports Med* 1998; 19: S129–S132.
133 Moses FM, Singh A, Smoak B *et al.* Alterations in intestinal permeability during prolonged high intensity running. *Gastroenterology* 1991; 100: A472.
134 Oektedalen O, Lunde OC, Aabakken PK *et al.* Changes in the gastrointestinal mucosa after long-distance running. *Scand J Gastroenterol* 1992; 27: 307–313.
135 Brouns F, Beckers E. Is the gut an athletic organ? Digestion, absorption and exercise. *Sports Med* 1993; 15: 242–257.
136 Brouns F. *Food and fluid related aspects in highly trained athletes.* Haarlem, Netherlands, de Vrieseborch, 1988.
137 Dressendorfer RH, Scaff JH, Wagner JO *et al.* Metabolic adjustments to marathon running in coronary patients. *NY Acad Sci* 1977; 301: 466–483.
138 Kavanagh T, Shephard RJ, Pandit V. Marathon running after myocardial infarction. *JAMA* 1974; 229: 1602–1605.
139 Saltin B. Aerobic work capacity and circulation at exercise in man; with special reference to the effect of prolonged exercise and/or heat exposure. *Acta Physiol Scand* 1964; 62: 1–52.
140 Sawka MN, Burke LM, Eichner ER *et al.* Exercise and fluid replacement. *Med Sci Sports Exerc* 2007; 39(2): 377–390.
141 Bergström J, Hultman E. A study of the glycogen metabolism during exercise in man. *Scand J Clin Lab Invest* 1967; 19: 218–228.
142 Coombes JS, Hamilton KL. The effectiveness of commercially available sports drinks. *Sports Med* 2000; 29(3): 181–209.
143 Costill DL, Miller JM. Nutrition for endurance sport: carbohydrate and fluid balance. *Int J Sports Med* 1980; 1: 2–4.
144 Coyle EF. Fluid and fuel intake during exercise. *J Sports Sci* 2004; 22(1): 39–55.
145 Rodriguez NR, Di Marco NM, Langley S. American College of Sports Medicine position stand. Nutrition and athletic performance. *Med Sci Sports Exerc* 2009; 41(3): 708–730.
146 Coyle EF, Montain DJ. Carbohydrate and fluid ingestion during exercise: Are there trade-offs? *Med Sci Sports Exerc* 1992; 24(6): 671–678.

147 Below PR, Mora-Rodriguez R, González-Alonso J *et al.* Fluid and carbohydrate ingestion independently improve performance during 1 h of intensive exercise. *Med Sci Sports Exerc* 1995; 27(2): 200–210.

148 Dickinson AL, Haymes EM, Sparks KE *et al.* Effects of moderate caffeine ingestion on factors contributing to the quality of endurance performance. *Med Sci Sports Exerc* 1984; 16(2): 171.

149 Gant N, Leiper JB, Williams C. Gastric emptying of fluids during variable-intensity running in the heat. *Int J Sports Nutr Exerc Metab* 2007 17(3): 270–283.

150 Gonzálvez MAB, Nuño de la Rosa y Pozuelo JA *et al.* Estudio gammagráfico del ritmo de vaciado gástrico de bebidas de reposición en deportistas [Scintigraphic study of the rate of gastric emptying of replacement beverages in athletes]. *Rev Espanol Med Nucl Imag Mol* 2005; 24(1): 19–26.

151 Kavanagh T, Shephard RJ. On the choice of fluid for the hydration of middle-aged marathon runners. *Br J Sports Med* 1977; 11: 26–35.

152 Mitchell G, Costill DL, Houmard JA *et al.* Effects of carbohydrate ingestion on gastric emptying and exercise performance. *Med Sci Sports Exerc* 1988; 20(2): 110–115.

153 Mitchell JB, Costill DL, Houmard JA *et al.* Gastric emptying: influence of prolonged exercise and carbohydrate concentrations. *Med Sci Sports Exerc* 1989; 21(3): 269–274.

154 Murray R, Eddy DE, Bartoli WP *et al.* Gastric emptying of water and isocaloric solutions consumed at rest. *Med Sci Sports Exerc* 1994; 26(6): 725–732.

155 Murray L, Bertoli WP, Eddy DE *et al.* Gastric emptying and plasma deuterium accumulation following ingestion of water and two carbohydrate-electrolyte beverages. *Int J Sports Nutr* 1997; 7(2): 144–153.

156 Näveri H, Tikkanen H, Kairento AL *et al.* Gastric emptying and serum insulin levels after intake of glucose-polymer solutions. *Eur J Appl Physiol* 1989; 58: 661–665.

157 Neufer PD, Costill DL, Fink WJ *et al.* Effects of exercise and carbohydrate composition on gastric emptying. *Med Sci Sports Exerc* 1986; 18(6): 658–662.

158 Rehrer NJ, Wagenmakers AJM, Beckers E *et al.* Gastric emptying, absorption, and carbohydrate oxidation during prolonged exercise. *J Appl Physiol* 1992; 72(2): 468–475.

159 Sole CC, Noakes TD. Faster gastric emptying for glucose-polymer and fructose solutions than for glucose in humans. *Eur J Appl Physiol* 1989; 58: 605–612.

160 Vist GE, Maughan RJ. Gastric emptying of ingested solutions in man: effect of beverage glucose concentration. *Med Sci Sports Exerc* 1994; 26(10): 1269–1273.

161 Zachwieja JJ, Costill DL, Beard GC *et al.* The effects of a carbonated carbohydrate drink on gastric emptying, gastrointestinal distress, and exercise performance. *Int J Sport Nutr* 1992; 2(3): 239–250.

162 Maughan RJ, Shirreffs SM, Leiper JB. Rehydration and recovery after exercise. *Sport Sci Exch* 1996; 9: 1–5.

163 Hill RJ, Bluck LJC, Davies PSW. Using a non-invasive stable isotope tracer to measure the absorption of water in humans. *Rapid Commun Mass Spectrom* 2004; 18: 701–706.

164 Hill RJ, Bluck LJC, Davies PSW. The hydration ability of three commercially available sports drinks and water. *J Science Med Sport* 2008; 11: 116–123.

165 Wheeler KB, Banwell JG. Intestinal water and electrolyte flux of glucose-polymer electrolyte solutions. *Med Sci Sports Exerc* 1986; 18(4): 436–439.

166 Gisolfi CV, Summers RW, Lambert GP *et al.* Effect of beverage osmolality on intestinal fluid absorption during exercise. *J Appl Physiol* 1998; 85(5): 1941–1948.

167 Rehrer NJ, Brouns F, Beckers E *et al.* The influence of beverage composition and gastrointestinal function on fluid and nutrient availability during exercise. *Scand J Med Sci Sports* 1994; 4: 159–172.

70   *Optimizing gastro-duodenal function*

168 Vist GE, Maughan RJ. The effect of osmolality and carbohydrate content on the rate of gastric emptying of liquids in man. *J Physiol* 1995; 486(2): 523–531.
169 Galloway SDR, Wootton SA, Murphy JL *et al.* Exogenous carbohydrate oxidation from drinks ingested during prolonged exercise in a cold environment. *J Appl Physiol* 2001; 91(2): 654–660.
170 Moodley D, Noakes TD, Bosch AN *et al.* Oxidation of exogenous carbohydrate during prolonged exercise: the effects of the carbohydrate type and its concentration. *Eur J Appl Physiol* 1992; 64: 328–334.
171 Lambert GP, Lanspa SJ, Welch R *et al.* Combined effects of glucose and fructose on fluid absorption from hypertonic carbohydrate-electrolyte solutions. *J Exerc Physiol On-Line* 2008; 11(2): 46–55.
172 Jeukendrup AE, Moseley L. Multiple transportable carbohydrates enhance gastric emptying and fluid delivery. *Scand J Med Sci Sports* 2010; 20: 112–121.
173 El Sayed MS, MacLaren D, Rattu A. Exogenous carbohydrate utilisation: Effects on metabolism and exercise performance. *Comp Biochem Physiol* 1997; 118A(3): 789–803.
174 Jeukendrup AE, Jentjens R. Oxidation of carbohydrate during prolonged exercise. Current thoughts, guidelines and directions for future research. *Sports Med* 2000; 29(6): 407–424.
175 Rowlands DS, Clarke J. Lower oxidation of a high molecular weight glucose polymer vs glucose during cycling. *Appl Physiol Nutr Metab* 2011; 36: 298–306.
176 Leiper JB, Maughan RJ. The effect of luminal hypotonicity on water absorption from a segment of the intact human jejunum. *J Physiol* 1986; 378: 95P.
177 Hunt JB, Elliott EJ, Farthing MJ. Efficacy of a standard United Kingdom oral rehydration solution (ORS) and a hypotonic ORS assessed by human intestinal perfusion. *Aliment Pharmacol Therap* 1989; 3(6): 565–571.
178 Wapnir RA, Lifshitz F. Osmolality and solute concentration – Their relationship with oral rehydration solution effectiveness: An experimental assessment. *Pediatr Res* 1985; 19: 894–898.
179 Gisolfi C, Lambert GP, Summers RW. Intestinal fluid absorption during exercise: role of sport drink and [Na⁺]. *Med Sci Sports Exerc* 2001; 33(6): 907–915.
180 van Loon LJC. Is there a need for protein ingestion during exercise? *Sports Med* 2014; 44 (Suppl. 1): 105–111.
181 Seifert J, Harmon J, DeClercq P. Protein added to a sports drink improved fluid retention. *Int J Sport Nutr Exerc Metab* 2006; 16: 420–429.
182 Ivy JL, Res PT, Sprague RC *et al.* Effect of a carbohydrate-protein supplement on endurance performance during exercise of varying intensity. *Int J Sport Nutr Exerc Metab* 2003; 13: 382–395.
183 Saunders M, Kane M, Todd M. Effects of a carbohydrate-protein beverage on cycling endurance and muscle damage. *Med Sci Sports Exerc* 2004; 36(7): 1233–1238.
184 Breen L, Tipton K, Jeukendrup A. No effect of carbohydrate-protein on cycling performance and indices of recovery. *Med Sci Sports Exerc* 2010; 42(6): 1140–1148.
185 van Essen M, Gibala MJ. Failure of protein to improve time trial performance when added to a sports drink. *Med Sci Sports Exerc* 2006; 38(8): 1476–1483.
186 Baty JJ, Hwang H, Ding Z *et al.* The effect of a carbohydrate and protein supplement on resistance exercise performance, hormonal response, and muscle damage. *J Strength Cond Res* 2007; 21(2): 321–329.
187 Valentine RJ, Saunders MJ, Todd MK *et al.* Influence of carbohydrate-protein beverage on cycling endurance and indices of muscle disruption. *Int J Sport Nutr Exerc Metab* 2008; 18: 363–378.

188 Minehan MR, Riley MD, Burke LM. Effect of flavor and awareness of kilojoule content of drinks on preference and fluid balance in team sports. *Int J Sport Nutr Exerc Metab* 2002; 12(1): 81–92.

189 Lambert GP, Bleiler TL, Chang RT *et al.* Effects of carbonated and noncarbonated beverages at specific intervals during treadmill running in the heat. *Int J Sports Nutr* 1993; 3(2): 177–193.

190 Ryan AJ, Navarre AE, Gisolfi CV. Consumption of carbonated and noncarbonated sports drinks during prolonged treadmill exercise in the heat. *Int J Sports Nutr* 1991; 1(3): 225–230.

191 Sun WM, Houghton LA, Read NW *et al.* Effect of meal temperature on gastric emptying of liquids in man. *Gut* 1988; 29: 302–305.

192 Bernier JJ. L'état postprandial, vidange gastrique et rôle du duodénum [The postprandial state, gastric emptying and the role of the duodenum]. *Cahiers Nutr Diét* 1985; 20(1): 13–17.

193 Holt S, Reid J, Taylor TV. Gastric emptying of solids in man. *Gut* 1982; 23: 292–296.

194 Meyers JH, MacGregor LL, Gueller R *et al.* 99mTc tagged chicken liver as a marker of solid food in the human stomach. *Am J Dig Dis* 1975; 21: 296–303.

195 Moore JG, Christian BE, Coleman RE. Gastric emptying of varying meal weight and composition. *Dig Dis Sci* 1981; 26: 16–22.

196 Shephard RJ. How fast must you trot? Vigorous exercise and diarrhoea. *Health Fitness J Canada* 2015; 8(1): 32–52.

197 Martin D. Physical activity benefits and risks on the gastrointestinal system. *South Med J* 2011; 104(12): 831–837.

198 Peters HP, Zweers M, Backx FJ *et al.* Gastrointestinal symptoms during long-distance walking. *Med Sci Sports Exerc* 1999; 31: 767–773.

199 Peters HP, Akkermans LM, Bol E *et al.* Gastrointestinal symptoms during exercise. The effect of fluid supplementation. *Sports Med* 1995; 20: 65–76.

200 Peters HP, de Vries WR, Vanberg-Henegouwen GP *et al.* Potential benefits and hazards of physical activity and exercise on the gastrointestinal tract. *Gut* 2001; 48: 435–439.

201 van Nieuwenhoven MA, Brouns F, Brummer RM. Gastrointestinal profile of symptomatic athletes at rest and during physical exercise. *Eur J Appl Physiol* 2004; 91: 429–434.

202 Riddoch C, Trinick T. Gastrointestinal disturbances in marathon runners. *Br J Sports Med* 1988; 22(2): 71–74.

203 Morton DP, Aragon-Vargas LF, Callister R. Effect of ingested fluid composition on exercise-related transient abdominal pain. *Int J Sport Nutr Exerc Metab* 2004; 14: 197–208.

204 van Nieuwenhoven MA, Brouns F, Kovac EM. The effect of two sports drinks and water on GI complaints and performance during an 18 km run. *Int J Sports Med* 2005; 26: 281–285.

205 Shi X, Horn MK, Osterberg KL *et al.* Gastro-intestinal discomfort during intermittent high-intensity exercise. *Int J Sport Nutr Exerc Metab* 2004; 14(6): 673–683.

4 Physical activity and peptic ulcers

Introduction

Gastric and duodenal ulcers are both relatively common conditions, although there is some disagreement as to their prevalence. Self-reports suggest that in any given year as many as 3% of the population are affected by peptic ulcers,[1] whereas the annual incidence of physician-diagnosed lesions is much lower, in the range 0.10–0.19%.[2] Endoscopy of symptomless Louisiana volunteers found a prevalence between these two extremes, 1.1% for gastric ulcers and 1.8% for duodenal ulcers.[3,4] Ulceration is apparently associated with endogenous factors such as heredity, an excessive secretion of gastric acid and pepsin and an impaired mucosal blood flow, as well as exogenous influences that include Helicobacter pylori infection, smoking, excessive alcohol consumption, stress and an overuse of non-steroidal anti-inflammatory drugs.[5,6] However, interactions between these several predisposing factors hamper a determination of the dominant aetiology.[4]

The potential impact of habitual physical activity upon peptic ulceration has as yet received little attention, and data linking human peptic ulceration and habitual physical activity are particularly limited. After reviewing the available empirical data, we will explore mechanisms whereby regular physical activity could modify the known risk factors for peptic ulceration (see Table 4.1).

Empirical data on physical activity and peptic ulcers

Much of the available empirical information on physical activity and the risk of peptic ulceration has been collected on racehorses, sled dogs and laboratory animals. Such studies point consistently to an adverse effect of very prolonged, vigorous and repeated bouts of physical activity, with a specific association between periods of race participation and a high prevalence of ulceration.

There have been suggestions that vigorous abdominal exercises such as "crunches" may increase the risk of perforation of an existing ulcer in humans, but there is a lack of good evidence on this specific issue. In terms of ulcer prevention, there have been a few cross-sectional human investigations based upon the comparison of groups differing in occupational or leisure activity, and in contrast to the animal data, these studies provide some basis for believing that regular moderate exercise may reduce the risk of peptic ulceration.

Physical activity and peptic ulcers in animals

The prevalence of gastric ulcers in racehorses is very high. One French study found that outside of the main racing season, 48% of high-level endurance racehorses had gastric ulcers, and that 93% were affected at times of the year when the animals were competing frequently.[7] Other investigations in New Zealand, North America and Sweden have all shown a high prevalence of peptic ulcers among race-horses.[8-12] Peptic ulcers seem somewhat more frequent in trotters than in pacers[13] and although the number of lesions usually decreases during periods of detrain-ing,[14] a substantial risk remains,[15] with a continuing adverse impact upon the animal's maximal oxygen consumption and physical performance.[16]

Suggested factors leading to the high incidence of peptic ulceration in the racehorse include a tensing of the abdominal muscles that pushes the acidic gastric contents into the proximal part of the stomach when galloping,[17] exercise-induced increases in concentrations of gastrin and thus acid secretion,[18] the repeated administration of hypertonic electrolytes,[19] and the stress of transport-ing the animals in horseboxes over long distances to and from the sites of competition.[20] The importance of acid secretion to the causation of gastric ulcers

Table 4.1 Risk factors for peptic ulceration, and their potential modification by regular physical activity

Factor	Possible influence of habitual physical activity
Genetic characteristics	No likely effect of physical activity
Excessive secretion of gastric acid and pepsin	Reduced by moderate physical activity, but response may differ with established ulceration
Impaired mucosal blood flow	Mucosal blood flow can be reduced by excessive use of NSAIDs and by the visceral ischaemia associated with prolonged and intensive exercise
Helicobacter pylori infection	Moderate physical activity may enhance and vigorous exercise suppress immune responses
Smoking	Regular physical activity associated with healthy lifestyle and may facilitate smoking withdrawal
Excessive alcohol consumption	Regular physical activity associated with healthy lifestyle
Stress/anxiety	Moderate physical activity tends to relieve anxiety, but high level athletic competition may increase stress/anxiety
Overuse of NSAIDs	Athletic competition may increase use of NSAIDs
Socio-economic status	Low socio-economic status associated with low habitual leisure physical activity

Abbreviation: NSAIDs = non-specific anti-inflammatory drugs.

is suggested by the effectiveness of H_2-antagonists[21,22] and proton-pump inhibitors[23-27] in the treatment of affected animals. Benefit has also been found from administration of sucralfate – a combination of sucrose, sulphate and aluminium. This medication inhibits pepsin and increases prostaglandin levels, although protection against peptic ulceration probably derives mainly from its action in provoking an increased production of mucin.[28]

Dogs that are involved in long-distance sled races such as the "Iditarod" also seem very vulnerable to peptic ulcers.[29,30] Races such as the Iditarod can require the animals to cover distances of 160 km/day for 1–2 weeks. They are recognized to increase the permeability of the gut to intestinal toxins,[31] worsen any existing peptic ulceration,[30] and sometimes even lead to death of the animals during the event.[32]

Excessive running in an exercise wheel has also caused peptic ulceration in laboratory rats. The likelihood of developing an ulcer can be reduced by chemical erosion of a part of the rat brain known as the ventro-medial hypothalamus.[33] The authors of this report suggested that the ventro-medial hypothalamus plays a crucial role, causing the rats to engage in excessive running when they are exposed to stress.[33]

Human occupational activity and the risk of peptic ulceration

An individual's choice of occupation influences his or her level of habitual physical activity, but there are other potential concomitants of occupation that influence the risk of developing a peptic ulcer, including the worker's socio-economic status, exposure to industrial toxins, stress levels, and requirements of shift and night-time work. All of these covariates must be taken into account when making activity comparisons in the risk of peptic ulceration based upon occupational title. The prevalence of peptic ulcers is particularly high among night and shift workers, and in this category of employees stress and irregular meals rather than unusual levels of physical activity seem the main culprits.[34,35]

Doll *et al.*[36] compared the incidence of peptic ulcers between London bus drivers and conductors. In many respects, this seemed an ideal occupational study. The two types of worker had in many respects similar working conditions, comparable socio-economic status, but there was a large inter-group difference in their volume of daily physical activity. The drivers remained comfortably seated in the cabs of their vehicles for the most of the day, but the conductors had to scramble to the upper deck to inspect tickets and collect fares twice along each mile of the bus route. The bus drivers and conductors had similar rates of peptic ulceration, and the prevalence of ulcers was higher than that seen in agricultural workers (who in the era of Doll's study commonly had high average rates of energy expenditure and little exposure to toxic agricultural chemicals, but did not face the considerable stress of operating a safe passenger service in the dense traffic of central London).

Other early reports linked peptic ulcers to what were apparently sedentary tasks: professional employment, being a supervisor or holding a responsible position.[36–39] However, these results were not controlled for possible differences in leisure activity, or, in the case of air-traffic controllers,[37] for the demands of shift work. A study from Northern Norway found a high prevalence of peptic ulcers in fishermen and land and sea transport workers[40]; here, it was speculated that the stresses of dangerous work, irregular hours and heavy smoking might be causal factors.

More recent data have found the highest rates of peptic ulcers in unskilled workers[41–44] who are generally engaged in physical tasks, but also have the other characteristics associated with a low socio-economic status. It has been suggested that the current high prevalence of ulcers among migrant workers may reflect their predominant employment in physically demanding jobs (although they also face many stresses not encountered by the general population), and that the secular decline in the incidence of peptic ulcers in some populations could be linked to a progressive reduction in the average energy demands of industrial work.[44]

The most recent analysis[45] found that even after adjusting for the covariates of age, smoking habits and social class, the risk of a recent diagnosis of duodenal ulcer was 1.3 for those who were engaged in moderate physical work, and 3.6 for individuals with a high level of occupational activity.

Human leisure-time physical activity and the risk of peptic ulceration

Cheng *et al.*[46,47] made a cross-sectional analysis of data for 8529 men and 2884 women who were attending health evaluations at the Cooper Fitness Center in Dallas, Texas. Study participants were placed into 1 of 3 habitual activity categories: "active" (those who reported walking or running for more than 16 km/ week), "moderately active" (those who engaged in some deliberate walking or running, but covered less than 16 km/week) or "inactive". A proportional hazards model that made statistical adjustments for age, smoking, alcohol use, body mass index, and self-reported "tension" found no impact of habitual physical activity upon the incidence of physician-diagnosed gastric ulcers, but there were significant exercise-related differences in the prevalence of duodenal ulcers among men only (relative hazards of 0.38 for those who were "active" and of 0.54 for those who were "moderately active" relative to those who were classed as "inactive"). This study made no specific allowance for socio-economic status, but given the exclusive nature of the Cooper Fitness Center, most of the study participants were likely to have been relatively wealthy individuals. In discussing the apparent absence of influence of physical activity upon the risk of duodenal ulcers in women, the authors of this report suggested that the physical activity patterns of the women may have differed from that of the men, both in type and intensity (with less of a focus upon running); they also noted that the statistical power of the analysis for women was limited because only a very small number of females had developed peptic ulcers. One might comment further that most current physical activity questionnaires have been designed primarily for men, and that they fail to capture some of the physical tasks that fall to women, such as childcare and the support of elderly relatives.

A random sampling of 2416 Danish adults used a 3-level self-report of habitual physical activity and a national registry of chronic diseases to examine relationships between leisure activity and the incidence of peptic ulcer over a 12-year period. A multivariate logistic analysis of the data included as covariates many of the traditional risk factors for peptic ulceration such as the detection of Helicobacter antibodies, smoking, an excessive alcohol consumption, and the use of NSAIDs and gastro-intestinal drugs, although it did not consider inter-individual differences of socio-economic status. Participants classed themselves as "sedentary", "ambulatory" or "active", and inclusion of this simple activity measure in the analysis captured a significantly lower risk of gastric ulcer in those who described themselves as "ambulatory" rather than "sedentary" (odds ratio 0.4). However, the trend to benefit for those who classed themselves as "active" (odds ratio 0.70) was not significant relative to sedentary individuals, and neither of the 2 more active categories of individual had any apparent advantage over those who were sedentary with respect to duodenal ulcers.[48]

Conclusions

Animal studies suggest that a combination of prolonged, high intensity exercise and competitive stress can increase the risk of peptic ulceration. In contrast, human data based upon both occupational comparisons and leisure activity suggest that regular leisure activity of moderate intensity may offer some protection, particularly against duodenal ulcers, but there is little protection from heavy occupational activity.

Physical activity and endogenous risk factors for peptic ulcers

Of the common endogenous risk factors for peptic ulceration, there is little possibility of modifying inherent genetic susceptibility. However, mucosal blood flow and gastric secretions are both influenced by vigorous exercise. It has further been argued that the supply of bicarbonate to the stomach and thus gastric acidity is totally dependent upon local perfusion, and is thus susceptible to the drastic reductions of visceral blood flow that are induced by bouts of prolonged and vigorous exercise.

Reduction of mucosal blood flow

Both the formation and the healing of peptic ulcers are strongly influenced by any changes in the local blood flow to the gastric mucosa.[49] Among other functions, the local circulation supplies oxygen and bicarbonate ions, and removes any excess of hydrogen ions.[50] Mucosal blood flow may be compromised either by an accumulation of the vasoconstrictor endothelin caused by the administration of excessive doses of NSAIDs (see below),[51] or by the visceral ischaemia that is an immediate consequence of prolonged and vigorous endurance physical activity.[52]

When the circulatory system is faced with an extreme challenge, such as the completion of an ultra-triathlon event, the reduction of local blood flow to the gut can be severe enough to damage the integrity of the gastro-intestinal endothelium, with plasma antibodies signalling the absorption of intestinal endo-toxins.[53] However, an adverse effect upon endothelial function is unlikely unless environmental conditions are unfavourable (hot and humid weather) and the activity is prolonged and is undertaken at an intensity >75% of the individual's maximal oxygen intake (as in a marathon or an ultramarathon run). Regular doses of more moderate physical activity during training sessions should enhance the physical condition of an individual, thus lessening the likelihood that any given bout of vigorous physical activity will exceed the threshold fraction of maximal oxygen intake where endothelial function is compromised.

Changes in gastric secretions

The amount of gastric acid that an individual secretes seems an important factor influencing the genesis and particularly the healing of peptic ulcers, although the relationship is far from simple.[54] In horses, at least, acid secretion is increased by a starch diet,[7] and peptic ulceration is alleviated by the administration of H_2 antagonists and proton-pump inhibitors (above). Early human experiments sug-gested that vigorous exercise decreased both basal acid output and the amounts of acid secreted in response to a meal or histamine administration. Moreover, these effects were independent of vagal innervation, and cross-transfusion experiments suggested that a hormone was responsible.[55–57] The exercise-induced inhibition of acid secretion persisted into the recovery period,[58,59] was inversely related to the individual's level of aerobic fitness and was exacerbated by competition.[60]

More recent studies of this issue have been inconsistent, with some authors finding reductions in basic acid secretion and the secretory response to 5% glucose during or following a bout of physical activity,[58,59,61,62] and others seeing no change in acid secretion with physical activity at an intensity demanding up to 75% of the individual's maximal aerobic power.[63–65] Two authors compared responses in healthy individuals and in those with peptic ulcers. Zach et al.[59] found that cycling at 50% of maximal heart rate reduced acid secretion in healthy individuals and in those with gastric ulcers, but it increased acid secretion in those with duodenal ulcers. Likewise, Canalles et al.[61] reported that physical activity at an intensity falling into the recommended training zone (60–70% of maximal oxygen intake) decreased basal acid secretion in healthy individuals, but increased it in those with peptic ulcers.

Zach et al.[59] found that an hour of cycle ergometer exercise at 50% of the individual's maximal heart rate reduced both the volume of gastric secretion and its electrolyte content. Oektedalen et al.[66] also noted a decrease in meal-stimulated gastrin secretion during an arduous four-day military exercise. The secretion of gastro-intestinal hormones (gastrin, motilin, glucagon, pancreatic polypeptide and vasoactive intestinal peptide) seem to be unaffected by exercise at intensities of up to 90% of $\dot{V}O_{2max}$,[67,68] although increases in the serum gastrin response to feeding have been observed in endurance racehorses following rigorous training.[18] Interval training also increases levels of the appetite controlling hormones ghrelin and leptin, at least in horses.[69]

We may conclude that moderate exercise either has no effect or reduces gastric secretions in healthy individuals, but this pattern of response is less clearly established for those with established peptic ulcers. There is no information on the effects of very vigorous exercise, although an associated accumulation of lactate may decrease gastric mucosal pH.[70]

Physical activity and exogenous risk factors for peptic ulcers

Of the exogenous risk factors for peptic ulceration, an increase of habitual physical activity may modify the extent of Helicobacter pylori infections, influence smoking habits and alcohol consumption, modulate stress, and alter the usage of NSAIDs. Levels of habitual physical activity also vary with socio-economic status, another risk factor for peptic ulceration.

Helicobacter pylori infection

Helicobacter pylori infection was once thought to be the prime cause of peptic ulcers, and indeed one study found no relapses in patients where the ulcer had healed and this microorganism had been eliminated by antibiotic therapy.[71]

Could patterns of physical activity modulate the risk of infection by Helicobacter pylori? There is good evidence that a single bout of prolonged endurance exercise or a period of very rigorous training has at least a short-lived adverse effect upon some components of the immune system, leading to a temporary increase in the risk of upper respiratory infections.[72-74] There is also less substantial evidence that regular moderate physical activity has a beneficial effect upon immune responses, increasing one of the first lines of defence (immunoglobulin A levels[75,76]) and thus reducing the risk of respiratory infections.[77] Interestingly, the levels of immunoglobulin A that are found in saliva and gastric juice correlate well with the individual's level of protection against Helicobacter pylori infections.[78,79]

However, direct proof of benefit from an action of moderate physical activity upon the risk of Helicobacter pylori infections is difficult to establish, since both the likelihood of such an infection and an individual's level of habitual physical activity are linked to socio-economic status, and it is difficult to eliminate all of the resulting covariation from statistical analyses.

Cigarette smoking and alcohol consumption

Cigarette smoking is associated with an increased risk of developing gastric and particularly duodenal ulcers,[80] with adverse effects arising from an accumulation of free radicals, a decrease of mucosal nitric oxide synthase activity and resulting decreases in mucosal blood flow. Likewise, an excessive consumption of alcohol is linked to gastric metaplasia, reduced mucosal integrity, and an increased risk of Helicobacter pylori infection, with an increased likelihood of developing a peptic ulcer.[81] However, there are again problems of data interpretation, as heavy cigarette consumption and the abuse of alcohol are related to several risk factors for peptic ulceration, including stress, anxiety and a low socio-economic status.

Regular exercisers are usually non-smokers, and there is some evidence that involvement in exercise classes can help in smoking cessation programmes.[82–85] However, the pattern of any association between excessive alcohol consumption and sport participation is less clear cut.[85] Regular moderate physical activity may relieve stress and thus contribute to abstinence from alcohol, but on the other hand some athletic clubs consume large amounts of alcohol following a successful match, and an association between exercise and problem drinking may also arise because alcoholics tend to increase their physical activity in an attempt to avoid weight gain.[86]

Levels of stress and anxiety

Stress and/or anxiety seem linked to peptic ulceration. In some studies, the prevalence of ulcers has been as much as three times greater in those individuals reporting stress[87] or frequent tranquillizer use.[48] Stress could also increase a person's likelihood of adopting other adverse health behaviours such as smoking and consuming an excessive amount of alcohol. Analyses looking at the effects of stress have often controlled data statistically for reports of "current smoking",[87] or cumulative tobacco consumption,[48] but generally such adjustments have not allowed for the number of cigarettes consumed in recent weeks (which may have increased due to a period of increased stress).

Participation in regular physical activity sessions has a small but positive effect upon an individual's anxiety level. One early study found that 20 minutes of exercise at 70% of a person's self-imposed maximal heart rate reduced state anxiety by an amount equal to 20 minutes of formal meditation.[88] A more recent analysis of 159 reports concluded that trait anxiety was lower in fit individuals, and state anxiety could be reduced by aerobic exercise.[89] Involvement in competitive exercise, on the other hand, can substantially increase both anxiety and stress.

Frequent administration of NSAIDs

Empirical studies looking at the habitual use of NSAIDs and the risk of peptic ulcers have yielded conflicting results,[90] but it seems likely that prostaglandin inhibition by the administration of NSAIDs may compromise certain gastroduodenal defences, including local mucosal blood flow, mucus secretion and bicarbonate levels. The risks of peptic ulceration are thus likely to be increased in high-intensity exercisers who make frequent use of NSAIDs.[91] One U.S. study found that 15% of high-school football players were taking NSAIDs on a daily basis,[92] and figures are probably even higher in professional competitors and highly committed amateur athletes.

Socio-economic status

A low socio-economic status is commonly considered a risk factor for peptic ulceration, although the observed association arises in part because individuals with a low socio-economic status are more likely to face a poor diet, shift work, exposure to industrial toxins, and stresses both at work and at home, with a greater probability of smoking, consuming excessive quantities of alcohol and developing Helicobacter pylori infections. Even in the twenty-first century, individuals with low socio-economic status may still have a physically demanding job, but another adverse factor is that from a young age their participation in voluntary leisure activity is substantially lower than that of people in the upper echelons of society.[93,94]

Practical implications for prevention and management

Given the prevalence of peptic ulcers in the general population, there has been surprisingly little study of the place of habitual physical activity in either preventive programmes addressing the likely risk factors for ulceration or in the optimal management of affected individuals. Studies in racehorses and other animals involved in demanding running events seemingly point towards a negative effect of prolonged and intensive exercise upon the risks of Helicobacter pylori infections and peptic ulceration, although application of these findings to humans must be tempered by recognition of specific factors adversely affecting the horses, including dietary changes, the administration of hypertonic fluids and medications, prolonged travel in horseboxes and other stressors associated with the participation of such animals in high-level competition.[19,20]

Human studies of the relationship between peptic ulcer and habitual physical activity also have their problems. When looking at occupational studies, it is difficult to eliminate associations between involvement in heavy physical work and such covariates as a low socio-economic status, an increased risk of Helicobacter pylori infection, a high prevalence of smoking, an excessive consumption of alcohol, and a greater likelihood of shift work. Given the growing automation of most employment, further occupational studies seem unlikely to provide useful information on the relationship between physical activity and ulceration.

It is remarkable that to date there have been only two studies of leisure activity and human peptic ulceration.[46–48] One of these investigations was uncontrolled for socio-economic status,[48] and although participants in both studies were classified into three categories of habitual physical activity, neither report was able to obtain a very precise description of the types and volumes of activity that were undertaken. Nevertheless, both investigations pointed towards some benefit from engagement in regular moderate leisure activity. One study found a helpful effect upon gastric ulcers, and the other a reduction of duodenal ulcers in men only. There remains a need for further study of both recreational exercisers and athletes involved in high performance sport to clarify these discrepancies. But, as with other facets of health, combining available information from human leisure and occupational studies with animal investigations seems to suggest that there may be a J-shaped relationship between physical activity and benefit, with moderate physical activity reducing the risks of peptic ulceration and very vigorous activity increasing its prevalence.

The benefit obtained from administering proton inhibitors to racehorses points to possible effects from moderating gastric acid secretion. Moderate physical activity could also enhance immune function and thus reduce the risk of Helicobacter pylori infection, although any activity-induced changes in immune response are generally small and short-lived. Some benefit may come from an activity-based relief of anxiety or an improvement of lifestyle. Finally, regular physical activity enhances an individual's overall physical condition, so that when a given heavy task must be undertaken it is less likely to demand a large fraction of the individual's maximal oxygen intake and thus compromise blood flow to the gastric mucosa.

Areas for further research

There are suggestions that regular moderate physical activity may reduce the risk of peptic ulcers in humans. However, this topic has as yet received only very limited study, and substantial further research on the benefits of various patterns and intensities of leisure activity is warranted. There have been suggestions that vigorous exercise that raises intra-abdominal pressures may indeed increase both the likelihood of developing a peptic ulcer and the risk of its perforation, although good epidemiological evidence on this question is as yet lacking. Information on the shape of the dose–response relationship in particular is very limited; there may be a J-shaped relationship between the intensity and/or the volume of physical activity and benefit, with a moderate dose reducing the risks of peptic ulceration and very vigorous activity increasing the incidence of ulcers. However, it is important for those managing patients at a high risk of peptic ulcers that this conclusion be verified, and that the nadir of risk be established for those at various levels of initial physical condition. Further study of the mechanisms underlying any benefits from moderate physical activity may also help in maximizing the benefit yielded by preventive exercise programmes.

Conclusions

There is a high prevalence of peptic ulceration in racehorses and sled dogs, particularly during periods of competition. Some older occupational comparisons suggested that there was also an increased risk of peptic ulcers among manual workers, but it remains difficult to separate the effects of a high work-related energy expenditure from the covariates of social class and attendant influences of smoking, excessive alcohol consumption, shift work and other stressors. Two studies of leisure activity point to some protection from moderate physical activity, one finding a reduced risk of gastric ulcers, and the other a reduced risk of duodenal ulcers in men only. Moderate physical activity could certainly have a favourable impact upon a number of the risk factors underlying peptic ulceration. It could reduce gastric secretions and enhance immune function, with the latter reducing the risk of Helicobacter pylori infection. It might also reduce anxiety, and encourage the adoption of a healthy lifestyle, with avoidance of smoking and an excessive consumption of alcohol. On the other hand, there is some evidence that ultra-endurance exercise and/or excessive training has a negative impact, suppressing immune function, reducing mucosal blood flow, and calling for frequent administration of NSAIDs. As with other aspects of exercise medicine, there may thus be a J-shaped relationship between dose and response, with a favourable response to bouts of moderate physical activity, but increasingly negative effects as the volume and intensity of exercise becomes excessive. Further research is recommended to explore the nature of this relationship, to clarify the location of the nadir of risk for various classes of individual, and to explore mechanisms and antidotes.

References

1　Sonnenberg A, Everhart JE. Prevalence of self-reported peptic ulcer in the United States. *Am J Publ Health* 1996; 86(2): 200–205.
2　Sung JJY, Kuipers EJ, El-Serag HB. Systematic review: the global incidence of peptic ulcer disease. *Aliment Pharm Therap* 2009; 29(3): 938–946.
3　Adkamar K, Ertan A, Agrawal N *et al.* Upper gastrointestinal endoscopy in normal asymptomatic volunteers. *Gastrointest Endosc* 1986; 32(2): 78–80.
4　Duggan JM, Duggan AE. *Epidemiology of Alimentary Diseases*. New York, NY: Springer, 2006.
5　Konturek SJ, Bielański W, Płonka M *et al.* Helicobacter pylori, non-steroidal anti-inflammatory drugs and smoking in risk pattern of gastroduodenal ulcers. *Scand J Gastroenterol* 2003; 38: 923–930.
6　Sonnenberg A. Factors which influence the incidence and course of peptic ulcer. *Scand J Gastroenterol* 1988; 23 (Suppl. 155): 119–140.
7　Tamzali Y, Marguet C, Priyemko N *et al.* Prevalence of gastric ulcer syndrome in high-level endurance horses. *Equine Vet J* 2011; 43(2): 141–144.
8　Bell RJ, Kingston JK, Mogg TD *et al.* The prevalence of gastric ulceration in racehorses in New Zealand. *NZ Vet. J* 2007; 55(1): 13–18.
9　Dionne RM, Vrins A, Doucet MY *et al.* Gastric ulcers in standardbred racehorses: prevalence, lesion description, and risk factors. *J Vet Intern Med* 2003; 17(2): 218–222.
10　Jonsson H, Egenval A. Prevalence of gastric ulceration in Swedish Standardbreds in race training. *Equine Vet J* 2006; 38(3): 209–213.
11　Nieto JE, Snyder JR, Beldomenico P *et al.* Prevalence of gastric ulcers in endurance horses – a preliminary report. *Vet J* 2004; 167(1): 33–37.
12　Vatistas NJ, Snyder JR, Carlson G *et al.* Cross-sectional study of gastric ulcers of the squamous mucosa in thoroughbred racehorses. *Equine Vet J* 1999; 29 (Suppl.): 34–38.
13　Roy M-A, Vrins A, Beauchamp G *et al.* Prevalence of ulcers of the squamous gastric mucosa in standardbred horses. *J Vet Intern Med* 2005; 19(5): 744–750.
14　De Graaf-Roelfsema E, Keizer HA, Wijnberg ID *et al.* The incidence and severity of gastric ulceration does not increase in overtrained Standardbred horses. *Equine Vet J* 2010; 42 (Suppl 38.): 56–61.

15 Luthersson N, Nielsen KH, Harris P *et al.* The prevalence and anatomical distribution of equine gastric ulceration syndrome (EGUS) in 201 horses in Denmark. *Equine Vet J* 2009; 41(7): 619–624.

16 Nieto JE, Snyder JR, Vatistas NJ *et al.* Effect of gastric ulceration on physiologic responses to exercise in horses. *Am J Vet Res* 2009; 70(6): 787–795.

17 Lorenzo-Figueras M, Merritt AM. Effects of exercise on gastric volume and pH in the proximal portion of the stomach of horses. *Am J Vet Res* 2002; 63(11): 1481–1487.

18 Furr M, Taylor L, Kronfeld D. The effects of exercise training on serum gastrin responses in the horse. *Cornell Vet* 1994; 84(1): 41–45.

19 Holbrook TC, Simmons RD, Payton ME *et al.* Effect of repeated oral administration of hypertonic electrolyte solution on equine gastric mucosa. *Equine Vet J* 2005; 37(5): 501–504.

20 McClure SR, Carithers DS, Gross SJ *et al.* Gastric ulcer development in horses in a simulated show or training environment. *J Am Vet Assoc* 2005; 227(5): 775–777.

21 Buchanan BR, Andrews FM. Treatment and prevention of equine gastric ulcer syndrome. *Vet Clin North Am Equine Pract* 2003; 19(3): 575–597.

22 Lester GD, Smith RL, Robertson ID. Effects of treatment with omeprazole or ranitidine on gastric squamous ulceration in racing thoroughbreds. *J Am Vet Assoc* 2005; 227(10): 1636–1639.

23 Andrews FM, Sifferman RL, Bernard W *et al.* Efficacy of omeprazole paste in the treatment and prevention of gastric ulcers in horses. *Equine Vet J* 1999; 29 (Suppl): 81–86.

24 Doucet MY, Vrins AA, Dionne R *et al.* Efficacy of a paste formulation of omeprazole for the treatment of naturally occurring gastric ulcers in training standardbred racehorses in Canada. *Can Vet J* 2003; 44(7): 581–585.

25 Endo Y, Tsuchiya T, Sato F *et al.* Efficacy of omeprazole paste in the prevention of gastric ulcers in 2 years old Thoroughbreds. *J Vet Med Sci* 2012; 74(8): 1079–1081.

26 Orsini JA, Haddock M, Stine L *et al.* Odds of moderate or severe gastric ulceration in racehorses receiving antiulcer medications. *J Am Vet Med Assoc* 2003; 223(3): 336–339.

27 White G, McClure SR, Sifferman R *et al.* Effects of short-term light to heavy exercise on gastric ulcer development in horses and efficacy of omeprazole paste in preventing gastric ulceration. *J Am Vet Med Assoc* 2007; 230(11): 1680–1682.

28 Shea-Donohue T, Steel L, Montcalm E *et al.* Gastric protection by sucralfate. Role of mucus and prostaglandins. *Gastroenterology* 1986; 91(3): 660–666.

29 Davis MS, Willard MD, Nelson SL *et al.* Prevalence of gastric lesions in racing Alaskan sled dogs. *J Vet Intern Med* 2003; 17(3): 311–314.

30 Davis M, Willard M, Williamson K *et al.* Temporal relationship between gastrointestinal protein loss, gastric ulceration or erosion, and strenuous exercise in racing Alaskan sled dogs. *J Vet Intern Med* 2006; 20(4): 835–839.

31 Davis MS, Willard MD, Williamson KK *et al.* Sustained strenuous exercise increases intestinal permeability in racing Alaskan sled dogs. *J Vet Intern Med* 2005; 19(1): 34–39.

32 Dennis MM, Nelson SN, Cantor GH *et al.* Assessment of necropsy findings in sled dogs that died during Iditarod Trail sled dog races: 23 cases (1994–2006). *J Am Vet Med Assoc* 2008; 232(4): 564–573.

33 Iwamoto Y, Nishihara M, Takahashi M. VMH lesions reduce excessive running under the activity-stress paradigm in the rat. *Physiol Behav* 1999; 66(5): 803–808.

34 Costa G. The impact of shift and night work on health. *Appl Ergon* 1996; 27(1): 9–16.

35 Knutsson A, Bøggild H. Gastrointestinal disorders among shift workers. *Scand J Work Environ Health* 2010; 36(2): 85–95.

36 Doll R, Avery Jones F, Buckatzsch MM. *Occupational factors in the aetiology of gastric and duodenal ulcers with an estimate of their incidence in the general population*. London, UK: Her Majesty's Stationery Office, 1951.

37 Cobb S, Rose RM. Hypertension, peptic ulcer, and diabetes in air traffic controllers. *JAMA* 1973; 224: 489–492.

38 Dunn JP, Cobb S. Frequency of peptic ulcer among executives. *J Occup Med* 1962; 4: 343–348.

39 Monson RR, MacMahon B. Peptic ulcer in Massachusetts physicians. *N Engl J Med* 1969; 281: 11–15.

40 Ostensen H, Burhol PG, Størmer J et al. The incidence of peptic ulcer disease related to occupation in the northern part of Norway. A prospective epidemiological and radiological study. *Scand J Gastroenterol* 1985; 20: 79–82.

41 Langman MS. *The epidemiology of chronic digestive disease*. London, UK: Edward Arnold, 1979.

42 Pulvertaft CN. Comments on the incidence and natural history of gastric and duodenal ulcers. *Postgrad Med J* 1968; 44: 497–502.

43 Sonnenberg A, Sonnenberg GS. Occupational mortality from gastric and duodenal ulcer. *Br J Industr Med* 1986; 43: 50–55.

44 Sonnenberg A, Haas J. Joint effect of occupation and nationality on the prevalence of peptic ulcer in German workers. *Br J Industr Med* 1986; 43: 490–493.

45 Katchinsk BD, Logan RFA, Edmond M et al. Physical activity at work and duodenal ulcer risk. *Gut* 1991; 32: 983–986.

46 Cheng Y, Macera CA, Davis DR et al. Physical activity and peptic ulcers. Does physical activity reduce the risk of developing peptic ulcers? *West J Med* 2000; 173(2): 101–107.

47 Cheng C, Macera CA, Davis DR et al. Does physical activity reduce the risk of developing peptic ulcers? *Br J Sports Med* 2000; 34: 116–121.

48 Rosenstock S, Jørgensen T, Bonnevie O et al. Risk factors for peptic ulcer: a population-based prospective cohort study comprising 2416 Danish adults. *Gut* 2003; 52: 186–193.

49 Sato N, Kawano S, Tsuji S et al. Gastric blood flow in ulcer diseases. *Scand J Gastroenterol* 1995; 208 (Suppl.): 14–20.

50 Sørbe H, Svanes K. The role of blood flow in gastric mucosal defence, damage and healing. *Dig Dis* 1994; 12(5): 305–317.

51 Whittle BJR, Espluges JV. Induction of rat gastric damage by the endothelium-derived peptide, endothelin. *Br J Pharmacol* 1988; 95: 1011–1013.

52 Johnson JM. Endurance exercise and the regulation of visceral and cutaneous blood flow. In: Shephard RJ and Åstrand P-O, (eds). *Endurance in Sport*. Oxford, UK: Blackwell Science, 2000; pp. 103–117.

53 Bosenberg AT, Brock-Utne JC, Gaffin DL et al. Strenuous exercise causes systemic endotoxemia. *J Appl Physiol* 1988; 65: 106–108.

54 Calam J, Baron JH. Pathophysiology of duodenal and gastric ulcer and gastric cancer. *BMJ* 2001; 323(7319): 980–982.

55 Campbell JMH, Mitchell G, Powell ATW. The influence of exercise on digestion. *Guy's Hosp Rep* 1928; 78: 279–283.

56 Hammar S, Öbrink KJ. The inhibitory effect of muscular exercise on gastric secretion. *Acta Physiol Scand* 1953; 28(2–3): 151–162.

57 Sullivan SN. The effect of running on the gastrointestinal tract. *J Clin Gastroenterol* 1984; 6: 461–465.

58 Markiewicz K, Cholewa M, Gorski L *et al.* Effect of physical exercise on gastric basal secretion of healthy men. *Acta Hepatogastroenterol* 1977; 24: 377–380.

59 Zach E, Markiewicz K, Lukin M *et al.* Das Verhalten der basalen Magensäure-Sekretion während des Trainings und Restitution in chronischen Magen- und Zwölffingerdarmgeschwür Patienten [The behaviour of basal gastric secretion during exercise and restitution in chronic gastric and duodenal ulcer patients]. *Dtsch Z Verdau Stoffwechselkr* 1982; 42(2–3): 53–63.

60 Hellebrandt FA, Miles MM. The effect of muscular work and competition on gastric acidity. *Am J Physiol* 1932; 102: 258–266.

61 Canalles P, Diago M, Tomé A *et al.* El ejercicio físico y la secreción de ácido gástrico [Physical exercise and gastric acid secretion]. *Rev Esp Enferm Dig* 1990; 77(3): 179–184.

62 Ramsbottom N, Hunt JN. Effect of exercise on gastric emptying and gastric secretion. *Digestion* 1974; 10: 1–8.

63 Feldman M, Nixon JV. Effect of exercise on postprandial gastric secretion and emptying in humans. *J Appl Physiol* 1982; 53(4): 851–854.

64 Fordtran JS, Saltin B. Gastric emptying and intestinal absorption during prolonged severe exercise. *J Appl Physiol* 1967; 23: 331–335.

65 van Nieuwenhoven MA, Brouns F, Brummer RJ. The effect of physical exercise on parameters of gastrointestinal function. *Neurogastroenterol Motil* 1999; 11: 431–439.

66 Oektedalen O, Flaten P, Opstad PK. LPP and gastric response to a liquid meal and oral glucose during prolonged severe exercise, caloric deficit and sleep deprivation. *Scand J Gastroenterol* 1982; 19: 619–624.

67 Soffer EE, Merchant RK, Duethman G *et al.* The effect of graded exercise on esophageal motility and gastroesophageal reflux in trained athletes. *Gastroenterology* 1991; 100: A497 (abstr.).

68 Soffer EE, Wilson J, Duethman G *et al.* Effect of graded exercise on esophageal motility and gastroesophageal reflux in nontrained subjects. *Dig Dis Sci* 1994; 39: 193–198.

69 Gordon ME, McKeever KH, Bokman S *et al.* Interval exercise alters feed intake as well as leptin and ghrelin concentrations in standardbred mares. *Equine Vet J* 2008; 36 (Suppl): 596–605.

70 Friedman G, Berlot G, Kahn RJ *et al.* Combined measurements of blood lactate concentrations and gastric intramucosal pH in patients with severe sepsis. *Crit Care Med* 1995; 23(7): 1184–1193.

71 Rauws E, Tytgat GN. Cure of duodenal ulcer associated with eradication of Helicobacter pylori. *Lancet Oncol* 1990; 335(8700): 1233–1235.

72 Gleeson M. Immune function in sport and exercise. *J Appl Physiol* 2007; 103(2): 693–699.

73 Nieman DC. Is infection risk linked to exercise workload? *Med Sci Sports Exerc* 2000; 32(7 Suppl.): S406–S411.

74 Shephard RJ. Special feature for the Olympics: Effects of exercise on the immune system: overview of the epidemiology of exercise immunology. *Immunol Cell Biol* 2000; 78: 485–495.

75 Klentrou P, Cieslak T, Macera CA *et al.* Effect of moderate exercise on salivary immunoglobulin A and infection risk in humans. *Eur J Appl Physiol* 2002; 87: 153–158.

76 Shimizu K, Kimura F, Akimoto T *et al.* Effect of free-living daily physical activity on salivary secretory IgA in elderly. *Med Sci Sports Exerc* 2007; 39: 593–598.

77 Nieman DC. Exercise, upper respiratory tract infection, and the immune system. *Med Sci Sports Exerc* 1994; 26(2): 128–139.

78 Goto T, Nishizono A, Fujioka T *et al.* Local secretory immunoglobulin A and postimmunization gastritis infection after oral vaccination of mice. *Infect Immun* 1999; 67(5): 2531–2539.

79 Wirth HP, Vogt P, Ammann R *et al.* IgA-antibodies against Helicobacter pylori in gastric secretions: gastric secretory immune response or salivary contamination? *Schweiz Med Wochenschr* 1993; 123: 1106–1110.

80 Ostensen H, Gudmundsen TE, Ostensen M *et al.* Smoking, alcohol, coffee, and familial factors: any associations with peptic ulcer disease? A clinically and radiologically prospective study. *Scand J Gastroenterol* 1985; 20(10): 1227–1235.

81 Ko K, Cho CH. Alcohol drinking and cigarette smoking: a "partner" for gastric ulceration. *Zhonghua Yi Xue Za Zhi* (Taipei). 2000; 63(12): 845–854.

82 Marcus BH, Albrecht AE, Niaura RS *et al.* Exercise enhances the maintenance of smoking cessation in women. *Addict Behav* 1995; 20(1): 87–92.

83 Nagaya T, Yoshida H, Takahashi H *et al.* Cigarette smoking weakens exercise habits in healthy men. *Nicotine Tob Res* 2006; 9(10): 1027–1032.

84 Ussher MH, Taylor AH, Faulkner G. Exercise interventions for smoking cessation. *Cochrane Database Syst Rev* 2008; 8(4): CD002295.

85 Wankel LM, Sefton JM. Physical activity and other lifestyle behaviors. In: Bouchard C, Shephard RJ, Stephens T, (eds). *Physical activity, fitness and health*. Champaign, IL: Human Kinetics, 1994; pp. 530–550.

86 El-Sayed MS, Ali N, El-Sayed Ali Z. Interaction between alcohol and exercise. Physiological and haematological implications. *Sports Med* 2005; 35(3): 257–269.

87 Räihä I, Kemppaininen H, Kaprio J *et al.* Lifestyle, stress, and genes in peptic ulcer disease: a nationwide twin cohort study. *Arch Intern Med* 1998; 158: 698–704.

88 Bahrke MS, Morgan WP. Anxiety reduction following exercise and meditation. *Cogn Therap Res* 1978; 2(4): 323–333.

89 Landers DM, Petruzello SJ. Physical activity, fitness and anxiety. In: Bouchard C, Shephard RJ, Stephens T, (eds). *Physical activity, fitness and health*. Champaign, IL: Human Kinetics, 1994; pp. 868–882.

90 Pawlik T, Konturek PC, Konturek JW *et al.* Impact of Helicobacter pylori and nonsteroidal anti-inflammatory drugs on gastric ulcerogenesis in experiments on animals and humans. *Eur J Pharmacol* 2002; 449: 1–2.

91 Hawkey CJ. Nonsteroidal anti-inflammatory drug gastropathy. *Gastroenterology* 2000; 119(2): 521–535.

92 Warner DC, Schnepf G, Barrett MS *et al.* Prevalence, attitudes and behaviors related to the use of nonsteroidal anti-inflammatory drugs (NSAIDs) in student athletes. *J Adolesc Health* 2002; 30(3): 150–153.

93 Drenowatz C, Eisenmann JC, Pfeiffer KA *et al.* Influence of socio-economic status on habitual physical activity and sedentary behavior in 8- to 11-year old children. *BMC Public Health* 2010; 10: 214.

94 Shephard RJ, Bouchard C. Associations between health behaviours and health related fitness. *Br J Sports Med* 1996; 30(2): 94–101.

5 Physical activity and the risk of gastro-oesophageal cancers

Introduction

Gastric cancers are a common sequel to a peptic ulcer, and thus show a similar range of risk factors. Nearly a million cases of gastric cancer are diagnosed world-wide each year. Moreover, gastric neoplasms are the second most common cause of cancer deaths[1] and once a gastric tumour has been diagnosed, the prognosis is poor.[2] Squamous and adenomatous oesophageal cancers have a lower annual incidence, varying from 1–5 per 100,000 people in different countries.[3,4] Often, tumours of the oesophagus are preceded by a history of oesophageal reflux (see Chapter 2). Again, once an oesophageal cancer has been diagnosed, the prognosis is very poor. Malignant tumours of the duodenum account for only 0.3% of all gastro-intestinal tumours,[5] and there does not seem to be any information as to how their prevalence may be affected by physical activity. Thus, they will not be discussed further in the present chapter.

Until around 2013, physical activity was commonly regarded as having little impact upon the risk of developing either gastric or oesophageal cancers. An article published in 2014 suggested that only 5 of the 12 available reports had found an inverse relationship between physical activity and oesophageal cancer, and the same was true for only 8 of 21 studies of gastric cancer.[6] However, in the last four years, five systematic reviews and meta-analyses have dramatically changed this negative viewpoint. All 5 of the recent reports have presented evidence that regular physical activity is associated with a 20–30% decrease in the risk of gastro-oesophageal adenocarcinomas in humans that is statistically and clinically significant (see Table 5.1).

Factors affecting the physical activity/gastro-oesophageal cancer relationship

All five of the recent articles used the latest techniques (the PRISMA or the MOOSE research guidelines) in conducting their meta-analyses. One article dealt exclusively with oesophageal cancers,[7] and two analyses referred specifically to gastric cancers.[8,9] All of these meta-analyses were based on very large populations. As can be seen from Table 5.2, they had several key articles in

Table 5.1 Review articles and meta-analyses examining the possible influence of habitual physical activity upon the risk of gastric and/or oesophageal cancers

Author	Findings
Reviews conducted prior to 2013	
Balbuena and Casson[10]	Physical inactivity implicated as a risk factor for oesophageal carcinoma
Forman and Burley[11]	General review citing only 3 studies; in one investigation, physical activity increased the risk, in the 2 others, it had no effect
Hardman[12]	Review of physical activity and cancers – no mention of physical activity in relation to gastric cancer
Kelley and Duggan[13]	Review of gastric cancer epidemiology, no mention of possible value of physical activity
Lee[14]	General review. No suggestion that physical activity affected digestive tract cancers, no suggestion of any link between physical inactivity and oesophageal cancer
Lee[15]	Review of physical activity and cancer. No information cited in relation to gastric cancers
Lee and Derakhshan.[16]	General review, citing 4 studies. Heavy exercise increased risk in one, not in a second; 2 other reports show hazard ratios of 0.5 and 0.7 respectively for active individuals
Peters *et al.*[17]	Conclusion that data controversial for effect of physical activity upon gastric cancer
Rozen[18]	Obesity noted as risk factor for oesophageal cancer, but no mention of physical activity in relation to either oesophageal or gastric cancer
Wolin and Tuchman[19]	World Cancer Research Fund concluded insufficient evidence to evaluate association between gastric cancer and physical activity; only 4 of 16 studies showed benefit from physical activity, 1 showed negative effect

Reviews and meta-analyses conducted between 2013 and 2016

Abioye et al.[8]	Meta-analysis of 7944 cases of gastric cancer. Study quality assessed on Newcastle Ottawa scale, based on selection, comparability, exposure assessment and outcome ascertainment (but studies not rejected on grounds of quality). Age, BMI and smoking included as covariates. Analysis suggests physical activity has small protective effect in both cohort (risk ratio 0.82, 0.70–0.97) and case-control (risk ratio 0.83, 0.66–1.04) studies
Behrens et al.[6]	Systematic review and meta-analysis following PRISMA protocol, based on 15,745 cases, including age and sex as covariates, categorized studies by quality score based on selection bias, potential misclassification and additional covariates, and analysed data by anatomical site and type and timing of physical activity. Analysis suggests modest reduction in risk of oesophageal and gastric cancers, most marked in those engaging in moderate to vigorous physical activity 5 times/week (risk ratio 0.82, 0.74–0.90)
Chen et al.[20]	Meta-analysis based on case-control and cohort studies (984 oesophageal, 7087 gastric cancers), assessing study quality in terms of activity measurement, and inclusion of age and obesity as covariates. Analysis suggested modest protection against both oesophageal and gastric cancers (risk ratio 0.73 (0.56–0.97), 0.87 (0.78–0.97) respectively)
Singh et al.[7]	Systematic review and meta-analysis for 1871 oesophageal cancers following PRISMA protocol; decrease of risk lower in 6 high quality studies (odds ratio 0.86, 0.75–0.99) than for total series (odds ratio 0.71, 0.57–0.89)
Singh et al.[9]	Systematic review and meta-analysis for 11,111 gastric cancers following PRISMA protocol. Risk lower in most active vs least active. Average odds ratio 0.79 (0.71–0.87) was attenuated in high quality studies (odds ratio 0.86, 0.75–0.99)

Abbreviation: PRISMA = Preferred reporting items for systematic reviews and meta-analyses.

Table 5.2 An analysis of five recent systematic reviews and meta-analyses examining relationships between habitual physical activity and gastro-oesophageal cancer. The articles included in each author's analysis are marked by a cross, illustrating the overlap in the underlying data-base

Studies included	Authors of meta-analyses				
	Abioye et al.[8]	Singh et al.[9]	Behrens et al.[6]	Chen et al.[20]	Singh et al.[7] (oesophagus)
Case-control studies					
Balbuena and Casson[10]					x
Boccia et al.[28]		x	x		
Brownson et al.[29]		x	x	x	x
Campbell et al.[30]	x	x	x	x	
Chen et al.[31]				x	
Dar et al.[32]					x
Dosemeci et al.[33]		x	x	x	
Etemadi et al.[27] (oesophagus)			x	x	x
Huang et al.[34]		x	x		
Ibiebele et al.[35] (oesophagus)			x		
Jessri et al.[36] (oesophagus)			x		
Lam et al.[37]			x		
Parent et al.[38]	x	x	x	x	x
Suwanrungruang et al.[40]			x		
Vigen et al.[41]	x	x	x	x	x
Watabe et al.[39]			x	x	
Wen and Song[26]	x	x	x	x	

Cohort studies

Batty et al.[42]	x		x		
Huerta et al.[43]	x	x	x	x	x
Inoue et al.[23]	x	x	x	x	
Leitzmann et al.[24]	x	x	x	x	x
Paffenbarger et al.[44]			x		
Severson et al.[45]	x	x	x	x	
Sjödahl et al.[25]	x	x	x	x	
Wannamethee et al.[46]	x	x	x	x	x
Yun et al.[47]	x	x	x	x	x
OR or RR for physically active individuals (all studies)	0.78 (0.66–0.91)* 0.81 (0.69–0.96)**	0.79 (0.72–0.87)	0.82 (0.74–0.90)	0.87 (0.78–0.97)	0.71 (0.57–0.89)

Notes

* Case-control studies.

** Cohort studies.

Abbreviations: OR = odds ratio; RR = relative risk.

common. All of the meta-analyses made a formal assessment of the quality of the studies that were included in their calculations, although the criteria for acceptance of individual reports differed substantially between investigators. Statistical adjustment for covariates also varied between studies. Nevertheless, the five reports showed general agreement in terms of defining the protection associated with participation in regular physical activity. However, the 95% confidence limits of this benefit were quite broad (with the upper limit in some instances approaching a value of 1.00, i.e. implying a zero reduction of risk). Moreover, average effects were substantially smaller when the analysis was confined to higher quality studies, suggesting that artefacts from covariates had augmented the apparent benefit of exercise in some of the less well-designed evaluations. Nevertheless, the broad conclusion may be drawn that regular physical activity offers a significant protection against gastro-oesophageal cancers, not only in statistical terms, but also from a clinical point of view.

Methodological issues

The patient sample is now sufficiently large for the general conclusion that physical activity reduces the risk of gastric cancers to be beyond dispute. Even the most rigorous and selective of the 5 meta-analyses[8] was based upon 7944 cases of gastric cancer in a sample of 1,535,006 people. The method of disease diagnosis was also relatively precise (cancer registries or death records), although the assessment of habitual physical activity was less satisfactory, usually being based upon either validated or non-validated questionnaires, and typically sampling only recent rather than lifetime leisure behaviour. In some instances, cancers were correlated with occupational rather than leisure or total physical activity. Given the very long time course of the cancer process, it could be important to examine a person's physical activity over most of adult life, rather than simply looking at their recent past. In the case of gastric cancer, Behrens et al.[6] found comparable risk ratios for these two alternatives, but in the case of oesophageal cancers, the magnitude of associations seen with lifetime data were weakened when the focus was shifted to physical activity in the recent past.

   One potential complication when assessing the possible beneficial effects of physical activity upon any type of chronic disease is that socio-economic status (SES) can have a substantial impact upon the type and volume of leisure activity that a person undertakes.[21] Only 8 of the 15 trials that were introduced into the meta-analysis of Singh et al.[7] included SES as a covariate. Socio-economic status could potentially influence not only patterns of leisure activity, but also other cancer risk factors such as diet, overall lifestyle, H. pylori infection, area of residence, and exposure to industrial toxins.[22] However, in the 15 studies reported by Singh et al. the reductions of risk when active individuals were compared to those with a sedentary lifestyle were very similar with (0.79) or without (0.81) SES adjustment.

Optimal pattern of physical activity to reduce the risk of gastro-oesophageal cancer

How far do the available data allow us to identify an optimal pattern of physical activity in terms of a reducing a person's risk of gastro-oesophageal cancer? Abioye *et al.*[8] classed a person's physical activity as "adequate" if he or she reported meeting the current minimum World Health Organization recommendation (150 minutes of moderate aerobic activity, or 75 minutes of vigorous physical activity each week), and as "highly active" if they reported twice this volume of activity. In their analysis, the lower risk of gastro-oesophageal cancers was essentially similar for individuals who reported engaging in "adequate" or "vigorous" physical activity.

Singh *et al.*[9] related the risks of gastro-oesophageal cancer to the tertile of reported habitual physical activity. Benefit was statistically significant for those in the highest activity tertile. It was not significant for those in the middle tertile, although the difference of risk between the highest and middle activity tertiles was also not statistically significant.

A dose–response relationship is one well-accepted pointer towards the causal nature of an association between two variables. Chen *et al.*[20] found evidence of a statistically significant inverse dose–response relationship between the level of habitual physical activity and risk in four studies of gastric cancer,[23-26] and one study of oesophageal cancer.[27] Singh *et al.*[7] also reported a non-significant trend towards an inverse dose–response relationship in their studies of oesophageal cancer. Behrens *et al.*[6] plotted risk ratios against the reported frequency of moderate to vigorous physical activity, finding a J-shaped relationship, with the optimal response being seen among those who undertook five sessions of physical activity per week.

Chen *et al.*[20] found a slightly greater benefit from occupational than from recreational physical activity. This may imply that optimal benefit is obtained from a pattern of prolonged moderate physical activity rather than from shorter periods of more intensive effort, or it may merely reflect a better ascertainment of an individual's lifetime energy expenditures from an occupational classification rather than a physical activity questionnaire.

From a practical point of view, a reduction in the risk of gastro-oesophageal cancer seems to require meeting or exceeding the minimum public health recommendation for the weekly dose of physical activity.

Influence of cancer cell type and site

With one exception,[6] reports have considered the risk of cancers, without distinguishing between adenocarcinomas and squamous-cell tumours. There is thus a need for further studies to determine whether regular physical activity is equally effective against the two types of tumour. A large Indian study of 703 histologically confirmed cases of oesophageal squamous-cell cancer[32] reported a strong inverse relationship between occupational physical activity and the risk of this type of neoplasm. However, the authors of this report admitted that at least a part of the association that they observed may have reflected an incomplete allowance for the large socio-economic differences between heavy workers and those with sedentary employment.

Abioye *et al.*[8] noted a trend that physical activity was associated with a greater reduction of risk for distal gastric cancers (influenced by H. pylori and dietary factors) than for lesions of the cardia (mainly a male phenomenon, and influenced by the extent of gastro-oesophageal reflux). Chen *et al.*[20] reported a similar tendency. Likewise, Singh *et al.*[7] found a larger beneficial effect of physical activity at the distal site (odds ratio 0.63) than at the cardia (odds ratio 0.80), and Behrens *et al.*[6] reported a similar trend for adenocarcinomas (respective odds ratios non-cardia 0.72; cardia 0.83, oesophagus 0.79).

Potential mechanisms for reduced risk of gastro-oesophageal cancer with greater habitual physical activity

As might be expected from the frequent progression of peptic ulcers to cancers, potential mechanisms whereby physical activity might reduce the risk of gastro-oesophageal cancers are similar to those influencing the risk of peptic ulcers (Chapter 4). The benefits of physical activity might be mediated through a reduction of body fat and associated metabolic risk factors, an enhancement of immune function, an up-regulation of anti-oxidant mechanisms, protection against Helicobacter pylori infections and associated gastric ulceration, a reduced risk of gastro-oesophageal reflux, and a countering of the associations between a sedentary lifestyle, smoking and an excessive alcohol consumption.[11,16,18,48,49]

Influence of body fat content and metabolic risk factors

It is well recognized that the risk of gastric cancer is substantially higher in obese individuals than those with a normal body mass, particularly if there has been a visceral accumulation of fat.[50–53] Visceral fat can liberate adipokines and cytokines that lead to hyperinsulinaemia and an increased secretion of the cancer-promoting insulin-like growth factor,[54] processes that are reversed as an increase of habitual physical activity reduces the burden of visceral fat.[55] In athletes, a high body mass index (BMI) may reflect muscular development, but in the average individual it is a useful surrogate for the accumulation of body fat. Abnet and associates[56] found that any increase of BMI, even within the normal range, increased the risk of developing an oesophageal adenocarcinoma. A meta-analysis by Kubo and Corley[57] also demonstrated a significant increase in the risk of oesophageal cancers as BMI increased, with a possible parallel association for cancers of the gastric cardia. A meta-analysis by Chen and colleagues[58] confirmed an association between cancers of the gastric cardia and BMI, but found no such relationship for cancers elsewhere in the stomach.

However, any impact of physical activity upon BMI and thus the risk of gastro-oesophageal cancer is relatively small. In their meta-regression analysis,

Abnet et al.[56] found that in those who were taking "adequate" activity, there was a just significant beta coefficient for the influence of BMI upon the risk of cancer, and there was no significant effect in those whose activity was classed as "vigorous". Behrens et al.[6] also noted that the inverse association between physical activity and gastro-oesophageal cancer risk was only attenuated modestly in studies where statistical allowance was made for the individual's adiposity, and Cook et al.[59] saw no evidence that BMI was a confounder of the physical activity/cancer relationship. Three of the 15 studies analysed by Singh et al.[7] did not adjust for obesity or BMI, and in these reports, the average reduction of risk for the active individuals (0.89) was actually less than in the remaining 12 analyses that made such an adjustment.

Two studies controlled for evidence of diabetes mellitus,[23,47] and interestingly, in these two investigations the advantage to active individuals was relatively small after adjusting for this factor (respective risk ratios of 0.93 and 0.91 versus sedentary individuals).

Enhanced immune function

Moderate physical activity is thought to have a small positive effect upon many aspects of both innate and acquired immune function, but on the other hand either a single bout of very severe exercise such as a marathon or an ultramarathon run or a period of very heavy training can depress various components of the immune response.[60] Potential benefits from regular moderate physical activity include a reduced secretion of pro-inflammatory cytokines such as interleukin-6 (IL-6) and tumour necrosis factor-α (TNF-α),[55] and possibly an overall increase of immune function. These changes could counter Helicobacter pylori infections and allow a closer surveillance of cells for cancerous change.[61]

High IL-6 concentrations are known to have an adverse effect upon prognosis in colo-rectal cancer,[62] and a programme of regular physical activity has been shown to reduce adipose tissue inflammation and circulating levels of inflammatory cytokines in obese, over-fed mice.[63] However, as yet there have been no studies where the risk of gastro-oesophageal cancers have been controlled for cytokine levels, and investigations to date have suggested that regular physical activity has little impact upon the risk of Helicobacter pylori infections.

Up-regulation of anti-oxidant mechanisms

Physical activity may decrease the risk of carcinogenesis by up-regulating anti-oxidant systems, decreasing inflammation and oxidative stress and up-regulating DNA repair mechanisms.[61] Such adaptations to regular physical activity are well established,[64] but there has as yet been no examination of their possible role in the relationship between physical activity and the prevention of gastro-oesophageal cancers. This seems a topic that merits further investigation.

Control of Helicobacter pylori infection and a reduced incidence of gastric ulceration

Helicobacter pylori infection has traditionally been considered as the main cause of peptic ulceration worldwide, although its practical importance has declined in the developed world, apparently as socio-economic conditions have improved.[22] A gastric ulcer in turn increases the individual's risk of developing a gastric cancer,[65] thus suggesting the possibility that regular physical activity might influence the risk of carcinogenesis by countering H. pylori infections and the formation of peptic ulcers. However, Abioye *et al.*[8] and Huerta *et al.*[43] found no association between the protective effects of physical activity and a reduced risk of Helicobacter pylori infections. No other studies have as yet controlled for this factor.

No studies of physical activity and gastro-oesophageal cancer have as yet compared patients with and without a previous history of peptic ulcer, but protection against ulceration gained from moderate physical activity could account also for some of the reduction in risk of gastro-oesophageal tumours.

Physical activity-related decrease of gastro-oesophageal reflux

Gastro-oesophageal reflux causes local mucosal damage (see Chapter 2) that predisposes to oesophageal and proximal gastric cancers.[66,67] Reflux is increased by a high BMI, particularly a visceral accumulation of body fat, mainly because this increases intra-abdominal pressures.[66,68] Plainly, there is potential for regular physical activity to reduce visceral fat and thus gastro-oesophageal reflux, with a positive impact upon the risk of oesophageal and proximal gastric cancers. However, this issue has not been examined in the analyses conducted to date.

Adverse overall lifestyle

The effect of physical activity upon the risk of gastro-oesophageal cancer tends to be smaller in men than in women (a trend noted by[6,8] but not by[20]). This could reflect the long-term carcinogenic effects of an adverse personal lifestyle, since until recently a higher proportion of men than women have smoked and abused alcohol.[8] Another factor favouring the experience of the women could be a negative effect of oestrogens upon the growth of gastric tumours.[69,70]

Smoking is an important risk factor in the causation of peptic ulcers,[71] and it substantially increases the risk of gastro-oesophageal cancers. Smoking was the one factor that yielded a substantial and statistically significant beta coefficient in the meta-regression analysis of Abioye *et al.*[8] looking at the influence of physical activity upon gastro-oesophageal cancers. Continued smoking also appears to attenuate the risk reduction normally associated with participation in regular physical activity. Possibly, smoking counters the effect of moderate exercise in reducing inflammatory responses.[72] Almost all studies of the association between physical activity and gastric cancer have made statistical adjustments for smoking habits. Of the two exceptions, Huang *et al.*[34] found a relatively typical risk ratio of 0.77 for physically active individuals, while Boccia *et al.* (who included no covariates in their analyses) reported no significant reduction of gastro-oesophageal cancer risk among active individuals (a risk ratio of 0.98).[28]

Alcohol consumption did not exert a significant effect in the meta-regression of Abioye *et al.*[8] In the meta-analysis of Singh *et al.*,[7] only 8 of 15 authors made statistical adjustments for alcohol consumption; discounting the outlying result of Severson *et al.*,[45] the average risk ratio for physically active individuals was rather similar whether calculated with (0.77) or without (0.79) adjustments for alcohol consumption.

An active lifestyle tends to increase a person's exposure to sunlight, and an increase in circulating levels of vitamin D could be a further factor depressing the proliferation of cancer cells in those who choose to exercise out of doors.[73]

Practical implications for the prevention of gastro-oesophageal cancers

There now seems relatively strong evidence of an association between engaging regularly in physical activity and a reduced risk of developing both gastric and oesophageal cancers. A clinically significant reduction in risk of 20–30% has been demonstrated repeatedly and consistently in differing populations from many parts of the world, and the benefit has persisted after statistical adjustment for a multitude of extraneous risk factors. Several reports have also documented an inverse dose–response relationship for both gastric[23-26] and oesophageal[27] cancers. The main weaknesses in terms of establishing a causal relationship between physical activity and a diminution of risk[74] are lack of evidence for a strong, over-arching mechanism, and the absence of randomized controlled trials in animals or in humans showing that the adoption of regular physical activity can indeed inhibit subsequent tumour formation.

Nevertheless, there are many plausible interlocking mechanisms that could contribute to the lower risk of gastric and oesophageal cancers that is seen in physically active individuals. Regular physical activity could reduce body fat and metabolic risk factors, enhance immune function, up-regulate anti-oxidant mechanisms, protect against Helicobacter pylori infections and gastric ulceration, reduce gastro-oesophageal reflux, and encourage abstinence from smoking and an excessive alcohol consumption. There are several ways in which an exercise-induced reduction of BMI and visceral fat accumulation could also diminish the risk of carcinogenesis, but the limited evidence available to date suggests that their impact is relatively small. Smoking has a powerful carcinogenic influence on many organs, including the stomach, and a lower prevalence of smoking among physically active individuals could contribute to the reduced risk of gastro-oesophageal tumours. There are many good reasons for controlling both obesity and smoking, but in the context of reducing the risk of gastro-oesophageal cancers, the assumption of benefit from such initiatives must await greater evidence on the role of other possible causal mechanisms.

From the viewpoint of public policy, the precise magnitude of the risk associated with a sedentary lifestyle remains uncertain. The published risk ratios have quite broad 95% confidence limits, and the average values seem lower for high quality investigations than for more poorly designed studies.[7,9] On the other hand, many of the assessments of risk have been based on assessments of recent lifestyle behaviour, and where physical activity habits have been ascertained over a longer fraction of adult life, active individuals have had a substantially larger advantage over their sedentary peers.[6] As a final note of caution, the lower risk ratios have typically been observed in individuals who have adopted and maintained regular, moderate to vigorous physical activity over long periods, and there may be only a small proportion of the sedentary public who can be persuaded to follow the requisite pattern of activity. Nevertheless, the evidence is strong that this is an effective preventive health behaviour.

Areas for further research

In looking at the relationship between physical activity and gastro-oesophageal cancers, most investigators have failed to distinguish between adenocarcinomas and squamous-cell tumours, and there is a need to examine whether exercise is equally beneficial in protecting against both types of cancers. It is widely assumed that the protection against peptic ulceration gained from moderate physical activity explains at least a part of the reduced risk of gastro-oesophageal tumours among exercisers, but there remains a need for studies comparing the protective value of physical activity in patients with and without a history of peptic ulcer. There is also scope for more research on the mechanisms underlying benefit, looking at the influence of such factors as altered cytokine levels. a reduced prevalence of Helicobacter pylori infections, up-regulation of anti-oxidant systems, decreases of inflammation and oxidant stress and up-regulation of DNA repair mechanisms.[61] Plainly, there is potential for regular physical activity to reduce visceral fat and thus gastro-oesophageal reflux, with a positive impact on the risk of oesophageal and proximal gastric cancers, but again this issue has not been tested in the analyses conducted to date. Finally, there does not seem to be any information as to how the prevalence of malignant duodenal tumours may be affected by exercise.

Conclusions

Findings from several recent meta-analyses point to a reduced risk of gastric and oesophageal cancers in physically active individuals. In many published reports, moderate to vigorous physical activity has been associated with a clinically important 20–30% reduction in the risk of gastro-oesophageal adenocarcinomas, with a significant dose–response relationship. Mechanisms could include a reduction of visceral fat (with a lesser production of cancer promoting hormones and reduced gastro-oesophageal reflux) and/or a lesser likelihood of smoking and excessive alcohol consumption. Physical activity does not protect against Helicobacter pylori infections, but potential mechanisms related to the impact of physical activity upon immune function, anti-oxidant mechanisms, and gastro-oesophageal reflux remain to be explored. From the viewpoint of the practising clinician and the wellness counsellor, the main lesson seems that regular moderate to vigorous physical activity can significantly reduce the risk of cancer for the stomach and the oesophagus. The benefit among those who maintain an active lifestyle is of sufficient magnitude to provide one more strong reason to maintain a substantial weekly volume of moderate to vigorous physical activity. The necessary dose of exercise seems to match or exceed the minimal weekly volume proposed by public health agencies and the challenge for the practitioner is to persuade those who are currently sedentary to adopt such a lifestyle.

References

1　Ferlay J, Shin HR, Bray F *et al.* Estimates of worldwide burden of cancer in 2008: GLOBOCAN 2008. *Int J Cancer* 2010; 127: 2893–2917.
2　Crew KD, Neugut AI. Epidemiology of gastric cancer. *World J Gastroenterol* 2006; 12: 354–362.
3　Holmes RS, Vaughan TL. Epidemiology and pathogenesis of esophageal cancer. *Semin Radiat Oncol* 2006; 17: 2–9.
4　Lagergren J. Adenocarcinoma of oesophagus: what exactly is the size of the problem, and who is at risk? *Gut* 2005; 54 (Suppl. 1): i1–i15.
5　Fagniez P-L, Rotman N. Malignant tumors of the duodenum. In: Holzheimer RG, Mannick JA, (eds). *Surgical treatment: Evidence-based and problem-oriented.* Munich, Germany: Zuckschwerdt, 2001.
6　Behrens G, Jochem C, Keimling M, Ricci C *et al.* The association between physical activity and gastro-oesophageal cancer: systematic review and meta-analysis. *Eur J Epidemiol* 2014; 29: 151–170.
7　Singh S, Varayil JE, Devanna S *et al.* Physical activity is associated with reduced risk of gastric cancer: A systematic review and meta-analysis. *Cancer Prev Res* 2013; 7(1): 12–22.
8　Abioye AI, Odesanya MO, Abioye AI *et al.* Physical activity and risk of gastric cancer: a meta-analysis of observational studies. *Br J Sports Med* 2015; 49: 224–229.
9　Singh S, Devanna S, Varayil JE *et al.* Physical activity is associated with reduced risk of esophageal cancer, particularly esophageal adenocarcinoma: a systematic review and meta-analysis. *BMC Gastroenterol* 2014; 14: 101.
10　Balbuena L, Casson AG. Physical activity, obesity and risk for esophageal adenocarcinoma. *Future Oncol* 2009; 5(7): 1051–1063.
11　Forman D, Burley VJ. Gastric cancer: global pattern of the disease and an overview of environmental risk factors. *Best Pract Res Clin Gastroenterol* 2006; 20(4): 633–649.
12　Hardman AE. Physical activity and cancer risk. *Proc Nutr Soc* 2001; 60: 107–113.
13　Kelley JR, Duggan JM. Gastric cancer epidemiology and risk factors. *J Clin Epidemiol* 2003; 56: 1–9.
14　Lee I-M. Physical activity, fitness and cancer In: Bouchard C, Shephard RJ, Stephens T, (eds). *Physical activity, fitness and health.* Champaign, IL, Human Kinetics; 1994.
15　Lee I-M. Physical activity and cancer prevention – data from epidemiological studies. *Med Sci Sports Exerc* 2003; 35(11): 1823–1827.

16 Lee YY, Derakhshan MH. Environmental and lifestyle risk factors of gastric cancer. *Arch Iran Med* 2013; 16(6): 358–365.
17 Peters HPF, De Vries WR, Vanberge-Henegouwen GP *et al.* Potential benefits and hazards of physical activity and exercise on the gastro-intestinal tract. *Gut* 2001; 48: 435–439.
18 Rozen P. Cancer of the gastrointestinal tract: early detection or early prevention? *Eur J Cancer Prev* 2004; 13(1): 71–75.
19 Wolin KY, Tuchman H. Physical activity and gastrointestinal cancer prevention. *Recent Results Cancer Res* 2011; 186: 734–100.
20 Chen Y, Yu C, Li Y. Physical activity and risks of esophageal and gastric cancers: a meta-analysis. *PLoS One* 2014; 9(2): e88082.
21 Shephard RJ, Bouchard C. Principal components of fitness: Relationship to physical activity and lifestyle. *Can J Appl Physiol* 1994; 19: 200–214.
22 Rosenstock SJ, Jørgensen T, Bonnevie O *et al.* Does Helicobacter pylori infection explain all socio-economic differences in peptic ulcer incidence? Genetic and psycho-social markers for incident peptic ulcer disease in a large cohort of Danish adults. *Scand J Gastroenterol* 2004; 39: 823–829.
23 Inoue M, Yamamoto S, Kurahashi N *et al.* Daily total physical activity level and total cancer risk in men and women: results from a large-scale population-based cohort study in Japan. *Am J Epidemiol* 2008; 168: 391–403.
24 Leitzmann MF, Koebnick C, Freedman ND *et al.* Physical activity and esophageal and gastric carcinoma in a large prospective study. *Am J Prev Med* 2009; 36: 112–119.
25 Sjödahl K, Jia C, Vatten L *et al.* Body mass and physical activity and risk of gastric cancer in a population-based cohort study in Norway. *Cancer Epidemiol Biomarkers Prev* 2008; 17(1): 135–140.
26 Wen X-Y, Song F-M. Salt taste sensitivity, physical activity and gastric cancer. *Asian Pacific J Cancer Prev* 2010; 11: 1473–1478.
27 Etemadi A, Golozar A, Kamangar F *et al.* Large body size and sedentary lifestyle during childhood and early adulthood and esophageal squamous cell carcinoma in a high-risk population. *Ann Oncol* 2012; 23(6): 1593–1600.
28 Boccia S, Perdsiani R, La Torre G *et al.* Sulfotransferase 1A1 polymorphism and gastric cancer risk: a pilot case-control study. *Cancer Letters* 2005; 229: 235–243.
29 Brownson RC, Chang JC, Davis JR *et al.* Physical activity on the job and cancer in Missouri. *Am J Publ Health* 1991; 81(5): 639–642.
30 Campbell PT, Sloan M, Kreiger N. Physical activity and stomach cancer risk: The influence of intensity and timing during the lifetime. *Eur J Cancer Prev* 2007; 43: 593–600.
31 Chen M-J, Wu D-C, Lin J-M *et al.* Etiologic factors of gastric adenocarcinoma among men in Taiwan. *World J Gastroenterol* 2009; 15(43): 5472–5480.
32 Dar NA, Shah IA, Bhat GA *et al.* Socioeconomic status and esophageal squamous cell carcinoma risk in Kashmir. *India Cancer Sci* 2013; 104(9): 1231–1236.
33 Dosemeci M, Hayes RB, Vetter R *et al.* Occupational physical activity, socioeconomic status, and risks of 15 cancer sites in Turkey. *Cancer Causes Control* 1993; 4: 313–321.
34 Huang XE, Hirose K, Wakai K *et al.* Comparison of lifestyle risk factors by family history for gastric, breast, lung and colorectal cancer. *Asian Pac J Cancer Prev* 2004; 5: 419–427.
35 Ibiebele TI, Hughes MC, Whiteman DC *et al.* Dietary patterns and risk of oesophageal cancers: a population-based case-control study. *Br J Nutr* 2012; 107(8): 1207–1216.
36 Jessri M, Rashidkhani B, Hajizadeh B *et al.* Adherence to dietary recommendations and risk of esophageal squamous cell carcinoma: a case-control study in Iran. *Ann Nutr Metab* 2011; 59(2–4): 166–175.

37 Lam TH, Ho SY, Hedley AJ *et al.* Leisure time physical activity and mortality in Hong Kong: case-control study of all adult deaths in 1998. *Ann Epidemiol* 2004; 14(6): 391–398.

38 Parent M-E, Rousseau M-C, El-Zein M *et al.* Occupational and recreational physical activity during adult life and the risk of cancer among men. *Cancer Epidemiol* 2011; 35: 151–159.

39 Watabe K, Nishi M, Miyake H. Lifestyle and gastric cancer: a case-control study. *Oncol Rep* 1998; 5(5): 1191–1194.

40 Suwanrungruang K, Sriamporn S, Wiangnon S *et al.* Lifestyle-related risk factors for stomach cancer in northeast Thailand. *Asian Pac J Cancer Prev* 2008; 9(1): 71–75.

41 Vigen C, Bernstein L, Wu AH. Occupational physical activity and risk of adenocarcinomas of the esophagus and stomach. *Int J Cancer* 2006; 118: 1004–1009.

42 Batty GD, Shipley MJ, Marmot M *et al.* Physical activity and cause-specific mortality in men: further evidence from the Whitehall study. *Eur J Epidemiol* 2001; 17(9): 863–869.

43 Huerta JM, Navarro C, Chiriaque M-D *et al.* Prospective study of physical activity and risk of primary adenocarcinomas of the oesophagus and stomach in the EPIC (European Prospective Investigation into Cancer and Nutrition) cohort. *Cancer Causes Control* 2010; 21: 657–669.

44 Paffenbarger RS, Hyde RT, Wing AL. Physical activity and incidence of cancer in diverse populations: a preliminary report. *Am J Clin Nutr* 1987; 45(1)(1 Suppl): 312–317.

45 Severson RK, Nomura AMY, Grove JS *et al.* A prospective analysis of physical activity and cancer. *Am J Epidemiol* 1989; 130: 522–529.

46 Wannamethee SG, Shjaper AG, Walker M. Physical activity and risk of cancer in middle-aged men. *Br J Cancer* 2001; 85(9): 1311–1316.

47 Yun YH, Lim MK, Won Y-J *et al.* Dietary preference, physical activity, and cancer risk in men: National Health Insurance Corporation Study. *BMC Cancer* 2008; 8: 366.

48 Thiagarajan P, Jankowski JA. Why is there a change in patterns of GE cancer? *Recent Results Cancer Res* 2012; 196: 115–140.

49 Bonequi P, Meneses-Gonzalez F, Correa P *et al.* Risk factors for gastric cancer in Latin America: a meta-analysis. *Cancer Causes Control* 2013; 24: 217–231.

50 Bianchini F, Kaaks R, Vainio H. Overweight, obesity, and cancer risk. *Lancet Oncol* 2002; 3: 565–574.

51 MacInnis RJ, English DR, Hopper JL *et al.* Body size and the risk of gastric and oesophageal adenocarcinoma. *Int J Cancer* 2006; 118: 2628–2631.

52 O'Doherty MG, Freedman ND, Hollenbeck AR *et al.* A prospective cohort study of obesity and risk of oesophageal and gastric adenocarcinoma in the NIH-AARP Diet and Health Study. *Gut* 2012; 1261–1268.

53 Yang P, Zhou Y, Chen B *et al.* Overweight, obesity and gastric cancer risk: results from a meta-analysis of cohort studies. *Eur J Cancer Prev* 2009; 45: 2867–2873.

54 Inoue M, Tsugane S. Insulin resistance and cancer: epidemiological evidence. *Endocr Relat Cancer* 2012; 19: F1–F9.

55 McTiernan A. Mechanisms linking physical activity with cancer. *Nat Rev Cancer* 2008; 8: 205–211.

56 Abnet C, Freedman ND, Hollenbeck AR *et al.* A prospective study of BMI and risk of oesophageal and gastric adenocarcinoma. *Eur J Cancer* 2008; 44: 465–471.

57 Kubo A, Corley DA. Body mass index and adenocarcinomas of the esophagus or gastric cardia: A systematic review and meta-analysis. *Cancer Epidemiol Biomarkers Prev* 2006; 15(5): 872–878.

58 Chen Y, Liu L, Wang X *et al.* Body mass index and risk of gastric cancer: A meta-analysis of a population with more than ten million from 24 prospective studies. *Cancer Epidemiol Biomarkers Prev* 2013; 22(8): 1395–3408.

59 Cook MB, Mathews CE, Gunga MZ *et al.* Physical activity and sedentary behavior in relation to esophageal and gastric cancers in the NIH-AARP cohort. *PLoS One* 2013 Dec 19; 8(12): e84805.

60 Shephard RJ. *Physical activity, training and the immune response.* Carmel, IN: Cooper Publications, 1997.

61 Friedenreich CM, Neilson HK, Lynch BM. State of the epidemiological evidence on physical activity and cancer prevention. *Eur J Cancer* 2010; 46: 2593–2604.

62 Belluco C, Nitti D, Frantz M *et al.* Interleukin-6 blood level is associated with circulating carcinoembryonic antigen and prognosis in patients with colorectal cancer. *Ann Surg Oncol* 2000; 7: 133–138.

63 Bradley RL, Jeon JY, Liu FF *et al.* Voluntary exercise improves insulin sensitivity and adipose tissue inflammation in diet-induced obese mice. *Am J Physiol* 2008; 295(3): E586–E594.

64 Alesio H, Goldfarb H. Lipid peroxidation and scavenger enzymes during exercise: adaptive responses to training. *J Appl Physiol* 1988; 64: 1333–1336.

65 Molloy RM, Sonnenberg A. Relation between gastric cancer and previous peptic ulcer disease. *Gut* 1997; 40: 247–252.

66 Hampel H, Abraham NS, El-Serag HB. Meta-analysis: Obesity and the risk for gastro-esophageal reflux disease and its complications. *Ann Intern Med* 2005; 143(3): 199–211.

67 Rubenstein JH, Taylor JB. Meta-analysis: the association of oesophageal adenocarcinoma with symptoms of gastro-oesophageal reflux. *Aliment Pharmacol Therap* 2010; 32: 1222–1227.

68 Derakhshan MH, Robertson EV, Fletcher J *et al.* Mechanism of association between BMI and dysfunction of the gastro-oesophageal barrier in patients with normal endoscopy. *Gut* 2012; 61: 337–343.

69 Ueo H, Matsuoka H, Sugimachi K *et al.* Inhibitory effects of estrogen on the growth of a human esophageal carcinoma cell line. *Cancer Res* 1990; 50(22): 7212–7215.

70 Wakui S, Motohashi M, Muto T *et al.* Sex-associated difference in estrogen receptor beta expression in N-methyl-N'-nitro-N-nitrosoguanidine-induced gastric cancers in rats. *Comp Med* 2011; 61(5): 412–418.

71 Rosenstock SJ, Jankowski JA, Bonnevie O *et al.* Risk factors for peptic ulcer disease: a population based prospective cohort study comprising 2416 Danish adults. *Gut* 2003; 52: 186–193.

72 Lee J, Taneja V, Vassallo R. Cigarette smoking and inflammation: cellular and molecular mechanisms. *J Dent Res* 2012; 91: 142–149.

73 Deeb KK, Trump DL, Johnson CS. Vitamin D signalling pathways in cancer: potential for anticancer therapeutics. *Nat Rev Cancer* 2007; 7: 684–700.

74 Hill BA. *Principles of medical statistics*, 9th ed. New York, NY: Oxford University Press, 1971.

6   Physical activity and large bowel function

Constipation, diarrhoea and rectal bleeding

Introduction

Some of the methods used in examining function of the small intestine were discussed in Chapter 3. In this chapter, we will focus upon how acute and chronic physical activity modifies the transit of materials through the large intestine, and how this may influence such clinical problems as constipation, athlete's diarrhoea, occult bleeding and rectal haemorrhage. Issues relating to physical activity in the prevention and management of chronic inflammatory disease, benign and malignant, and tumours of the colon are deferred to the three following chapters.

Methods of studying large intestinal transit

Empirical data on physical activity and gastro-intestinal motility have shown substantial variation from one survey to another, reflecting differences of methodology, differences in the reported data (oro-anal, oro-caecal or colonic transit times), differences in the intensity of the exercise that is performed, differences in the population studied (particularly its age) and studies that have focussed upon the acute versus the chronic effects of physical activity. Harrison et al.[1] suggested that there are also marked inter-individual differences in response, with exercise programmes speeding transit in individuals where bowel movements were previously slow, but having the opposite effect in individuals whose bowel movements were normally rapid.

Many studies have looked at the effects of physical activity upon gastric and small intestinal motility, using a breath hydrogen estimate of oro-caecal transit (Chapter 3). But from the viewpoint of exercise-induced diarrhoea, a more important factor is the time that food takes to pass through the colon. This is usually deduced from the displacement of radioactive or radio-opaque markers.[2] Such markers can be ingested continuously over a period of several weeks, which is a rather inconvenient technique from the viewpoint of the subject, or (with a reduction in precision of the data) the markers can be fed as a single dose.[3] Account can also be taken of the average mass and consistency of the faeces, the number of defaecations per day, and any haemoglobin or occult blood that may be present in the stools.

Acute effects of physical activity upon colonic transit

Half-emptying of the stomach occurs in two and a half to three hours, and half-emptying of the small intestine requires a similar time. However, transit through the colon proceeds much more slowly, taking 30–40 hours or longer.

Oro-caecal transit. Six reports have examined the acute effects of moderate and vigorous aerobic exercise upon the oro-caecal transit time (see Table 6.1). Three investigations found a slowing of oro-caecal transit with exercise,[7,8,10] one a speeding of gastric emptying but no change in small intestinal behaviour,[4] one no change in motility,[9] and one a speeding of transit[6] (although this last outcome possibly reflected more rapid gastric emptying rather than altered intestinal behaviour).

Meshkionpour et al.[7] reported that 60 minutes of treadmill walking at a speed of 4.5 km/h slowed the mouth to caecal transit time for a lactulose solution from an average of 55 minutes at rest to 89 minutes during this light form of physical activity. Moses and associates[8] found that more vigorous effort, a 2-hour treadmill run at a speed demanding 65% of the individual's maximal oxygen intake, also delayed the transit of both water and a glucose polymer solution relative to resting conditions. Likewise, van Nieuwenhoven et al.[10] noted that 90 minutes of cycling or running at 70% of the subject's maximal aerobic power increased oro-caecal transit time, the changes being greater with running than with cycling. Ollerenshaw et al.[9] used ^{99}Tc labelled resin beads to study the effects of three differing patterns of physical activity upon the speed of small intestinal transit. The most vigorous activity in this study involved three 20-minute periods of cycling at a heart rate of 160 beats/min, interspersed with five 20-minute periods of walking. Small intestinal transit times did not differ between what were classed as "minimal", "moderate" and "strenuous" patterns of physical activity. Cammack et al.[4] had subjects ingest a meal containing a combination of radioactive technetium (a measure of gastric emptying) and breath hydrogen excretion (a measure of small intestine transit) to study the passage of a solid meal. Six hours of cycle ergometer exercise at a pulse rate of 120/min cut the half-time of gastric emptying from 1.5 to 1.2 hours, but the small intestinal transit time remained unchanged. The one discordant result was that of Keeling and Martin;[6] they compared breath hydrogen estimates of the oro-caecal transit time when walking up a 2% grade at 5.6 km/h versus seated rest. They observed a decrease in transit time when exercising, greatest amongst those with the slowest resting transit time. However, a speeding of gastric emptying rather than a change of intestinal behaviour could account for their findings.

Colonic transit. Transit through the gut is stimulated by migrating motor complex contractions. Most of the experimental data relate to such intestinal activity (see Table 6.1). Holdstock et al.[14] noted that mass movements in the colon were increased and a call to defaecate was initiated by a combination of eating breakfast, a change of posture, and modest walking around the hospital. Several studies have suggested that various levels of physical activity increase the likelihood of precipitating defaecation.

Early pressure measurements from dogs with caecostomies[17] found increased colonic motility in response to a bout of vigorous physical activity. In more recent research, an hour of treadmill running decreased colonic migrating motor complexes in the dog, but at the beginning of exercise a giant migrating complex often initiated defaecation.[12] A human radio-telemetry study[13] compared 10 exercisers with 10 controls, finding that contractions in the proximal jejunum were roughly halved in those taking a 4-hour, 12-mile walk. On the other hand, one hour of treadmill running at 70–80% of maximal heart rate for increased colonic contractions (as measured by a catheter containing a pressure transducer) from an irregular 1–4 cycles/min at rest to a regular 3–9 cycles/min during exercise. Five of the six individuals who showed increased colonic activity reported that they were also susceptible to athlete's diarrhoea.[11] Another report noted that during graded cycle ergometer exercise to 75% of the individual's maximal oxygen intake, colonic phasic activity was decreased, reducing resistance to colonic flow, and that following such exercise an increase of propagated activity in the gut wall led to expulsion of the colonic contents.[16] Finally, Lampe *et al.*[15] found that participation in a marathon run increased the total gut transit time of 15 women by 21%, with significant decreases in stool weight and the frequency of defaecation.

Chronic effects of physical activity upon colonic transit

Ten studies have looked at the chronic effects of physical activity upon the intestines, most investigators looking at total or colonic transit times. Four investigations found no effect of chronic physical activity upon gastro-intestinal transit, but the other six investigations observed a speeding of transit through the gut after a period of training (see Table 6.2).

Coenen *et al.*[18] found no difference in the speed of oro-anal transit when data were compared between three days of moderate jogging and three days of sedentary living, although the weight of the stools was increased when their subjects were exercising. Likewise, moderate exercise (one hour of treadmill walking at 4.5 km/h on three days) had no significant effect on either total or colonic transit time in sedentary men.[19] Bingham and Cummings[2] again found no changes in colonic or overall intestinal transit time when sedentary subjects undertook a 6–9 week programme of progressive aerobic training. Finally, Seboué *et al.*[20] observed no differences of colonic transit time in a cross-sectional comparison between 11 soccer players who were training 15 h/wk and 9 relatively inactive radiology technicians.

In contrast, Cordain *et al.*,[21] using the less reliable carmine dye method to estimate gastro-intestinal transit times, found a speeding of transit following six weeks of aerobic running. Likewise, the colonic transit time of elderly men was almost doubled when recreationally active individuals were asked to remain temporarily inactive[22]; this response was due largely to a slowing of passage through the right and left segments of the colon. Song *et al.*[23] used accelerometers to make a three-level cross-sectional classification of habitual physical

Table 6.1 Acute effects of vigorous physical activity upon oro-caecal and colonic transit

Author	Subjects	Methodology	Exercise	Findings
Oro-caecal transit				
Cammack et al.[4]	1 M, 6 F	Breath hydrogen analysis and [99]Tc	60 min cycle ergometry at heart rate of 117/min	Gastric emptying speeded, but no change of small intestinal transit time for solid meal (average 300 min)
Kayaleh et al.[5]	8 M runners	Breath hydrogen	1-h run (9.6 km) vs rest	No change in mouth to caecum transit time
Keeling and Martin[6]	12 M	Breath hydrogen analysis	120 min treadmill walk at 5.6 km/h up 2% grade vs sitting	Liquid meal, decrease of oro-caecal transit from 66 to 44 min with exercise
Meshkinpour et al.[7]	7 M, 14 F	Breath hydrogen analysis	60 min treadmill walk at 4.5 km/h	Liquid meal. Increase of oro-caecal transit time 58 to 89 min with exercise
Moses et al.[8]	10 M	Breath hydrogen analysis	120 min treadmill run at 65% maximal oxygen intake	Oral-caecal transit delayed relative to rest with either water or glucose/polymer meal
Ollerenshaw et al.[9]	9 M	^{99}Tc-tagged resin beads	Comparison of mild, moderate walking and strenuous exercise (at heart5 rate to160/min)	Water+lunch, small intestinal transit 240–300 min, no significant difference between 3 exercise patterns
van Niewenhoven et al.[10]	10 symptomatic, 10 asymptomatic athletes	Breath hydrogen	90 min of cycling or running at 70% of maximal power	Exercise increased oro-caecal transit time, greater effect from running than from cycling

Colonic transit

Study	Subjects	Method	Exercise	Result
Cheskin et al.[11]	5 M, 5 F	Pressure sensitive catheter in colon	1 h jogging at 70–80% of maximal heart rate	Colonic contractions increased in 6/10 subjects, including 5 with exercise-induced diarrhoea
Dapoigny and Sarna[12]	6 dogs	9 strain gauge transducers	1-h treadmill run, 5 km/h, 5% slope	Exercise decreased colonic migrating motor complexes, but at beginning of exercise giant migrating complexes followed by defaecation
Evans et al.[13]	20 healthy volunteers (10 exercise, 10 controls)	Pressure sensitive radio-telemetry capsule in proximal jejunum	4 h, 12-mile walk	Decreased migrating motor complex contractions by about a half
Holdstock et al.[14]	13 M, 14 F (19/27 had irritable colon syndrome)	^{51}Cr capsules in colon	Modest walking vs sitting	Exercise increases mass movements of colon and urge to defaecate
Lampe et al.[15]	15 women	Radio-opaque pellets	Participation in marathon event	21% increase of total transit time, decrease of stool weight and defaecation frequency
Rao et al.[16]	Untrained subjects (6 M, 6 F)	Solid state probe placed by colonoscopy	Graded cycle ergometer exercise to 75% maximal oxygen intake	Colonic phasic activity decreased during exercise, (intensity-dependent response) increase of propagated activity after exercise

Note
M = male, F = female.

Table 6.2 Chronic effects of physical activity upon gastro-intestinal transit

Authors	Subjects	Methods	Findings	Comments
Bingham and Cummings[2]	14 sedentary men and women	Radio-opaque markers	6–9 weeks of progressive aerobic training	Gains of fitness but no consistent change in colonic or overall transit time
Coenen et al.[18]	20 healthy M	Radio-opaque markers	3 days of easy sports activity (jogging) vs 3-day pause	No significant change in oro-anal transit time, but increased weight of stools
Cordain et al.[21]	Not available	Carmine dye estimate of gastro-intestinal transit time	6 weeks of aerobic running	Speeding of daily transit time
De Schryver et al.[24]	5 M and 20 F (intervention) vs 2 M, 16 F (controls)	Radiographic markers	12-wk physical activity (30 min brisk walk + 11 min home activities) vs controls	Total colon transit time decreased from 79.2 to 58.4 h, recto-sigmoid transit 17.5 to 9.6 h. Indices of constipation also lessened
Koffler et al.[25]	7 older untrained M	Breath hydrogen and radio-opaque markers	13-wk strength training programme	No change of mouth–caecum time, but whole bowel transit speeded from 41 to 20 h
Liu et al.[22]	9 elderly M	Breath hydrogen analysis, radio-opaque marker	Recreationally active individuals ceased physical activity	Oro-caecal time unchanged, colonic transit increased from 10.9 to 19.5 h
Oettlé[3]	6 M, 4F	Radio-opaque markers	1 h of running or cycling/day at 50% maximal oxygen intake for 1 wk vs sitting	Whole gut transit decreased from 51.2 h (rest) to 36/6h (cycling) or 34.0wh (jogging)
Rao et al.[27]	11 F athletes (6 with GI symptoms)	pH telemetry	Athletes with exercise-induced diarrhoea vs those free of problems	No difference of small intestinal or colonic transit times if prone to exercise-induced diarrhoea
Robertson et al.[19]	16 sedentary M	Radio-opaque markers	Rest vs 3 days of treadmill walking (60 min/d at 4.5 km/h, 0% slope)	No significant change of total or colonic transit time
Seboué et al.[20]	11 soccer players, 9 radiology technicians	Radio-opaque markers	Soccer players training 15h/wk + soccer game	No difference of colonic transit time
Song et al.[23]	24 M, 25 F	Radio-opaque markers	3-level accelerometer classification of habitual physical activity	In women, but not men, colonic transit faster in medium and high activity groups

Abbreviations: F = female; GI = gastro-intestinal; M = male.

activity; in women, but not in men, moderate and high levels of activity were associated with a faster colon transit time than that seen in less active individuals. De Schryver et al.[24] had half of a group of middle-aged and previously inactive subjects with a tendency to constipation engage in a daily regimen that included a 30-minute walk and 11 minutes of home-based exercises; the initiation of this amount of exercise was sufficient to halve their colonic transit times. Further, Koffler et al.[25] noted that although a 13-week strength training programme that resulted in 41–45% increases in muscle strength had no effect upon the oro-caecal transit time, it doubled the speed of whole bowel transit.

Biological basis of activity-related changes in colonic transit

Decreases in colonic transit time associated with increased physical activity have been attributed to dietary factors, a reduction of visceral blood flow, altered concentration of certain hormones, neurogenic influences, or simply the mechanical effects of gut movement during the exercise bouts.

Dietary influences. Cross-sectional comparisons of colonic transit times between athletes and sedentary individuals are partially confounded by differences in general lifestyle and diet. A comparison of 93 randomly selected runners with 95 controls found that the runners had more frequent bowel movements, often loose and urgent, but they also ate more dietary fibre.[26] Most athletes also eat a greater bulk of food than sedentary people, and they frequently consume large quantities of vitamins and other dietary supplements that can affect intestinal motility. Offering some support to the notion that colonic motility is altered by the "runner's diet", Bingham and Cummings[2] noted that the allocation of subjects to a moderate exercise programme (jogging for an hour per day) produced no consistent change in large bowel function as traced by radioactive markers, provided that those allocated to the jogging programme continued to eat a similar diet to the sedentary controls (as assured by residence in a nutritional laboratory where food intake was strictly controlled).

Dietary fibre certainly increases the bulk of the colonic contents and thus tends to speed gastro-intestinal transit. Moreover, as intestinal transit becomes faster, this decreases water absorption, increasing the likelihood of defaecation.[28] Sometimes, vigorous exercise can also slow the absorption of minerals and sugars, thus causing an active secretion of fluids into the gut, with further modifications to the consistency of the faeces.

Fordtran and Saltin[29] reported that one hour of exercise at 70% of an individual's maximal oxygen intake caused no impairment of jejunal or ileal absorption. In contrast, Barclay and Turnberg[30] found that cycle ergometer exercise at only 45–50% of maximal oxygen intake halved the jejunal absorption of water, sodium, potassium and chlorine. Likewise, Maughan et al.[31] demonstrated a slowing in the absorption of deuterated water when subjects were exercising at 80% of their maximal oxygen intake relative to findings with exercise at 42% or 61% of their maximal aerobic power. Isaacs[32] made direct observations on five patients with ileostomies, finding evidence of mild salt depletion when his subjects were running a marathon. Changes of electrolyte balance, whether caused by altered mineral absorption or heavy sweating can irritate the colon and increase its motility.[33]

Reduced visceral blood flow. During prolonged and vigorous endurance exercise, particularly in a warm and humid environment, an increased activity of the sympathetic nervous system diverts up to 80% of the visceral blood flow to the skin and working muscles.[26,34-37] If the decrease in blood flow to the gut is sufficiently severe, visceral ischaemia can cause a temporary or even a permanent derangement of intestinal function. This danger is increased if the exerciser incurs a fluid loss equivalent to more than 4% of body mass,[38] and the problem is further exacerbated by any exercise-induced changes in erythrocyte deformability, blood viscosity or platelet aggregation.[39,40]

Altered hormone concentrations. The concentrations of various hormones that affect colonic secretions, motility and local blood flow are increased by vigorous physical activity,[41-49] partly as a consequence of visceral ischaemia, partly in response to mechanical stimulation of the gut wall, and partly through exercise-induced changes in metabolism (see Table 6.3).

There is a substantial release of **opioids** with prolonged aerobic exercise. These substances act on opioid receptors in the gut wall, and as with the ingestion of opioid medication, they generally slow intestinal transit,[4,50] although opioids can also enhance contractions of the gastric antrum and thus speed oro-caecal transit.[51] **Gastrin and motilin** concentrations are increased during exercise.[46] Gastrin primarily controls gastric emptying, but it also influences the action of the ileo-caecal valve. Motilin stimulates migratory motor complexes and contraction of the intestinal muscle.[52] Mechanical stimulation causes the release of **vasoactive intestinal polypeptide (VIP)** from the gut wall, and blood levels of this substance can rise to high levels if endurance exercise is combined with dehydration. VIP decreases the small intestinal absorption of fluids and sodium, and stimulates the secretion of water, sodium, chloride and bicarbonate into the gut.[53-55] It also increases colonic contraction.[55,56] VIP and peptide histidine isoleucine both decrease internal anal sphincter pressures, facilitating defaecation.[57] **Secretin** provokes the release of a watery secretion from the pancreatic and bile duct epithelia. **Pancreatic polypeptide** also modifies intestinal secretions and induces relaxation of the colon.[58,59] **Neurokinin A** stimulates smooth muscle. Colonic relaxation is also stimulated by an exercise-induced fall in **insulin** levels. Increases in the concentrations of several **prostaglandins**, including PGE_1, PGF_1 and 6-keto PGF, are also found after running a marathon.[60] They are released in response to a mechanical stimulation of the jejunal mucosa, and cause a trans-mucosal shift of water.[61] PGE and PGF also accelerate intestinal transit and decrease colonic contraction. PGE_2 initiates the giant migrating contractions of the colon that are often associated with defaecation.[62] Splanchnic vasoconstriction finally increases the production of **peptide YY**, which increases small intestine motility and contraction.[63]

Neurogenic influences. The effects of anxiety and mental stress upon bowel function are well recognized in the phrase "my bowels are turned to water".

Table 6.3 Hormones secreted during vigorous aerobic exercise that affect the motility of the gastro-intestinal tract

Hormone	Function
Opioids	Slows intestinal transit, although stimulating gastric antrum
Gastrin	Controls gastric emptying and modulates action of ileo-caecal valve
Motilin	Stimulates migratory motor complexes and contraction of intestinal muscle
Vasoactive intestinal polypeptide (VIP)	Decreases intestinal absorption of fluids and sodium, stimulates secretion of water, sodium, chloride and possibly bicarbonate into the gut, increases colonic contraction, decrease internal anal sphincter pressure
Secretin	Provokes a watery secretion from pancreas and bile duct
Pancreatic polypeptide	Modifies intestinal secretions, causes colonic relaxation
Neurokinin A	Stimulates smooth muscle
Decreased insulin levels	Causes colonic relaxation
Prostaglandins	PGE and PGF speed intestinal transit but decrease colonic contractions; PGE2 initiates giant migrating contractions associated with defaecation, and also causes trans-mucosal shift of water into gut
Peptide YY	Increases small intestine motility and contraction

Although stress generally delays oro-caecal transit,[64] it also increases colonic motility.[65] Thus, in rats, the stress of restraint slows passage through the small intestine, but speeds movement through the large intestine; it also initiates gastro-intestinal secretory responses.[66] This reaction may be initiated by **corticorelin** (corticotrophin-releasing factor).

Anxiety can exacerbate the shift of blood flow away from the intestines, increasing the extent of visceral ischaemia during vigorous physical activity. Moreover, many athletes develop intestinal symptoms before they begin to exercise, and a third of them report similar symptoms when they are emotionally distressed.[67]

Moderate physical activity increases parasympathetic nerve activity, stimulating colonic motility. However, problems of exercise-induced diarrhoea appear at higher intensities of effort, when the sympathetic component of autonomic nerve activity is dominant.[4,68] A combination of exercise and stress decreases parasympathetic tone, accelerating passage of the colonic contents. In support of the involvement of autonomic factors, the extent of sympathetic nerve activity is less at any given absolute intensity of effort after training, and this could explain why participation in a training programme can reduce the intestinal symptoms of athletes.

Mechanical factors. Accelerometer studies have confirmed that the abdomen undergoes greater physical movement during running than during cycling,[69] and the impact of this mechanical stimulation upon the gut (either directly or via changes in hormone secretion) is shown by a greater speeding of intestinal transit with running than with cycling[3] or other forms of exercise that cause little mechanical stimulation of the abdomen. Studies using an accelerometer have confirmed that there is a greater movement of the abdomen during running than when cycling at a similar intensity of effort.

Constipation and a sedentary lifestyle

Constipation implies that the passage of faeces is infrequent, and difficult because of hardness of the stools. It can progress to an impaction of the faeces and a total bowel obstruction. It is often a major factor leading to a deterioration in the quality of life for an elderly person, and indeed faecal soiling secondary to the impaction of faeces can be a factor leading to the institutionalizing of a senior citizen. There have been suggestions that the problem is linked to a sedentary lifestyle and that it can be corrected by an increase of daily physical activity.[70] We will offer brief comments on this issue, based upon available studies.

The problem of constipation. A systematic review found that the estimated prevalence of constipation in North America ranged from 1.9% to 27.2%, with higher rates in women; among the elderly living in care homes, rates may rise as high as 50–75%.[71] In the United States, purchases of medications to counter constipation exceed $250 million per year.

Role of physical activity in countering constipation. The value of regular physical activity as a means of countering constipation is a very controversial topic, with some authors finding considerable benefit from an increase of physical activity, and others little or no effect. Indeed, a position statement on constipation issued by the American Gastroenterological Association[72] makes no mention of the possible merits of treating this problem by an increase of daily physical activity. The divergent views may reflect in part a wide variety in the causes and definitions of constipation,[72,73] and in part the fact that many studies have been conducted in elderly people, where it is difficult to ascertain levels of physical activity, compliance with any exercise intervention is usually poor, and the range of physical activity within a given sample is typically too small to test the effect of differences in exercise habits upon bowel function. There is also a need to distinguish more clearly between problems arising from a slowing of colon transit and those associated with a slowing of rectal transit.

Nevertheless, several major cross-sectional studies have shown an association between an adequate level of habitual physical activity and a reduced risk of constipation (see Table 6.4). Thus, where appropriate, it seems preferable to treat constipation by an increase of physical activity and simple dietary measures, rather than by medication and other more drastic measures.

Effects of acute physical activity. There have only been three small-scale studies examining the acute effects of increased physical activity upon constipation (see Table 6.4). None of these investigations has shown any striking response to exercise-based interventions. In one investigation, the introduction of a jogging programme had no acute effect on oro-anal transit time or the frequency of defaecation, although it did increase the stool weight from an average of 600 g to 743 g.[18] In another report, the bowel habits of eight elderly people with chronic idiopathic constipation were compared during two weeks of rest and four subsequent weeks of a pedometer-monitored increase of physical activity (one hour per day, five days per week).[74] This intervention was successful in increasing the daily walking distance somewhat, from 2.9 to 5.2 km, but there was only a minor reduction in the constipation index (from a score of 9.1 to 8.6). Finally, Robertson *et al.*[19] had 16 health-care workers walk on a treadmill for an hour at a speed of 4.5 km/h on each of three days. This caused only a non-significant trend to a reduction in the total gastro-intestinal transit time (from 24.5 to 20.9 hours).

Effects of chronic physical activity. Cross-sectional surveys looking at long-term associations between physical inactivity and constipation present a more consistent picture of benefit from an active lifestyle (see Table 6.4). Six reports showed a clear inverse relationship between physical activity and constipation, in two other studies there was a non-significant trend, and there were only three investigations where constipation was unrelated to habitual physical activity.

Campbell *et al.*[75] examined factors associated with constipation in 778 people aged 70 years or older. Those who were constipated were significantly less likely to take deliberate exercise, although they were not more likely than their peers to report extremely low levels of physical activity. Cara *et al.*[76] found a non-significant trend to more frequent defaecation in those who were taking regular exercise. De Schryver *et al.*[24] divided a group of adults over the age of 45 years into two sub-groups, conducting a cross-over trial that examined responses to 12 weeks of moderately increased physical activity (30 minutes of bi-weekly brisk walking and an 11-minute daily home programme). Both groups showed a substantial decrease of their constipation score on the standard ROME criteria, and one of the two groups also showed substantial decreases in recto-sigmoid and total colon transit times (17.5 to 9.6 hours and 79.2 to 58.4 hours, respectively) when they were engaged in the active phase of the trial. Dukas *et al.*[77] made a cross-sectional analysis of findings for a large sample of 62,036 women aged 36–61 years. Constipation, defined as a bowel movement two times or less per week, was reported by 5.4% of the sample, and in a multivariate analysis the prevalence ratio dropped from the reference value of 1.0 to 0.56 among those who reported engaging in daily exercise. Huang *et al.*[78] questioned a large sample of Hong Kong adolescents; 15.6% of this group reported constipation; the odds ratio for such a finding was increased from the reference value of 1.0 to 1.26 among those who were taking insufficient exercise, and 1.25 among those who reported excessive sedentary time. Furthermore, the association of constipation with physical inactivity showed a significant dose–response relationship. Sandler *et al.*[80] examined data for 15,014 U.S. subjects aged 12–74 years. After adjusting data for age, sex and race, constipation was associated with daily inactivity and the taking of little deliberate leisure exercise. Moreover, this association was seen across each of three age groups, and applied to both recreational and non-recreational activity. Song *et al.*[23] correlated the colon transit time with

Table 6.4 Associations between lack of physical activity and constipation

Author	Sample	Methodology	Findings	Comments
Acute effects of exercise				
Coenen et al.[18]	20 healthy men	Radio-opaque markers	Jogging had no significant effect on oro-anal transit (39 vs 48 h) or stool frequency; stool weight increased (743 vs 600 g)	
Meshkinpour et al.[74]	8 elderly with chronic idiopathic constipation	Pedometer and constipation questionnaire	Increase of daily walking from 2.9 to 5.2 km causes only small decrease in constipation index (9.1 to 8.6)	
Robertson et al.[19]	16 health-care workers	Radio-opaque markers	3 days walking for 1 h on treadmill at 4.5 km/h did not change total gastro-intestinal transit time	
Chronic effects of exercise				
Annells and Koch[73]	90 community-dwelling elderly	Constipation survey	Subjects divided on whether exercise was helpful	Some unable to exercise because of physical disabilities
Campbell et al.[75]	778 people aged >70 yrs	Structured questionnaire and interview	174 had infrequent bowel movements or straining. Constipated individuals less likely to take exercise	Many with constipation were using constipating drugs
Cara et al.[76]	414 Spanish aged >50 yrs, 4.4% with constipation	Lifestyle questionnaire	n.s. trend to more frequent defecations in those taking regular exercise	
de Schryver et al.[24]	43 adults >45 yr. Cross-over trial of 12 weeks of physical activity (brisk walking 30 min twice/wk and 11 min daily home programme)	Radiographic single marker technique	Criteria of constipation decreased with exercise, recto-sigmoid and total colonic transit speeded	ROME criteria of constipation used

Study	Subjects	Method	Results	Comments
Dukas et al.[77]	62,036 women aged 36–61 yrs	Questionnaire	5.4% reported constipation. Daily physical activity had lower prevalence ratio (0.56 in multivariate analysis)	Part of Nurses' Health Study; constipation=2 bowel movements/wk or less
Huang et al.[78]	33,692 secondary school students	Questionnaire	Constipation in 15.6%; odds ratio 1.26 insufficient exercise, 1.25 excessive sedentary behaviour	Dose–response relationship seen
Paw et al.[79]	157 subjects aged 64–94 yrs	Questionnaire	6-month resistance training programme did not increase activity or affect constipation	
Sandler et al.[80]	15,014 subjects aged 12–74 yrs	Questionnaire	Constipation associated with taking little exercise	Association seen for recreational and non-recreational activity, and present in each of 3 age categories
Simmons and Schnelle[81]	89 nursing home residents	Observed frequency of bowel movements	32-week programme attempted to increase exercise 4 times/day; no change in bowel frequency	Some improvements of function and strength
Song et al.[23]	49 adults	Radio-opaque capsules and accelerometer	In women (but not men) colon transit time shorter in more active subjects	Average colon transit time low in male subjects
Tuteja et al.[82]	1069 employees of Veterans Affairs	Questionnaire (Kaiser activity scale)	19.4% reported constipation; reported physical activity did not differ from other members of group	

Abbreviation: n.s.=non-significant.

habitual physical activity as estimated by 7-day accelerometer data in a sample of 49 adults. In the women, colon transit time was significantly shorter in those with a high level of habitual physical activity. This association was not seen in the men, but this was perhaps because all of the men in their sample had a very low colon transit time.

Two of the three negative reports were in quite elderly individuals, and in at least one of these trials there was difficulty in increasing levels of physical activity. Paw et al.[79] evaluated a group of 157 people aged 64–94 years. These were distributed between resistance, functional and combined training and control groups. However, accelerometer measurements showed that over six months, there was little change of physical activity in any of the four groups, and not surprisingly none of the groups showed any change in their bowel habits. A 32-week programme that attempted to increase the activity patterns of 89 nursing home residents on four occasions each day achieved some improvements of function and strength relative to controls, but it also was insufficient to change the frequency of bowel movements.[81] Tuteja et al.[82] questioned 1069 employees of Veterans Affairs, aged 24–77 years; 19.4% of this group reported constipation, but it was not associated with either total physical activity or any of the physical activity sub-scales as assessed by the Kaiser physical activity scale.

Athlete's diarrhoea

Runner's diarrhoea, or the "athlete's trots", was first described by Scobie[83] and Fogoros.[84] The association between the performance of vigorous physical activity and an urgent need to defaecate is now a well-recognized problem among endurance runners. Perhaps the best-known example is Paula Radcliffe, a female record holder for marathon events. When leading the women's pack at the twenty-second mile of the 2005 London marathon, she was forced to stop by the roadside and pass a loose motion in full view of the television cameras. Her symptoms had begun at mile 15, and she blamed the incident on eating too much, including a dinner of grilled salmon that she had enjoyed the previous evening.[85] A second "poster child" for the condition is the Grand Rapids-based writer, editor and journalist Lindsay Patton-Carson. She knew that she often had to defaecate after completing a training run, but when participating in the local marathon, all went well until she reached the nineteenth mile. There, she drank some pickle juice, expecting it to ease a cramp. Five minutes later, she failed to reach the next track-side "port-a-potty" before she had an uncontrollable bowel movement.[86] Many competitors have faced a similar irresistible urge in the latter part of a long distance run. Sometimes, the outcome has been a frank diarrhoea, with or without rectal bleeding, and in other instances the runner has passed very loose faeces, at the soft upper end of the Bristol scale of stool consistency.[87]

The problem is not confined exclusively to endurance athletes. Many men who have undergone extensive abdominal irradiation for the treatment of prostatic cancer also suffer from a persistent diarrhoea, particularly if radiotherapy has been supplemented by the administration of androgen-suppressant drugs.

It is less widely recognized that for the survivor of prostate cancer the problem is exacerbated by quite modest bouts of moderate endurance exercise, and indeed any form of physical activity that increases intra-abdominal pressures. Individuals with inflammatory bowel disease and irritable bowel syndrome are also particularly vulnerable to athlete's diarrhoea (see Chapter 7).

Apart from the immediate social embarrassment of public defaecation, the condition of athlete's diarrhoea has the unfortunate potential of discouraging affected individuals from taking the amount of physical activity that they would like, and it may prevent them from meeting the minimum volume of physical activity currently recommended for the maintenance of good health. Despite its prevalence, the topic of exercise-induced diarrhoea has received relatively little scientific attention, and is given only brief mention in a recent major textbook on diarrhoea.[88]

Prevalence

Runners who are affected by exercise-induced diarrhoea usually report a departure from normal bowel habits throughout the day; in particular, the stools are looser and defaecations more frequent than in the general population.[67] Specific problems may arise just prior to, during and immediately following an athletic event, with both an urge to defaecate and episodes of frank diarrhoea.[33] Abdominal distress, cramps, and the involuntary passage of stools may occur unless the runner has an opportunity to stop and defaecate.[102] For some competitors, the onset of urgency has become a predictable issue – they recognize that bowel problems are likely to develop after covering a specific distance, such as 2, 4 or 10 miles.[33] Peters *et al.*[103] found that the runner's urge to defaecate was commonly correlated with abdominal symptoms such as nausea, cramps and flatulence.

Published reports on the prevalence of exercise-induced diarrhoea vary quite widely (see Table 6.5). When seeking accurate data, two immediate issues are a low response rate of athletes to post-race questionnaires (with the possibility of a selective response from those most vulnerable to the condition), and differences in methods of reporting the numbers of those affected, ranging from competitors who developed diarrhoea during a recently completed event to those who have experienced exercise-related diarrhoea just once during a running career. The samples questioned have also varied in age, sex, level of training and the range and intensity of the sports performed. The problem seems to be more common in young than in older competitors,[33] and in women than in men.[33,89,96] Often, the condition is precipitated by a recent increase in training mileage or a particularly strenuous work-out,[84] and problems are three times more common in elite athletes than in recreational exercisers.[104] Some observers have found a direct relationship between bowel problems and the intensity of effort[33,98] or its duration,[92] but others have not.[93,101] Complaints are most prevalent among distance runners. Cases have also been described in swimmers,[105] cyclists[106] and skiers,[90] but the prevalence is roughly half as great in cycling and swimming as in running.[92,104] Finally, the condition seems to be more common in those with irritable bowel syndrome or lactose intolerance.[93]

Table 6.5 Reported prevalence of diarrhoea and involuntary defaecation during and immediately following vigorous exercise

Author	Sample	Exercise	Findings	Comments
Halvorsen et al.[89]	279 leisure-time marathon runners	Training and marathon running, particularly if fast-paced	GI disturbances in 34%. 20% sufficient to affect performance	Long-lasting GI problems in 25%, improved in 41% with regular training; diarrhoea in 15% during run, 6% post-event; blood in stools in 3/279
Keefe et al.[33]	707 marathon runners responding to questionnaire (41.6% response rate)	Hard runs and races	Bowel movements in 35%, diarrhoea in 19% after running "occasionally or frequently"	Races occasionally interrupted by bowel movement (18%) or diarrhoea (9%). Bloody diarrhoea in 1.2–1.8%
Kehl et al.[90]	41 cross-country skiers	Engadin ski marathon (42 km, with substantial changes of altitude)	8/41 had abdominal pains and/or diarrhoea during or after skiing	Faecal blood loss in 3/41
McCabe et al.[91]	125 runners	Marathon run	Abdominal cramps in 22/125, diarrhoea in 8/125 (6.4%) during or following event	Frank haematochezia in 6%. Questionnaire response rate 25%
Peters et al.[92]	199 runners, 197 cyclists, 210 triathletes	Running and cycling events	Lower abdominal symptoms in 69% M, 72% F when running, 60% M, 69% F during cycling; actual defaecation on only 4 occasions	Symptoms included cramps, bloating, urge to defaecate, defaecation, diarrhoea, flatulence and side-ache
Priebe and Priebe[93]	425 runners	Distance run	63% had experienced urge to defaecate, 51% an actual bowel movement with exercise, diarrhoea in 30%	Rectal bleeding in 12%. Some runners could control symptoms with prophylactic medication
Rehrer et al.[38]	114 previously untrained subjects	Marathon preparation	No cases of diarrhoea in a 25-km or a 42-km run	
Rehrer,[49] Rehrer et al.[94]	70 runners	67-km alpine marathon	Intestinal cramps in 7.6% of men, 25% of women; diarrhoea in 4% of men, 25% of women	70 of 170 runners responded to questionnaire

Reference	Subjects	Event/activity	Findings	Comments
Rehrer et al.[95]	55 male triathletes	Half-triathlon	20% had severe GI complaints when running, 9% when cycling, but no data on defaecation	Symptoms may be related to fermentation of fibre in lower GI tract
Riddoch and Trinick[96]	471 runners	Belfast marathon	42% had urge for bowel movement, 27% had diarrhoea "occasionally or frequently"	? respondent bias (27% response rate)
Sullivan[97]	57 Canadian recreational and competitive running club		30% had urge for bowel movement, diarrhoea in 25%	
Sullivan et al.[98]	109 distance running club members	Training and running events	On occasion, 12% incontinent while running, 62% had stopped to defaecate while training; in 3 of 109, happened on every run, for 17 of 109 at least once/month	43% had nervous diarrhoea before a competition
Sullivan et al.[67]	93 runners, 95 controls	Need for bowel movement was a common reason for runner to interrupt an event	Runners had more frequent bowel movements, more often loose and urgent	Runners ate more fibre than controls
ter Steege et al.[99]	1281 long-distance runners, Enschede marathon	11% had serious GI complaints during running, 2.7% 24 h after run	Urge to defaecate and diarrhoea in less than 1% of runners	62% response rate to 2076 questionnaires. Bloody stools in <0.5%. Complaints more frequent in females and younger runners
Worme et al.[100]	67 recreational triathletes	Triathlon	Incontinence 2/67, diarrhoea 12/67	
Worobetz and Gerrard[101]	70 multisport athletes	800-m swim/25-km cycle/5-km canoe/12-km run	43/70 (61%) had disturbing lower GI symptoms	Only 70/119 respondents may have exaggerated prevalence. Problems worst in first few weeks of training
Worobetz and Gerrard[101]	119 marathon runners	Marathon runs	54% had at some time felt need to defaecate, 44% had passed stools, 26% had diarrhoea while running	

Abbreviations: F = female; GI = gastro-intestinal; M = male.

Seventeen surveys on the prevalence of exercise-induced diarrhoea have been conducted by 12 laboratories (see Table 6.5). Most investigators have questioned long-distance runners, but there have also been studies of skiers,[90] cyclists,[92] tria-thletes[92,95,100] and multi-sport competitors.[101] Among those reporting a high inci-dence of defaecation during competition,[33,89,96,101] the question posed was usually "have you encountered such a problem occasionally or frequently?". Sullivan and Wong[98] obtained more precise information on a group of 107 recreational runners; 3 of this group had to stop their running to defaecate on almost every day, and in 17 this problem had recurred as frequently as once a month. However, other surveys have found quite low rates during a specific event.[38,99]

A number of reports have commented on the presence of blood in the stools, a factor important in determining the aetiology of bowel disorders. Again, the reported prevalence is quite varied (see Table 6.5), depending upon the intensity and duration of the activity performed, and also upon the criterion of blood loss, which has ranged from the detection of occult blood to the passage of overtly bloody faeces, either occasionally or frequently.[33,91,99] Estimations of the prevalence of overt blood loss have ranged from less than 0.5% of runners[99] to 6%[91] or even 12%.[93]

Causation

Various possible causes of exercise-induced diarrhoea have been suggested, including dietary issues, an acceleration of colonic transit, the development of visceral ischaemia, the mechanical effects of vigorous physical activity upon the intestines, activity-induced changes in hormone concentrations, development of an electrolyte imbalance, and autonomic and hormonal reactions to the stresses of competition. Ideally, the correct hypothesis should explain the greater preval-ence of problems in women and younger athletes, exacerbation of difficulties with a higher intensity of effort, and the lessening of issues as training is increased. Possibly, several of the suggested factors are implicated.

Dietary influences. The diet chosen by many athletes is one possible factor pre-disposing to diarrhoea. A comparison of 93 randomly selected runners with 95 controls found that the runners ate more dietary fibre than sedentary individuals, and they also had more frequent bowel movements, often urgent and with loose stools.[107] Athletes also eat a greater bulk of food than their sedentary peers, and many competitors consume large quantities of vitamins and other dietary supple-ments that can affect intestinal motility. Bingham and Cummings[2] noted that the allocation of subjects to a moderate exercise programme (jogging an hour per day) produced no consistent changes in large bowel function, provided that the active group continued to eat a diet that was identical to that of sedentary individuals (as assured by the residence of both groups in a nutritional laboratory). A high fibre intake certainly increases the bulk of the colonic contents and thus tends to speed transit. Moreover, as transit becomes faster, this decreases water absorption, further increasing the likelihood of defaecation.[28] However, one investigation of athletes who developed lower gastro-intestinal problems did not distinguish themselves by a high intake of either dietary fibre or milk.[107]

Many athletes and health-conscious members of exercise clubs ingest vitamins and other nutritional supplements at doses that are substantially above recommended daily limits, and this could predispose to both nausea and diarrhoea.[100,108,109] Doses of vitamin A >3000 mg/day, of vitamin C >2000 mg/day, of creatine >10 g/serving, and excessive intakes of magnesium, zinc, iron, bicarbonate and cysteine can all cause gastro-intestinal problems. A large intake of caffeine, possibly taken as an ergogenic aid, can also have a laxative effect.[110]

Sometimes, vigorous physical activity slows the absorption of water, minerals and sugars, with an active secretion of fluids into the gut. Fordtran and Saltin[29] reported that one hour of exercise at an intensity demanding 70% of maximal oxygen intake left gastric emptying unchanged, and caused no impairment of jejunal or ileal absorption that could increase the osmotic load in the intestines and thus predispose to diarrhoea. In contrast, another investigation found that cycle ergometer exercise at only 45–50% of maximal oxygen intake halved the jejunal intake of water, sodium, potassium and chlorine.[30] Likewise, Maughan *et al.*[31] demonstrated a slowing in the absorption of deuterated water when exercising at 80% of maximal oxygen intake relative to the absorption when the same person was exercising at 42% or 61% of maximal aerobic power, although their study failed to distinguish between effects that arose from a slowing of gastric emptying and those reflecting an action of exercise upon jejunal absorption. Isaacs[32] made direct observations on sodium absorption in five patients with ileostomies; he found evidence of sodium retention when his subjects were running a marathon.

Several authors have linked the urge to defaecate to a malabsorption of carbohydrate, with resulting changes in the volume of fluid in the gut,[38,93,103,111] and also a fermentation of carbohydrates in the large intestine.[108] Fordtran and Saltin[29] noted that nervous diarrhoea immediately before competition was often associated with lactose intolerance. Williams and associates had six healthy subjects walk for 4.5 hours at a speed of 4.8 km/h and an environmental temperature of 38°C. This caused no change of xylose absorption, but it did result in a slowing in the absorption and excretion of 3-O-methyl glucose.[111] Rehrer *et al.*[38] pointed out that sports drinks with >7–10% carbohydrate can impair osmotic water absorption and even draw water into the intestines. Foods with a high fibre content or a high glycaemic index have a similar effect.[38]

Accelerated gastro-intestinal transit. A general physical activity-induced speeding of gastro-intestinal transit would reduce the absorption of water from the gut, and thus would likely predispose to diarrhoea. More specific effects might be linked to increases of colonic motility and expulsive movements of the gut contents.

Opinions on the effect of chronic physical activity upon gut motility are divided, with almost a half of investigations showing no effect, and the remainder reporting a speeding of gastro-intestinal transit. Although in theory an increased speed of transit could contribute to exercise-induced diarrhoea, a telling argument against this viewpoint is the absence of any difference in either small intestinal or colonic transit times between athletes with exercise-induced diarrhoea and those without such problems.[27] However, one investigation suggested that athletes who develop lower gastro-intestinal problems during exercise did not distinguish themselves from their peers in terms of their intake of either dietary fibre or milk.[67]

Visceral ischaemia. A reduction of intestinal blood flow during prolonged exercise can cause intestinal damage, with resultant abdominal pain, diarrhoea and rectal bleeding.[112] In support of the visceral ischaemia hypothesis, training increases the visceral blood flow at any given absolute intensity of exercise[34] and this could explain why the risk of exercise-induced diarrhoea is decreased with training and/or a decrease in the relative intensity of effort.[84] However, several factors argue against ischaemic damage as being the primary cause of exercise-induced diarrhoea. Defaecation often occurs before a runner is exhausted. Only a small proportion of those affected report bloody stools (as would be anticipated with visceral injury to the gut wall), and in some instances the runner has gone on to complete his or her event despite the unwanted defaecation. Nevertheless, a lesser degree of visceral hypoxia could be a contributing factor, reducing the absorption from the intestines of fluids and carbohydrates such as methyl glucose and xylose, and causing such substances to accumulate in the colon.[99]

Hormonal changes. We have already noted the many hormonal changes that occur during exercise, and their potential impact upon intestinal motility (see Table 6.3). It is less clear how far these and other exercise-induced changes contribute to the onset of runner's diarrhoea,[113] although one could envisage a number of hormonal mechanisms leading to diarrhoea. In particular, a mechanical stimulation of the intestines may cause the release of hormones such as prostaglandins and vasoactive intestinal polypeptide (VIP), and the resulting secretions may increase the individual's propensity to a watery diarrhoea.[114–116] A mechanical contribution of this type is suggested by the greater prevalence of athlete's diarrhoea in running than in cycling or swimming.[98]

Neural influences. Moderate exercise increases parasympathetic nerve activity, thus stimulating colonic motor activity. However, exercise-induced diarrhoea usually appears at high intensities of effort, when sympathetic nerve activity is the dominant mode in the autonomic system.[4,68] Sympathetic nerve activity at any given absolute intensity of effort is decreased after training, and this might explain why conditioning programmes reduce intestinal symptoms in some athletes. On the other hand, emotional stress and an increase of sympathetic activity are unlikely to explain the diarrhoea that some runners encounter during normal training sessions.

Differential diagnosis

If an athlete reports diarrhoea, before dismissing this as a normal side-effect of prolonged endurance exercise, it is important to eliminate the possibility of other more serious pathologies. The diagnosis of athlete's diarrhoea is essentially reached by a process of exclusion (see Table 6.6). Ho[117] has published an algorithm to help in the process of differential diagnosis. Particularly if the diarrhoea is a unique event of recent onset, it is likely to have been incurred through the ingestion of contaminated water or food. Indeed, this is one of the commonest issues confronting health professionals who are providing medical coverage at international competitions.[118–121] Problems may also arise from swimming in infected water,[122,123] or from being splashed with contaminated mud.[124–126]

It is important to recognize that conditions such as inflammatory bowel disease and post-radiation colitis can be exacerbated by participating in high intensity exercise (see further, Chapter 7).

Management

Exercise-induced diarrhoea is generally regarded as more of a nuisance than a life-threatening condition. Nevertheless, if it is frequent, severe and accompanied by substantial bleeding, it not only reduces the quality of life, but can also contribute to athlete's anaemia, dehydration, heat injury and acute tubular necrosis of the kidneys.[84] Countermeasures include organizational preparations, modifications of diet and training, and specific medical treatment.

Organizational preparations. Perhaps the most important action of those organizing a competition or race is to ensure that an adequate number of toilet facilities are placed at the main site and along race routes. Provision of adequate opportunities for rehydration may also reduce the risk of visceral ischaemia.

Diet. Often, a simple dietary change can do much to minimize exercise-induced diarrhoea. Review of a runner's diet should look for an excessive intake of fibre and the use of dietary supplements that are liable to provoke diarrhoea. It may be helpful to eat a semi-hydrolyzed diet as competition approaches, particularly if the intestinal epithelium has been compromised by frequent bouts of visceral ischaemia.[127] If there is evidence of lactose intolerance, it may be necessary to switch to lactose-reduced or lactose-free milk and milk products.

Table 6.6 The differential diagnosis of exercise-induced diarrhoea

---

- Swimming in infected water
- Splashing with infected mud
- Atherosclerosis or infarction of mesenteric artery
- Mesenteric thrombosis
- Haemorrhoids, anal fissures and fistulae
- Inflammatory bowel disease
- Malabsorption syndromes
- Biliary and pancreatic disorders
- Irritable bowel syndrome
- Pseudomembranous colitis
- Colon cancer
- Traveller's diarrhoea
- General infections such as influenza
- Inappropriate diet, medications and supplements
- Thyrotoxicosis

The immediate pre-race food intake should be limited, and caffeine should also be avoided in preparation for an event.[128] Runners typically opt for a low fibre, low residue pre-race meal, and avoid gas-producing food items such as beans for as long as two to three days before competition.[117] One day before an event it is wise to restrict the intake of the sugar alcohols that are often found in sugar-free candies, gum and ice cream. Solid food should be avoided for two to five hours before competition,[33] and the colon should be emptied by defaecating shortly before competing.

Since feeding normally stimulates an increase of blood flow to the gut, the ingestion of small amounts of fluid may help to avert visceral ischaemia during an event. Dehydration can certainly exacerbate diarrhoea. If a competitor has a history of diarrhoea, it is wise to choose replacement fluids that take account of mineral losses in the faeces as well as in the sweat. Energy gels and energy bars should be used cautiously, as these appear to produce diarrhoea in some people.

Training. If exercise is consistently provoking diarrhoea, the intensity of training should be reduced for a period of one to two weeks.[28,128,129] Cross-training by an alternative type of activity may be helpful in building up physical condition without provoking diarrhoea. For example, a runner may add cycling, swimming or rowing to his or her conditioning regimen. Heat acclimation may also be helpful. Diarrhoea may be precipitated by contraction of the abdominal muscles, for example when climbing a steep slope. Clothing that fits too tightly around the waist may also increase the risk of diarrhoea.

Medical treatment. The medical support team should undertake a careful differential diagnosis and look for factors predisposing to loose bowel movements such as inflammatory bowel disease, irritable bowel syndrome or a history of abdominal irradiation. In those with a history of inflammatory bowel disease, heavy exercise should be avoided at times when the disease is active.[117] The anti-androgen drug flutamide currently used in treating prostate cancer can induce diarrhoea, in part by provoking lactose intolerance. Abdominal irradiation may also induce a chronic colitis, with a tendency to loose stools. Irradiation damage can be minimized, at least in rats, by a high intake of glutamine and arginine both before and after irradiation.[130]

If the exercise-induced diarrhoea is severe, the stools should be checked for occult blood, and the haemoglobin level checked for anaemia. The use of NSAIDs such as ibuprofen may need to be curbed, particularly if the diarrhoea is bloody. Self-medication must be evaluated carefully. Riddoch and Trinick[96] noted that affected athletes often gave themselves a wide range of supposed remedies, including kaolin, morphine, codeine phosphate, antacid tablets and anti-diarrhoea tablets.

Some medically prescribed antispasmodic preparations such as Lomotil (diphenoxylate with atropine) have anticholinergic effects that inhibit sweating, thus increasing the risk of heat stress.[93] Low doses of Loperamide (Imodium) are effective in countering prostaglandin-induced diarrhoea in both acute and chronic cases.[131] Loperamide is a peripheral opioid agonist; it blocks the myenteric plexus, decreasing the tone of the intestinal wall, slowing gastro-intestinal transit and allowing more complete water absorption. It also suppresses colic mass movements and the gastro-colic reflex. At higher doses, it blocks cal-modulin, a calcium binding messenger protein with functions that include inflammation, metabolism, apoptosis, smooth muscle contraction and the intrac-ellular movement of minerals. Unlike other opioids, there is no evidence that tol-erance develops with prolonged use of loperamide. Histamine H_2 receptor antagonists and proton-pump inhibitors may also be effective treatments in athletes with bloody diarrhoea caused by hemorrhagic gastritis.[132]

Physical activity and intestinal bleeding

In a 6-year study of joggers on Rhode Island, Paul Thompson and his associ-ates[133] encountered 12 exercise-related deaths, an estimated 1 fatal incident per year for every 7620 joggers. As might be expected, 11 of the 12 deaths were due to coronary arterial disease, but one was attributed to acute gastro-intestinal haemorrhage. Unfortunately, it was unclear whether bleeding originated in the upper part of the gastro-intestinal tract (for instance, acute haemorrhage in a gastro-duodenal ulcer or cancer), from a colo-rectal adenoma or cancer, from rectal haemorrhoids, or from the abuse of non-steroidal anti-inflammatory drugs (NSAIDs). However, the Rhode Island report raises the question as to the extent of risk the recreational exerciser faces from both occult haemorrhage and overt intestinal bleeding secondary to visceral ischaemia and a severe decrease in oxygen supply to the intestines. This is the topic addressed in the present section of the text.

Visceral ischaemia

During a bout of vigorous physical activity, there are drastic reductions in vis-ceral blood flow in order to meet the demands of the working muscles and the cutaneous circulation.[36,134] Some decrease of visceral flow is seen with even a brief period of very vigorous physical activity, but the local ischaemia is much more drastic if the activity is prolonged, if it is undertaken in a hot and humid environment, if fluid losses are not replenished adequately, and if capillary blood flow is impeded by polycythaemia, hypercoagulability, or an accumulation of metabolites that cause vascular constriction.

There seems to be a dose–response relationship between the intensity of phys-ical activity and the overall decrease of visceral blood flow as the intensity of effort is increased. Studies of hepatic arterial flow, based upon circulatory clear-ance of the dye indocyanine, have shown flow reductions of ~ 40% at 40% of maximal oxygen intake ($\dot{V}O_{2max}$),[135] of 60–70% at 60–70% of $\dot{V}O_{2max}$,[136] and of 83% during near-maximal exercise.[137,138] Further, ultrasonographic studies of the mesenteric and coeliac circulations have shown activity-related decreases in intestinal flow that parallel the reduction of blood supply to the liver and other visceral organs. Perko *et al.*[139] noted that during sub-maximal cycle ergometry, a

43% reduction of overall splanchnic flow was accompanied by a 50% reduction in coeliac blood flow.

Modest reductions of visceral blood flow do not cause pathological change in the intestines, since local oxygen needs can be met by a two- or three-fold increase in the normal capillary extraction of oxygen from the arterial blood. But as the intensity of activity is further increased, the limits of this simple compensatory mechanism are reached.[140] Visceral ischaemia then develops. Acute mesenteric ischaemia is potentially a life-threatening condition. Less severe ischaemic incidents cause nausea, abdominal cramping, vomiting and occult or overt intestinal bleeding (detected by the anal passage of tarry stools (melaena) or the appearance of bright red blood (haematochezia)). There may also be a loss of integrity of the normal gastro-intestinal barrier, allowing the absorption of intestinal endotoxins into the circulation.[141]

Most authors have focussed upon the colonic damage caused by visceral ischaemia, but one report also found endoscopic evidence of injury to the stomach mucosa in five of nine runners after completion of a marathon run.[48] An hour of cycling at 70% of $\dot{V}O_{2max}$ is enough to cause temporary damage to the intestinal mucosa, as shown by increased plasma concentrations of fatty acid binding protein (I-FABP), markers of inflammation (myeloperoxidase and calprotectin), and an increased intestinal permeability of the gut wall to carbohydrates. However this intensity of exercise is insufficient to cause an increase in antibodies to bacterial endotoxins (which would provide a warning sign that these toxins had penetrated the gut wall).[142] Moore et al.[143] confirmed that endotoxaemia was not responsible for the abdominal symptoms seen in endurance cyclists following a 100-mile ride, but they found some increase of plasma endotoxin concentrations in contestants after their participation in an 83-km run,[144] and increases were also seen among those who had completed an ultra-distance triathlon.[145]

Recovery of resting visceral blood flow levels is quite rapid, even following a heavy bout of physical activity.[35,142] Indeed, perhaps because of the inflammation that develops post-exercise, ultrasound studies of human hepatic portal blood flow may show greater than normal values for a few hours following a bout of vigorous physical activity.[146]

Prevalence of occult and overt bleeding

Many endurance athletes have learned to dissociate the sensation of abdominal pain while competing. Some of those who develop an ischaemic colitis ignore their symptoms for as long as 24 hours after a race, and others fail to report symptoms.[98] It is thus difficult to be certain of the prevalence of visceral ischaemia and associated occult and overt bleeding among athletes. In runners, reported values for occult and overt bleeding during and immediately after an event range from 1.3% to 85% (see Table 6.7), with the highest figures being seen after completing a 100-mile ultramarathon.[147] The lowest prevalence was seen in a survey where subjects were asked to report stool abnormalities without objective monitoring.[148]

Table 6.7 Reports of rectal bleeding during or immediately following physical activity

Authors	Subjects	Exercise	Prevalence of blood loss	Comments
Surveys of runners				
Baska et al.[147]	34 M, 1 F participants	100-mile ultramarathon	29/34 runners became occult blood positive over event	No relationship to age or training. Greater use of NSAIDs by negative group
Baska et al.[132]	25 participants	100-mile ultramarathon	14/16 controls, 1/9 experimental group became occult blood positive	Observational trial shows apparent protection from cimetidine (800 mg × 2)
Halvorsen et al.[149]	63 runners	Drammen marathon	8/63 had positive occult blood test after event (13%)	No GI disease, no effect of age or training
McCabe et al.[91]	68 M, 57 F	Marine corps marathon	28/125 converted from negative to positive occult blood test over event (22%)	No relation to age, sex, running ability, use of NSAIDs or steak ingestion
McMahon et al.[150]	34 runners, sex not specified	Boston marathon	7/34 became guaiac positive (21%) over event	Affected younger and faster runners. No effect of NSAIDs
Moses et al.[151]	30 runners (15 M, 15F)	Marathon	7/27 became hemo-occult positive after run	No benefit from cimetidine in blind placebo-controlled trial
Øktedalen et al.[48]	9 M	Marathon	5/9 show bleeding (56%) after event	Endoscopy shows source of bleeding in stomach
Porter[148]	287 M, 12 F	Guilford marathon	4/299 demonstrated melaena after race (1.3%)	None of 4 had haemorrhoids
Robertson et al.[152]	6 M	37-km walk on 4 consecutive days	No increase of faecal haemoglobin	

continued

Table 6.7 Continued

Authors	Subjects	Exercise	Prevalence of blood loss	Comments
Robertson et al.[152]	43 M, 3 F (5 eliminated because high pre-race values)	Aberdeen marathon	Increase of faecal haemoglobin averaging 0.42 mg/g after event	Increase of haemoglobin rose to 0.87 mg/g in athletes taking drugs before race. Bleeding not related to age or training status
Schwartz et al.[153]	41 runners	Chicago marathon	9/41 developed occult bleeding over event (22%)	Only symptoms cramping and diarrhoea; no effect of age, sex or training. Injuries seen at endoscopy in 3 runners within 3 days of race
Stewart et al.[154]	24 runners, 24 matched controls	10–42-km run in different subjects	Faecal haemoglobin increased in 20/24 runners after event (83%)	Not related to NSAIDs use
Sullivan and Wong[98]	109 runners	Members of London, ON, running club	17/109 reported blood in stools after hard run (14 M, 3F) (16%)	In 2 subjects, bleeding recurred 4–6 times
Case Reports				
Beaumont and Teare[155]	1 F	Canterbury half-marathon, run on hot day	Bloody diarrhoea persisted 10 days	Inflamed transverse and descending colon, eventually required sub-total colectomy
Cantwell[156]	1 M, 1F	20 sets of 180-m dashes, 16-km run respectively	Dark red, bright red stools respectively	Both individuals able to return to running
Cohen et al.[157]	1 M	London marathon		CT scan revealed ischaemic colitis of caecum and ascending; required hemi-colectomy and ileostomy

Study	Sex/number	Activity	Symptoms	Comments
Dodds[164]	Sex not specified	23-km Fell race	Bloody diarrhoea	Subsequently ran without problems
Fisher et al.[158]	4 F	Competitive marathon runners	2 with red stools, 2 with occult blood	No definitive GI pathology detected
Fogoros[84]	1 M	Increased training in preparation for marathon	Dark red blood	No abnormality at procto-sigmoidoscopy or barium enema; subsequently ran without problems
Heer et al.[40]	1 F	15-km mountain race	Bloody red stools	Haemorrhagic lesions throughout colon at colonoscopy; no specific treatment required
Kyriakos et al.[159]	3 F	Marathon	Bloody diarrhoea	CT scan shows reversible ischaemic colitis
Lucas and Schroy[160]	1 F	Marathon	Several episodes of bloody diarrhoea after the 4-mile mark	Polycythaemia and hypercoagulability may have contributed
Moses et al.[161]	1 M	Running 11 miles	3 bloody stools	Multiple areas of oedema at colonoscopy; fluid replenishment, recovery over 2 weeks
Sanchez et al.[162]	3 F	Marathon race	Bloody diarrhoea	Individuals late in reporting symptoms; caecum or colon affected on CT scan
Schaub et al.[37]	1 person	Competitive marathons	3 episodes of bloody diarrhoea	Ischaemic lesion in caecum at colonoscopy
Thompson et al.[133]	1 man (no details given)	Rhode Island jogger	Death from acute GI bleeding	

Abbreviations: CT = computed tomography; F = female; GI = gastro-intestinal; M = male; NSAIDs = non-steroidal anti-inflammatory drugs.

Often, bleeding was seen on only one occasion, although in some individuals it occurred as many as four times.[98] The immediate precipitating factor was typically a distance or ultra-distance run, sometimes exacerbated by a hot day, but one reported case seems to have been initiated by a series of anaerobic dashes.[156] Robertson et al.[152] further noted that whereas a marathon run increased haemoglobin loss in the faeces, walking 37 km on each of four consecutive days had no such effect.

Although bleeding is typically detected at the end of a race, it is conceivable that the ischaemic colitis may have built up over the previous weeks of training.[40,160]

Ischaemic colitis can be diagnosed by computed tomography(CT)[163] or endoscopy.[37,153,161] The findings at CT include thickening of the bowel wall, fat stranding, ascites, air in the mesenteric or portal veins, and extra-luminal air.[159] If a colonoscopy or a computed tomography scan can be performed immediately after an event, there is often evidence of ischaemic colitis. However, recovery from a minor bleeding episode is typically rapid, and no abnormal findings are likely to be seen if laboratory examination is delayed.[153]

What are the risks of developing a more serious haemorrhage? One report suggested that 16% of marathoners presented with bloody stools on at least one occasion.[98] Most observers regard the anal passage of bright red blood as a much rarer occurrence, although some case reports have described a number of incidents (see Table 6.7). The most dramatic episode was the death reported by Thompson et al.,[133] but the details of this incident are so sparse that we cannot be sure that visceral ischaemia was the cause. Two other cases required a partial colectomy,[155,157] but many athletes with haematochezia were able to return to competitive running without specific treatment.

Prevention of intestinal bleeding

The data presented in Table 6.7 provide few clues as to potential preventive measures. Diversion of blood flow from the intestines to the muscles and skin is likely to be greatest if the competitor becomes dehydrated. Strict environmental temperature limits should thus be placed upon all competitions, and care taken to maintain the fluid balance of contestants during their events. Studies to date have shown little relationship between bleeding and the administration of NSAIDs, but in view of the propensity of such drugs to cause gastro-intestinal haemorrhage, their usage by athletes should be held to a minimum. Optimization of training will certainly increase the overall cardiac output at any given absolute level of physical activity, but the potential decrease of visceral ischaemia with training is likely to be dissipated in most competitive events, because a fit runner will simply run faster than his or her opponents. A history of previous episodes of bleeding may provide some warning, although for many competitors one episode of rectal haemorrhage does not predict the risk of further similar incidents.

In an observational trial, Baska et al.[132] examined the protective effects of 800 mg of the histamine H2 receptor antagonist cimetidine taken 1 hour before and at the 50-mile mark of a 100-mile ultramarathon. Fourteen of sixteen controls were haemoccult positive following the race, as compared with only one of nine experimental subjects. The physical performance of those taking cimetidine matched that of controls, and they experienced less nausea and vomiting. These results encouraged a blinded, placebo-controlled trial of cimetidine in 30 marathon runners during the following year; 14 competitors took 800 mg of this drug 2 hours before running, and 16 controls ingested a placebo.[151] In the latter trial, there were no differences of bleeding between experimental and control subjects. Certainly, caution must be shown if cimetidine is administered, as it can cause cardiac conduction defects and alterations in psychological status.

Management of intestinal bleeding

If an athlete presents with either overt or occult gastro-intestinal bleeding, it is first important to exclude other more serious pathologies (see Table 6.6), particularly a gastric ulcer or carcinoma, and a colonic adenoma or a carcinoma. The hasty cleansing of the anus because of diarrhoea during a race may also have provoked bleeding from pre-existing haemorrhoids. If the diagnosis of bleeding due to ischaemic colitis is confirmed, it usually responds quite rapidly to a tapering of training and supportive therapy.[40,160,162] McMahon *et al.*[150] found that in five of seven runners, bleeding ceased within 72 hours of an event, although it can occasionally persist for several weeks.[164]

The main risk from repeated incidents of an activity-induced intestinal bleeding is a progressive development of anaemia. The haemoglobin levels of athletes should be monitored on a regular basis, while taking due account of the haemodilution that is associated with the expansion of blood volume in well-trained individuals.[165] Fortunately, serious long-term effects of visceral ischaemia seem very rare. The penetration of gut endotoxins into the circulation may contribute to symptoms of collapse following an exhausting race, but there do not seem to be any published reports of such cases progressing to the more serious condition of sepsis. Over a period of 18 years, there have been two published reports of patients requiring a partial colectomy because of intestinal damage and persistent haemorrhage following exercise-induced visceral ischaemia.[155,157] Given the number of marathons and ultra-endurance events performed annually, serious sequelae to visceral ischaemia must be considered a very remote contingency.

Areas for further research

There remains a need to confirm that the faster colonic transit seen in athletes is caused by physical activity, and not by associated lifestyle and dietary choices. Further, a clearer distinction should be drawn between effects that are due to competitive anxiety and those arising from physical activity per se. Finally, many theories have been advanced as to the causes of exercise-related changes in colonic transit. Nevertheless, there remains an opportunity to distinguish between these possibilities, and to exploit them in the appropriate treatment of both constipation and athletic diarrhoea.

Although several large cross-sectional surveys have pointed to an association between physical inactivity and constipation, there remains a need for substantial controlled trials looking at responses to both acute bouts of vigorous exercise and habitual physical activity, testing whether a deliberate increase of daily energy expenditures can help in the treatment of constipation, and assessing whether those who are constipated have the ability and the motivation to achieve a sufficient level of physical activity to correct their problem. Such an investigation will require careful definition of the types of constipation that are evaluated, and objective monitoring of the increases in habitual physical activity that have been achieved through any exercise intervention.

The current prevalence of athlete's diarrhoea underlines the need for further research on the causes of this condition and it offers scope to discover effective countermeasures. Such studies will be facilitated by clearer definitions of the extent and frequency of unwanted bowel movements during competition.

Although exercise-related intestinal bleeding does not generally have any major long-term health implications, there is a need for more quantitative data on the extent to which visceral ischaemia can cause significant anaemia and allow the penetration of intestinal endotoxins into the circulation.

Practical implications for healthy bowel function

A large part of the total mouth to anus transit time is occupied by the passage of material through the colon and rectum. There is growing evidence that both an acute bout of vigorous physical activity and regular training can speed colonic transit and increase the urge to defaecation, with practical implications for those concerned with the management of both chronic constipation and athlete's diarrhoea.

Few studies have looked at the acute effects of physical activity upon constipation, but the majority of available reports point to the conclusion that constipation is associated with an insufficient volume of habitual physical activity. Many of those complaining of constipation are elderly, and it is as yet less clear whether such individuals can be persuaded to attain and maintain the levels of daily exercise required for a normalization of bowel function.

Exercise-induced diarrhoea is a potential problem for many highly active individuals, not only dedicated long-distance runners but also middle-aged adults who are involved in preventive health programmes. Difficulties are particularly likely for those who face clinical issues such as inflammatory bowel disease, the irritable bowel syndrome or the after-effects of treatment for prostate cancer. Although the diarrhoea usually does not have major health consequences, it can predispose to fluid and mineral imbalance and if untreated it can cause anaemia. Perhaps more importantly for many people, the resulting social embarrassment can have a strongly negative impact upon motivation to exercise. After excluding more serious underlying pathologies, management includes the optimization of diet, enhancement of physical condition and heat acclimation by cross-training, maintenance of hydration, and provision of adequate toilet facilities near to exercise sites. Moderate doses of loperamide may be considered for individuals with persistent problems, but it is important to avoid excessive use of medications that reduce either brain function (opioids) or sweating (atropine preparations). With appropriate countermeasures, difficulties can be minimized and most exercisers can reach their desired levels of physical activity.

The general public can achieve many of the health benefits to intestinal health that are associated with regular physical activity through a relatively modest commitment to aerobic exercise (30–60 minutes of daily activity in the aerobic training zone). However, a growing proportion of the world's population finds a personal challenge in preparing themselves for the greater demands of competitive events such as the marathon, ultramarathon and triathlon. It remains unclear how far such efforts add to the health benefits accruing from more modest levels of physical activity, and indeed there is some evidence that participation in very demanding events can have negative consequences for the gut. The development of visceral ischaemia and associated intestinal bleeding is one important area of concern. As many as a fifth of participants in very prolonged endurance races are likely to suffer some gastro-intestinal blood loss, and if this is repeated on many occasions it may cause an athlete's anaemia. On the other hand, persistent bleeding sufficient to require a partial colectomy and/or allow circulatory absorption of bacterial endotoxins are sufficiently rare contingencies that they should not influence decisions regarding the participation of a dedicated runner in ultra-endurance events.

Conclusions

Physical activity tends to increase the rate of colonic transit, with dietary influences, reduced visceral blood flow, hormonal factors, neurogenic and mechanical factors all contributing to the observed response. Constipation is frequently associated with low levels of habitual physical activity, although small-scale exercise intervention attempting to correct constipation have had only limited success, perhaps because of poor compliance and the limited ability of the elderly to reach the desired levels of activity.

Prolonged competitive endurance physical activity frequently provokes diarrhoea, sometimes with the passage of fresh or occult blood in the faeces. Provided that a watch is kept for anaemia, and more serious causes of bleeding are excluded, this is not a major health concern. Excessive exercise can occasionally cause a sufficient reduction of intestinal blood flow to damage the endothelium and permit the entry of bacterial endotoxins into the circulation, potentially with fatal consequences.

References

1 Harrison RJ, Leeds AR, Bolster NR *et al.* Exercise and wheat bran: Effect on whole gut transit. *Proc Nutr Soc* 1980; 39: 22A.
2 Bingham SA, Cummings JH. Effect of exercise and physical fitness on large intestinal function. *Gastroenterology* 1989; 97: 1389–1399.

3 Oettlé GJ. Effect of moderate exercise on bowel habit. *Gut* 1991; 32: 941–944.

4 Cammack J, Read NW, Cann PA *et al.* Effect of prolonged exercise on the passage of a solid meal through the stomach and small intestine. *Gut* 1982; 3: 957–961.

5 Kayaleh RA, Meshkinpour H, Avinashi A *et al.* Effect of exercise on mouth-to-cecum transit in trained athletes: a case against the role of runners' abdominal bouncing. *J Sports Med Phys Fitness* 1996; 36(4): 271–274.

6 Keeling WF, Martin BJ. Gastrointestinal transit during mild exercise. *J Appl Physiol* 1987; 63: 978–981.

7 Meshkinpour H, Kemp C, Fairshter R. Effect of aerobic exercise on mouth-to-cecum transit time. *Gastroenterology* 1989; 96(3): 938–941.

8 Moses FM, Ryan C, DeBolt J *et al.* Oral-cecal transit time during a 2 hr run with ingestion of water or glucose polymer. *Am J Gastroenterol* 1988; 83: 1055.

9 Ollerenshaw KJ, Norman S, Wilson CG *et al.* Exercise and small intestinal transit. *Nucl Med Comm* 1987; 8: 105–110.

10 van Nieuwenhoven MA, Brouns F, Brummer RJ. Gastrointestinal profile of symptomatic athletes at rest and during physical exercise. *Eur J Appl Physiol* 2004; 91: 429–434.

11 Cheskin LJ, Crowell MD, Kamal N *et al.* The effects of acute exercise on colonic motility. *Gastrointest Motil* 1992; 4: 173–177.

12 Dapoigny M, Sarna SK. Effects of physical exercise on colonic motor activity. *Am J Physiol* 1991; 260(4 Pt 1): G646–G652.

13 Evans DF, Foster GE, Hardcastle JD. Does exercise affect the migrating motor complex in man? In: Roman C (ed.). *Gatrointestinal motility*. Boston, MA, MTP Press, 1984.

14 Holdstock DJ, Misiewicz JJ, Smith T *et al.* Propulsion (mass movements) in the human colon and its relationship to meals and somatic activity. *Gut* 1970; 11: 91–99.

15 Lampe JW, Slavin JL, Apple FS. Iron status of active women and the effect of running a marathon on bowel function and gastrointestinal blood loss. *Int J Sports Med* 1991; 12(2): 173–179.

16 Rao SC, Beaty J, Chamberlin M *et al.* Effects of acute graded exercise on human colonic motility. *Am J Physiol* 1999; 276: G1221–1226.

17 de Young VR, Rice HA, Steinhaus AH. Studies in the physiology of exercise. VI. The modification of colonic motility induced by exercise and some indications for a nervous mechanism. *Am J Physiol* 1931; 99: 52–63.

18 Coenen C, Wegener M, Wedmann B *et al.* Does physical exercise influence transit time in healthy young men? *Am J Gastroenterol* 1992; 87(3): 292–295.

19 Robertson G, Meshkinour H, Vandenberg K *et al.* Effects of exercise on total and segmental colon transit. *J Clin Gastroenterol* 1993; 16(4): 300–303.

20 Seboué B, Arhan P, Devroede G *et al.* Colonic transit in soccer players. *J Clin Gastroenterol* 1995; 20(3): 211–214.

21 Cordain, L, Latin RW, Behnke JJ. The effect of an aerobic running program on bowel transit time. *J Sports Med Phys Fitness* 1986; 26: 101–104.

22 Liu F, Kondo T, Toda Y. Brief physical inactivity prolongs colonic transit time in elderly active men. *Int J Sports Med* 1993; 14(8): 465–467.

23 Song BK, Cho KO, Jo YJ *et al.* Colon transit time according to physical activity level in adults. *J Neurogastroenterol Motil* 2012; 18: 64–69.

24 De Schryver AM, Keulemans YC, Peters HP *et al.* Effects of regular physical activity on defecation pattern in middle-aged patients complaining of chronic constipation. *Scand J Gastroenterol* 2005; 40: 422–429.

25 Koffler KH, Menkes A, Redmond RA *et al.* Strength training accelerates gastro-intestinal transit in middle-aged and older men. *Med Sci Sports Exerc* 1992; 24(4): 415–419.

26 Sullivan SN. The effect of running on the gastrointestinal tract. *J Clin Gastroenterol* 1984; 6: 461–465.

27 Rao KA, Yazaki E, Evans DF *et al.* Objective evaluation of small bowel and colonic transit time using pH telemetry in athletes with gastrointestinal symptoms. *Br J Sports Med* 2004; 38: 482–487.

28 Brouns F, Becker E. Is the gut an athletic organ? *Sports Med* 1993; 15: 242–257.

29 Fordtran JS, Saltin B. Gastric emptying and intestinal absorption during prolonged severe exercise. *J Appl Physiol* 1967; 23: 331–335.

30 Barclay GR, Turnberg LA. Effect of moderate exercise on salt and water transport in the human jejunum. *Gut* 1988; 29: 816–820.

31 Maughan RJ, Leiper JB, McGaw A. Effects of exercise intensity on absorption of ingested fluids in man. *Exp Physiol* 1990; 75: 419–421.

32 Isaacs P. Marathon without a colon: salt and water balance in endurance running ileostomates. *Br J Sports Med* 1984; 18: 295–300.

33 Keeffe E, Lowe DK, Goss R *et al.* Gastrointestinal symptoms of marathon runners. *West Med J* 1984; 141: 481–484.

34 Clausen JP. Effect of physical training on cardiovascular adjustment to exercise in man. *Physiol Rev* 1977; 57: 779–815.

35 Qamar MI, Read AE. Effects of exercise on mesenteric blood flow in man. *Gut* 1987; 28: 583–587.

36 Rowell LB, Blackmon JR, Bruce RA. Indocyanine green clearance and estimated hepatic blood flow during mild to maximal exercise in upright man. *J Clin Invest* 1964; 43: 1677–1690.

37 Schaub N, Spichtin HP, Stalder GA. Ischamische Kolitis als Ursache einer Darmb-lutung bei Marathonlauf? [Ischemic colitis as a cause of intestinal bleeding after marathon running?]. *J Suisse Med* 1985; 115: 454–457.

38 Rehrer NJ, Janssen GME, Brouns F *et al.* Fluid intake and gastrointestinal problems in runners competing in a 25-km race and marathon. *Int J Sports Med* 1989; 10(Suppl. 1): S22–S25.

39 Vandewalle H, Lacombe C, Lelievre JC *et al.* Blood viscosity after a 1-h sub-maximal exercise with and without drinking. *Int J Sports Med* 1988; 9(2): 104–107.

40 Heer M, Repond F, Hany A *et al.* Acute ischaemic colitis in a female long distance runner. *Gut* 1987; 28: 896–899.

41 Banks RO, Gallavan RH, Zinner MJ *et al.* Vasoactive agents in control of the mesenteric circulation. *Fed Proc* 1985; 44: 2743–2749.

42 Bunt JC. Hormonal alterations due to exercise. *Sports Med* 1986; 3: 331–345.

43 O'Connor AM, Johnston CF, Buchanan KD *et al.* Circulating gastrointestinal hormone changes in marathon running. *Int J Sports Med* 1995; 16: 283–287.

44 Hilsted J, Galbo H, Sonne B *et al.* Gastroenteropancreatic hormonal changes during exercise. *Am J Physiol* 1980; 239: G136–G140.

45 Greenberg GR, Marliss EB, Zinman B. Effect of exercise on the pancreatic poly-peptide response to food in man. *Hormone Metab Res* 1986; 18: 194–196.

46 Sullivan SN, Champion MC, Christofides ND *et al.* Gastrointestinal regulatory peptide responses in long-distance runners. *Phys Sportsmed* 1984; 12(7): 77–82.

47 Martins C, Morgan LM, Bloom SR *et al.* Effects of exercise on gut peptides, energy intake and appetite. *J Endocrinol* 2007; 193: 251–258.

48 Øktedalen O, Lunde OC, Opstad PK *et al.* Changes in the gastrointestinal mucosa after long-distance running. *Scand J Gastroenterol* 1992; 27: 270–274.

49 Rehrer NJ. *Limits to fluid availability during exercise.* Maastricht, Netherlands: University of Limburg, Maastricht. PhD Thesis, 1990.

50 Chapman WP, Rowlands EN, Jones CM. Multiple balloon kymographic recording of the comparative action of demerol, morphine and placebos on the motility of the upper small intestine in man. *N Engl J Med* 1950; 243: 171–177.

51 Neely JL. The effect of analgesic drugs on gastrointestinal motility in man. *Br J Surg* 1969; 56: 925–929.

52 Rennie JA, Christophides ND, Bloom SR *et al.* Stimulation of human colonic activity by motilin. *Gut* 1979; 20: A912.

53 Kane MG, O'Dorisio TM, Krejs GJ. Production of secretory diarrhea by intravenous infusion of vasoactive intestinal polypeptide. *N Engl J Med* 1983; 309: 1482–1485.

54 Krejs GJ, Fordtran JS, Fahrenkrug J *et al.* Effect of VIP infusion on water and ion transport in the human jejunum. *Gastroenterology* 1980; 78(4): 722–727.

55 Mailman D. Effects of vasoactive intestinal polypeptide on intestinal absorption and blood flow. *J Physiol* 1978; 279: 121–132.

56 Eklund S, Jodal M, Lundgren O, Sjöqvist A. Effects of vasoactive intestinal polypeptide on blood flow, motility and fluid transport of the gastrointestinal tract of the cat. *Acta Physiol Scand* 1979; 105(4): 461–468.

57 Nurko S, Dunn BM, Rattan S. Peptide histidine isoleucine and vasoactive intestinal polypeptide cause relaxation of opossum internal anal sphincter via two distinct receptors. *Gastroenterology* 1989; 96: 403–413.

58 Galbo H. Gastro-entero-pancreatic hormones. In: Galbo H (ed.). *Hormonal and metabolic adaptation to exercise.* New York, NY: Thieme, 1983, pp. 59–61.

59 Tache Y. Nature and biological actions of gastro-intestinal peptides. *Clin Biochem* 1984; 17: 77–81.

60 Demers LM, Harrison TS *et al.* Effect of prolonged exercise on plasma prostaglandin levels. *Prostaglandins Med* 1981; 6(4): 413–418.

61 Beubler E, Juan H. PGE release, blood flow and transmucosal water movement after mechanical stimulation of the rat jejunal mucosa. *Naunyn Schmiedeberg's Arch Pharmacol* 1978; 305: 91–95.

62 Staumont G, Fioramonti J, Frexinos J *et al.* Changes in colonic motility induced by sennosides in dogs: evidence of prostaglandin mediation. *Gut* 1988; 29: 1180–1187.

63 Buell MG, Harding RK. Effects of peptide YY on intestinal blood flow distribution and motility in the dog. *Regul Pept* 1989; 24(2): 195–208.

64 O'Brien JD, Thompson GD, Holly J *et al.* Stress disturbs human gastrointestinal transit via a beta-1 adrenoceptor mediated pathway. *Gastroenterology* 1985; 88: 1520.

65 Barone FC, Deegan JF, Price WJ *et al.* Cold-restraint stress increases rat fecal pellet output and colonic transit. *Am J Physiol* 1990; 258(3 Pt.1): G329–G337.

66 Lenz HJ, Raedler A, Greten H *et al.* Stress-induced gastrointestinal secretory and motor responses in rats are mediated by endogenous corticotropin-releasing factor. *Gastroenterology* 1988; 95(6): 1510–1517.

67 Sullivan SN, Wong C, Heidenheim P. Does running cause gastrointestinal symptoms? A survey of 93 randomly selected runners compared with controls. *NZ J Med* 1994; 107(984): 328–331.

68 Read NW, Houghton LA. Physiology of gastric emptying and pathophysiology of gastroparesis. *Gastroenterol Clin North Am* 1989; 18: 359–373.

69 Rehrer NJ, Meijer CA. Biomechanical vibration of of the abdominal region during running and bicycling. *J Sports Med Phys Fitness* 1991; 31: 231–234.

70 Shephard RJ. Nutrition and physiology of aging. In: Young EA, (ed.). *Nutrition, aging and health.* New York, NY, Liss, 1986.
71 Higgins PDR, Johanson JF. Epidemiology of constipation in North America: A systematic review. *Am J Gastroenterol* 2004; 99(4): 750–759.
72 American Gastroenterological Association. Medical position statement: Guidelines on constipation. *Gastroenterology* 2000; 119: 1761–1778.
73 Annells M, Koch T. Constipation and the preached trio: diet, fluid intake, exercise. *Int J Nursing Stud* 2003; 40: 843–852.
74 Meshkinpour H, Selod S, Movahedi H *et al.* Effects of regular exercise in management of chronic idiopathic constipation. *Dig Dis Sci* 1998; 43(11): 2379–2383.
75 Campbell AJ, Busby WJ, Horwath CC. Factors associated with constipation in a community based sample of people aged 70 years and over. *J Epidemiol Comm Health* 1993; 47: 23–26.
76 Cara MAL, López PJT, Oliver MC *et al.* Constipation in the population over 50 years of age in Albacete province. *Rev Espan Enferm Dig* 2006; 98(6): 449–459.
77 Dukas L, Willett WC, Giovannucci EL. Association between physical activity, fiber intake, and other lifestyle variables and constipation in a study of women. *Am J Gastroenterol* 2003; 98(8):1790–1796.
78 Huang R, Ho S-Y, Lo W-S *et al.* Physical activity and constipation in Hong Kong adolescents. *PLos One* 2014; 9(2): e90193.
79 Paw MJMCA, van Poppel MNM, van Mechelen W. Effects of resistance and functional-skills training on habitual activity and constipation among older adults living in long-term care facilities: a randomized controlled trial. *BMC Geriatrics* 2006; 6: 9.
80 Sandler RS, Jordan MC, Shelton BJ. Demographic and dietary determinants of constipation in the US population. *Am J Publ Health* 1990; 80: 185–189.
81 Simmons SF, Schnelle JF. Effects of an exercise and scheduled-toileting intervention on appetite and constipation in nursing home residents. *J Nutr Health Aging* 2004; 8(2): 116–121.
82 Tuteja AK, Talley NJ, Joos SK *et al.* Is constipation associated with decreased physical activity in normally active subjects? *Am J Gastroenterol* 2005; 100: 124–129.
83 Scobie BA. Athletes' diarhoea. *NZ J Sports Med* 1970; 6: 31.
84 Fogoros N. "Runner's trots" Gastrointestinal disturbances in runners. *JAMA* 1980; 243: 1743–1744.
85 *The Scotsman.* Relief all round after Paula pauses on road to glory. 18 April 2005; www.scotsman.com/news/uk/relief-all-round-after-paula-pauses-on-road-to-glory-1-708248.
86 Patton-Carson L. It happened to me: I pooped myself running a marathon 13 February 2014; www.xojane.com/it-happened-to-me/runners-diarrhea.
87 Lewis SJ, Heaton KW. Stool form scale as a useful guide to intestinal transit time. *Scand J Gastroenterol* 1997; 32(9): 920–924.
88 Triezenberg D, Simons SM. Runner's diarrhea. In: Guandalini S, Vaziri H, (eds). *Diarrhea: Diagnostic and therapeutic advances.* New York, NY: Springer, 2010, pp. 425–430.
89 Halvorsen FA, Lyng J, Glomsaker T *et al.* Gastro-intestinal disturbances in marathon runners. *Br J Sports Med* 1990; 24: 266–268.
90 Kehl O, Jäger K, Münch R *et al.* Mesenteriale Ischamie als Ursache der Jogging-Anamie? [Mesenteric anemia as a cause of jogging anemia?]. *Schweiz Med Wochenschr* 1986; 116(29): 974–976.
91 McCabe ME, Peura DA, Kadakia SC *et al.* Gastrointestinal blood loss associated with running a marathon. *Dig Dis Sci* 1986; 31(11): 1229–1232.

92   Peters HP, Bos M, Seebregts L *et al.* Gastrointestinal symptoms in long-distance runners, cyclists and triathletes: prevalence, medication and etiology. *Am J Gastroenterol* 1999; 94: 1570–1581.

93   Priebe M, Priebe J. Runners diarrhea – prevalence and clinical symptomatology. *Am J Gastroenterol* 1984; 73: 872–878.

94   Rehrer NJ, Brouns F, Beckers EJ *et al.* Physiological changes and gastro-intestinal symptoms as a result of ultra-endurance running. *Eur J Appl Physiol* 1992; 64: 1–8.

95   Rehrer NJ, Kemenade MC, Meester TA *et al.* Nutrition in relation to GI-complaints in athletes. *Med Sci Sports Exerc* 1990; 22(2): S107.

96   Riddoch C, Trinick T. Gastrointestinal disturbances in marathon runners. *Br J Sports Med* 1988; 22(2): 71–74.

97   Sullivan SN. The gastrointestinal symptoms of running. *N Engl J Med* 1981; 30/4(15): 915 (letter).

98   Sullivan SN, Wong C. Runners' diarrhea. Different patterns and associated factors. *J Clin Gastroenterol* 1992; 14: 101–104.

99   Ter Steege RWF, Van der Palen J, Kolkman JJ. Prevalence of gastrointestinal complaints in runners competing in a long-distance run: An internet-based observational study in 1281 subjects. *Scand J Gastroenterol* 2008; 43: 1477–1482.

100 Worme JD, Doubt TJ, Singh A *et al.* Dietary patterns, gastrointestinal complaints and nutritional knowledge of recreational triathletes. *Am J Clin Nutr* 1990; 51: 690–697.

101 Worobetz LJ, Gerrard DF. Gastrointestinal symptoms during exercise and endurance athletes: prevalence and speculations of the etiology. *NZ Med J* 1985; 98: 644–646.

102 Brouns F. Etiology of gastrointestinal disturbances during endurance events. *Scand J Med Sci Sports* 1991; 1: 66–77.

103 Peters HP, Van Schelven FW, Verstappen PA *et al.* Gastrointestinal problems as a function of carbohydrate supplements and mode of exercise. *Med Sci Sports Exerc* 1993; 25(11): 1211–1224.

104 de Oliveira EP, Burini RC. The impact of physical exercise on the gastrointestinal tract. *Curr Opin Clin Nutr Metab Care* 2009; 12: 533–538.

105 Strauss RH, Lanese RR, Leizman DJ. Illness and absence among wrestlers, swimmers, and gymnasts at a large university. *Am J Sports Med* 1988; 16(6): 653–655.

106 Wilhite J, Mellion MB. Occult gastrointestinal bleeding in endurance cyclists. *Phys Sportsmed* 1990; 18(8): 75–78.

107 Sullivan SN, Wong C, Heidenheim P. Does running cause gastrointestinal symptoms? A survey of 93 randomly selected runners compared with controls. *NZ Med J* 1994; 10: 328.

108 Lanham-New S, Stear S, Shireffs S *et al.* Sport and exercise nutrition. Chichester, UK: Wiley/Blackwell, 2011.

109 Hoyt CJ. Diarrhoea from vitamin C. *JAMA* 1980; 244: 1674.

110 Putukian M. Don't miss gastrointestinal disorders in athletes. *Phys Sportsmed* 1997; 25(11): 80–94.

111 Williams JH, Mager M, Jacobson ED. Relationship of mesenteric blood flow to intestinal absorption of carbohydrates. *J Lab Clin Med* 1964; 63: 853–862.

112 Moses FM. Exercise-associated intestinal ischemia. *Curr Sports Med Rep* 2005; 4: 91–95.

113 Peters HPF, De Vries WR, Vanberge-Henegouwen GP *et al.* Potential benefits and hazards of physical activity and exercise on the gastrointestinal tract. *Gut* 2001; 48: 435–439.

114 Fahrenkrug J, Haglund U, Jodal M *et al.* Nervous release of VIP in the gastrointestinal tract of the cats: possible physiological implications. *J Physiol* 1978; 284: 291–305.

115 Hubel KA. Intestinal nerves and ion transport: stimuli, reflexes and responses. *Am J Physiol* 1985; 248: G261–G271.

116 Hossdorf T, Burger M, Karoff C *et al.* Radioimmunoassay for vasoactive intestinal polypeptide (VIP) in plasma before and during endoscopic examinations. *Hepatogastroenterol* 1982; 29(4): 146–150.

117 Ho GWK. Lower gastrointestinal distress in endurance athletes. *Curr Sports Med Rep* 2009; 8(2): 85–91.

118 Shephard RJ. Medical surveillance of endurance sport. In: Shephard RJ, Åstrand P-O (eds). *Endurance in Sport*, 2nd ed. Oxford, UK: Blackwell Scientific, 2000, pp. 653–666.

119 Tillett E, Loosemore M. Setting standards for the prevention and management of travellers' diarrhoea in elite athletes: an audit of one team during the Youth Commonwealth Games in India. *Br J Sports Med* 2009; 43(13): 1045–1048.

120 DuPont HL, Ericsson CD, Farthing MJ *et al.* Expert review of the evidence base for prevention of travelers' diarrhea. *J Travel Med* 2009; 16(3): 149–160.

121 Karageanes SJ. Gastrointestinal infections in the athlete. *Clin Sports Med* 2007; 26: 443–448.

122 van Asperen IA, Medema G, Borgdorff MW *et al.* Risk of gastroenteritis among triathletes in relation to faecal pollution of fresh waters. *Int J Epidemiol* 1998; 27(2): 309–315.

123 Weber CJ. Update on recreational water illnesses. *Urol Nurs* 2005; 25(4): 289–290.

124 Mexia R, Vold L, Heier BT *et al.* Gastrointestinal disease outbreaks in cycling events: are preventive measures effective? *Epidemiol Infect* 2013; 141(3): 517–523.

125 Griffiths SL, Salmon RL, Mason BW *et al.* Using the internet for rapid investigation of an outbreak of diarrhoeal illness in mountain bikers. *Epidemiol Infect* 2010; 138(12): 1704–1711.

126 Stuart T, Sandhu J, Stirling R *et al.* Campylobacteriosis outbreak associated with ingestion of mud during a mountain bike race. *Epidemiol Infect* 2010; 138(12): 1695–1703.

127 Bounos G, McArdle AH. Marathon runners: The intestinal handicap. *Med Hypotheses* 1990; 33: 261–264.

128 Murray R. Training the gut for competition. *Curr Sports Med Rep* 2006; 5: 161–164.

129 Butcher JD. Runner's diarrhea and other intestinal problems of athletes. *Am Fam Physician* 1993; 48(4): 623–627.

130 Ersin S, Tuncyurek P, Esassolak M *et al.* The prophylactic and therapeutic effects of glutamine- and arginine-enriched diets on radiation-induced enteritis in rats. *J Surg Res* 2000; 89: 121–125.

131 Lange AP, Secher NJ, Amery W. Prostaglandin-induced diarrhoea treated with loperamide or diphenoxylate: a double-blind study. *Acta Med Scand* 1977; 202(6): 449–454.

132 Baska RS, Moses FM, Deuster PA. Cimetidine reduces running-associated gastrointestinal bleeding. A prospective observation. *Dig Dis Sci* 1990; 35(8): 956–960.

133 Thompson PD, Funk EJ, Carleton RA *et al.* Incidence of death during jogging in Rhode Island from 1975 to 1980. *JAMA* 1982; 247: 2535–2538.

134 Rowell LB. *Human circulation: Regulation during physical stress.* New York, NY, Oxford University Press, 1986.

135 Busse M, Nordhusen D, Tegtbur U *et al.* Sorbitol clearance during exercise as a measure of hepatic and renal blood flow. *Clin Sportmed Internat* 2003; 1: 1–8.

136 Kemme MJ, Burggraaf J, Schoemaker RC *et al.* The influence of reduced liver blood flow on the pharmacokinetics and pharmacodynamics of recombinant tissue factor pathway inhibitor. *Clin Pharmacol Ther* 2000; 67: 504–511.

137 de Oliveira EP, Burini RC. Food-dependent exercise-induced gastrointestinal distress. *J Int Soc Sports Nutr* 2011; 8: 12.

138 Schoemaker RC, Burggraaf J, Cohen AF. Assessment of hepatic blood flow using continuous infusion of high clearance drugs. *Br J Clin Pharmacol* 1998; 45: 463–469.

139 Perko MJ, Nielsen HB, Skak C *et al.* Mesenteric, coeliac and splanchnic blood flow in humans during exercise. *J Physiol* 1998; 513(3): 907–913.

140 Otte JA, Oostveen E, Geelkerken RH *et al.* Exercise induces gastric ischemia in healthy volunteers: a tonometry study. *J Appl Physiol* 2001; 91: 866–871.

141 Derikx JP, Poeze M, van Bijnen AA *et al.* Evidence for intestinal epithelial and liver cell injury in the early phase of sepsis. *Shock* 2007; 18: 544–548.

142 van Wijck K, Lenaerts K, van Loon LJ *et al.* Exercise-induced splanchnic hypoperfusion results in gut dysfunction in healthy men. *PLosOne* 2011; 6: e22366.

143 Moore G, Holbein ME, Knochel JP. Exercise-associated collapse in cyclists is unrelated to endotoxemia. *Med Sci Sports Exerc* 1995; 27: 1238–1242.

144 Brock-Utne JG, Gaffin SL, Wells MT *et al.* Endotoxaemia in exhausted runners after a long-distance race. *S Afr Med J* 1988; 73(9): 533–536.

145 Bosenberg AT, Brock-Utne JG, Gaffin SL *et al.* Strenuous exercise causes systemic endotoxaemia. *J Appl Physiol* 1988; 65: 106–108.

146 Hurren NM, Balanos GM, Blannin AK. Is the beneficial effect of prior exercise on postprandial lipaemia partly due to redistribution of blood flow? *Clin Sci* 2011; 120: 537–548.

147 Baska RS, Moses FM, Graeber G *et al.* Gastrointestinal bleeding during an ultramarathon. *Dig Dis Sci* 1990; 35: 276–279.

148 Porter AMW. Do some marathon runners bleed into the gut? *Br Med J* 1983; 287: 1427.

149 Halvorsen FA, Lyng J, Ritland S. Gastrointestinal bleeding in marathon runners. *Scand J Gastroenterol* 1986; 21: 493–497.

150 McMahon LF, Ryan MJ, Larson DL *et al.* Occult gastrointestinal blood loss in marathon runners. *Ann Intern Med* 1984; 100: 846–847.

151 Moses FM, Baska RS, Peura DA *et al.* Effect of cimetidine on marathon-associated gastrointestinal symptoms and bleeding. *Dig Dis Sci* 1991; 36(10): 1390–1394.

152 Robertson JD, Maughan RJ, Davidson RJ. Faecal blood loss in response to exercise. *Br Med J* 1987; 295: 303–305.

153 Schwartz AE, Vanagunas A, Kamel PL. Endoscopy to evaluate gastrointestinal bleeding in marathon runners. *Ann Intern Med* 1990; 113: 632–633.

154 Stewart JG, Ahlquist DA, McGill DB *et al.* Gastrointestinal blood loss and anaemia in runners. *Ann Intern Med* 1984; 100: 843–845.

155 Beaumont AC, Teare JP. Subtotal colectomy following marathon running in a female patient. *J R Soc Med* 1991; 84: 439–440.

156 Cantwell JD. Gastrointestinal disorders of runners. *JAMA* 1981; 246(13): 1404–1405.

157 Cohen DC, Winstanley A, Engledow A, Windsor AC, Skipworth JR. Marathon induced ischemic colitis: why running is not always good for you. *Am J Emerg Med* 2009; 27(2): 255, e5–e7.

158 Fisher RL, McMahon LF, Ryan MJ *et al.* Gastrointestinal bleeding in competitive runners. *Dig Dis Sci* 1986; 31: 1226–1228.

159 Kyriakos R, Siewert B, Kato E *et al.* CT findings in runners' colitis. *Abdom Imaging* 2006; 31: 54–56.

160 Lucas W, Schroy PC. Reversible ischemic colitis in a high endurance athlete. *Am J Gastroeneterol* 1998; 93(11): 2231–2234.

161 Moses FM, Brewer TG, Peura DA. Running associated proximal hemorrhagic colitis. *Ann Intern Med* 1988; 108: 385–386.

162 Sanchez LD, Tracy JA, Berkhoff D *et al.* Ischemic colitis in marathon runners: A case-based review. *J Emerg Med* 200; 30(3): 321–326.

163 Wiesner W, Khurana B, Ji H *et al.* CT of acute bowel ischemia. *Radiology* 2003; 226: 635–650.

164 Dodds W. Subtotal colectomy following marathon running in a female patient. *J R Soc Med* 1992; 85: 304–305.

165 Chatard JC, Mujika I, Guy C *et al.* Anaemia and iron deficiency in athletes. Practical recommendations for treatment. *Sports Med* 1999; 27(4): 229–240.

7 Physical activity, chronic intestinal inflammation and coeliac disease

Introduction

The broad diagnosis of chronic inflammatory bowel disease (CIBD) includes individuals with both ulcerative colitis (UC) and Crohn's disease (CD). Together, these two conditions affect about 0.25% of the North American population, with a substantial direct economic cost (for example, an estimated $1.2 billion/year in Canada[1]). However, causes of the chronic inflammation are poorly understood; possibly, problems are related to inappropriately modulated immune responses.[2] Ulcerative colitis is a localized inflammation of the intestines, but Crohn's disease (CD) can also affect the mouth, oesophagus, stomach and anus.[3] Genetic predisposing factors apparently differ for the two conditions.[4] With appropriate management, the overall mortality for UC is close to population norms,[5] but the global mortality from CIBD remains a substantial 0.8/100,000.[6] Moreover, CIBD is a significant risk factor for the development of colonic cancer,[7,8] reducing the age at which this type of neoplasm develops.[9]

The normal functioning of the intestines is seriously disrupted by the various manifestations of chronic inflammatory bowel disease, including UC and CD. Given a limited understanding of causation, much of the treatment of CIBD is empirical, and health professionals often fail to consider the potential benefits of augmenting what are typically low levels of habitual physical activity. This chapter thus begins by documenting current patterns of habitual physical activity in CIBD, and assesses the impact of limited activity upon functional capacity. It then examines the safety and practicality of programmes designed to correct loss of function, and notes the potential role of regular physical activity in the prevention and treatment of CIBD. It concludes with a brief commentary on the role of physical activity in the management of patients with coeliac disease.

Habitual physical activity and functional status in CIBD

Current habitual activity

The level of habitual physical activity typical of individuals with CIBD has been assessed using occupational categorization, by the completion of interviews or physical activity questionnaires, and occasionally by the wearing of objective physical activity monitors such as accelerometers (see Table 7.1). Twelve of the 16 studies cited found lower levels of physical activity in patients with CIBD than in controls. With one exception,[13] differences were generally more marked for those with CD than for those with UC.[14,17,19] In the one study where the physical activity was similar to that of controls, the patients were children, and more had UC than CD.[12] In a second study, individuals with medical or psychiatric abnormalities were excluded, and despite similar accelerometer readings, muscle fatigue was greater in CD than in control subjects.[22] A third negative report[12] included more cases with UC than with CD, and diagnostic criteria were not standardized. In the fourth negative study,[21] although similar proportions of patients and controls reported high, moderate or low levels of physical activity, 23% of those with CD reported greater fatigue than controls, and 21% noted a reduction of leisure activities with CD.

It could be argued that in some patients, activity-induced diarrhoea or a substantial ileostomy made exercise a difficult undertaking,[26] accounting for low levels of physical activity. However, other surveys were conducted when patients were in remission,[24] and in at least one report[15] a lack of physical activity preceded development of the clinical illness.

Current functional capacity

As might be anticipated from the low levels of habitual physical activity, the functional capacity of those with CD is commonly impaired relative to age and sex matched controls or population norms (see Table 7.2), with an associated accumulation of body fat and a deterioration of bone health.

Aerobic capacity in CIBD has been reported by four groups of investigators. In two of the four studies[18,26] patients had received surgical treatment and one group was in remission.[2,27] Conclusions are based variously upon peak cycle ergometer or treadmill performance, gait speed measurements, and patient perceptions of reduced aerobic function, but all four studies agree in reporting some loss of aerobic function. Brevinge *et al.*[26] argued that impairment was limited in cases who had not undergone surgery, but that functional limitation increased progressively in relation to the extent of any intestinal resection that had been undertaken; this could, of course be simply a reflection of disease severity. Moreover, functional losses were greater than might have been predicted from the decrease of lean tissue,[26] possibly reflecting problems in the absorption of food, electrolyte imbalance and altered metabolism. Zaltman *et al.*[25] further commented that the extent of losses in aerobic function and grip strength was inversely related to habitual physical activity.

Lean tissue mass has been measured quite frequently in CIBD, usually by computed tomography or by bio-impedance techniques (see Table 7.2). In 13 out of 18 studies, values were lower than in controls, although (since the loss of lean tissue is greater in CD than in UC[34]), the average effect in individual studies was influenced by the relative proportions of UC and CD in the samples that were tested. As might be anticipated, a low lean tissue mass was often associated with a low level of habitual physical activity.[23,25,38]

Table 7.1 Current physical activity in patients with chronic inflammatory bowel disease

Author	Subjects	Activity determination	Findings	Comments
Boggild et al.[10]	Danes aged 20–59 yrs; analysis of 6296 first hospital admissions for CIBD	Physical activity at work, based on extended International Standard Classification of Occupations	Sedentary work increased risk of hospitalization from CIBD	All cases in Danish population register first admitted to hospital with CIBD
Boot et al.[11]	Children, 22 CD, 33 UC, unspecified controls	Interview	Mean physical activity not significantly less than in controls	Diagnoses made using Dutch consensus guidelines
Chan et al.[12]	177 cases of incident UC, 75 cases of incident CD among 300,724 participants in cancer survey	Questionnaire (5-level classification)	Reported physical activity of affected individuals developing UC or CD did not differ relative to 4 matched controls per case	Methods of case identification varied from one centre to another
Cucino and Sonnenberg[13]	2399 deaths from CD, 2419 deaths from UC as reported to U.S. National Center for Health Statistics, 1991–1996	U.S. Vital Statistics on occupational activity, expressed as proportional mortality ratios	Low risk in farmers, miners and labourers, high risk in sales persons and secretaries	Effects appear similar for UC and CD
Hlavaty et al.[14]	190 cases of CD, 148 cases of UC, 355 controls (case-control study); diagnosis based on clinical, endoscopic, radiologic and histological criteria	44-item questionnaire included question on sporting activities	Association of CIBD with <2 sporting activities/wk as a child (odds ratios 2.7 for CD, 2.0 for UC)	CD also associated with smoking
Klein et al.[15]	55 recent-onset cases of UC, 33 cases of CD referred by regional gastroenterologists, matched controls (76 orthopaedic clinic, 68 general population)	Questionnaire included item on time spent in various levels of physical activity	Physical activity of patients low, spent less time than controls in strenuous activity	Low activity level present before onset of clinical disease

Study	Sample	Method		
Lustyk et al.[16]	54 women (29 diagnosed, 25 suspected CIBD based on Rome criteria), 35 controls free of GI symptoms	1-month diary covering housework, mild, moderate and strenuous activity and 1-month symptom diary	CIBD group less active than controls, difference persisted when controlled for educational level	Among patients, symptoms (especially fatigue) inversely related to habitual physical activity
Mack et al.[17]	637 cases of self-reported UC, 474 CD, 113,685 control participants in Canadian Health Measures Survey	Questionnaire on health and time spent on 21 activities in previous 3 months	In CD, odds ratios to be classed as inactive (1.34) and active (0.69); similar but smaller effects and n.s. trends for UC	Most people with CD or UC did not meet public health guidelines for physical activity
Ojerskog et al.[18]	29 cases of UC, 1 case of CD, 1 case of familial polyposis before and after conversion to continent ileostomy	Interview by psychiatrist before and after conversion; leisure activity 1 of 11 topics	Hindrance of sport and bathing reported in 19/31 with traditional ileostomy, 4/30 with continent ileostomy	60% reported facilitation of leisure activities
Persson et al.[19]	152 cases CD, 145 cases UC (all new cases hospitalized in Stockholm county, Leonard-Jones score), random population sample of 305 controls	Postal questionnaire; single question on physical activity, 5 yrs ago and current	Relative risks with weekly and daily exercise: CD 0.6, 0.5, n.s. benefit in UC (RR 0.9)	"regular participation in any recreational, leisure or sports activity (e.g. long walks)"
Sonnenberg[20]	12,014 patients granted rehabilitation for CIBD (ICD classifications 555 and 556)	Occupation determined from 2-digit occupational code	Occupations involving physical exercise and work in open air have lower risk of CD and UC	Risk of CIBD also increased by irregular hours and shift work
Sorensen et al.[21]	106 cases of CD (adults, >1 yr duration), 75 age and sex matched previously healthy acute hospital admissions with illness of <28 days duration	Interview by principal investigator, 3-level classification of physical activity	Similar proportions of two groups classed as high, moderate or low physical activity	CD group had slightly higher SES than controls. Note: 23% of those with CD reported greater fatigue, and 21% noted reduced leisure activities

continued

Table 7.1 Continued

Author	Subjects	Activity determination	Findings	Comments
van Langenberg et al.[22]	27 cases of CD at CIBD clinic, 27 controls	Tri-axial accelerometer worn at waist for 7 days	Habitual physical activity similar in CD and controls	CD group had greater fatigue; those with medical or psychiatric co-morbidities excluded
Werkstetter et al.[23]	26 IBD in remission, 13 IBD mildly active (27 CD, 12 UC), 39 age and sex matched adolescent controls	Sense-wear arm band physical activity monitor	Trend to shorter duration of physical activity (0.44 h/d less activity >3 METs) and lower step count (−1339/day) in CD	Lean body mass also reduced in patients
Wiroth et al.[24]	41 adult cases of CD in remission (CD activity index <150) 26 healthy controls	Activity questionnaire (occupation, sport and leisure) and 7-day accelerometer record	Neither method showed difference of physical activity between 2 groups, but decreased sport index in CD	Strength of CD group lower than that of controls
Zaltman et al.[25]	23 women with UC, 23 age and BMI matched controls	Baecke physical activity questionnaire (score 3–15)	Physical activity 30% lower in patients with UC	Loss of lower limb strength and mobility associated with low level of physical activity

Abbreviations: CD = Crohn's disease; CIBD = chronic inflammatory bowel disease; ICD = international classification of diseases; METs = metabolic equivalents; n.s. = non-significant; SES = socio-economic status; UC = ulcerative colitis.

Table 7.2 Current aerobic capacity, lean tissue mass and muscle function in patients with CIBD

Author	Subjects	Measurement techniques	Findings	Comments
Aerobic capacity				
Brevinge et al.[26]	29 CD patients following proto-colectomy and 23 matched reference individuals	Supine cycle ergometry to voluntary exhaustion, questionnaire appraisal of perceived aerobic fitness	Maximal cycle ergometer loading reduced by 9% if no resection, rising to loss of 40% if extensive bowel resection	Loss of aerobic power greater than loss of lean tissue; patients unaware of loss of aerobic power unless extensive resection
D'Incà et al.[27]	6 cases of CD, 6 controls	Treadmill	Lower maximal oxygen intake in CD	
Ojerskog et al.[18]	29 UC, 1 CD, 1 familial polyposis before and after construction of continent ileostomy	Interview by psychiatrist	6/31 had reduction of working capacity with conventional ileostomy	13/27 had greater working capacity after continent ileostomy – fewer toilet visits, able to dress more freely
Zaltman et al.[25]	23 women with UC, 23 matched controls	4-metre gait speed	UC 17% slower gait than controls	Habitual physical activity and greater grip strength protect against slowing of gait
Lean tissue mass				
Bechtold et al.[28]	143 adolescent cases of CIBD (45 UC, 98 CD; ESPGHAN criteria), compared to anthropometry z-scores	Anthropometry and quantitated computed tomography and DXA	Mean muscle cross-sectional area significantly reduced in CIBD ($z=-1.1$)	Overall stunting of growth. Reduced bone cross-section linked to reduced muscle mass; history of steroids n.s. effect on muscle cross-section
Boot et al.[11]	Children, 22 CD, 33 UC, unspecified controls	Dual energy X-ray absorption and bio-impedance	Lean tissue mass lower than controls, CD > UC	35/55 cases had received steroid treatment, with negative effect on bone density

continued

Table 7.2 Continued

Author	Subjects	Measurement techniques	Findings	Comments
Brevinge et al.[26]	29 CD patients 1 yr or more after proto-colectomy and 23 matched reference individuals	Isotopic determinations of body water, body potassium and body nitrogen	Reduced lean tissue mass accounted for 74% of variation in maximal cycle ergometer loading	Total body N_2 shows 0.76 correlation with arm muscle circumference
Bryant et al.[29]	137 20–50-yr-old patients with CIBD (95 CD), 57% with active disease	Dual energy X-ray absorptiometry	21% of patients had lean body mass >1SD below population norms	59% of those with low lean mass also had low grip strength; odds ratio of sarcopaenia 2.03 if >12 months steroids
Capristo et al.[30]	18 cases of CD, 16 cases of UC, all in remission, 20 healthy volunteers	Bio-impedance	Fat-free mass tended to be lower in CD (n.s.)	Fat mass lower in CD than in UC and controls; no patients receiving steroids
Dubner et al.[31]	78 cases of incident CD in children	Quantitative computed tomography	Low initial muscle cross-sectional areas (z score=−0.96) improved over 12 months treatment	Low muscle values associated with impaired bone mineral density
Filippi et al.[32]	26 M, 28 F cases of CD in remission for >3 months, aged 18–70 yrs; 25 healthy controls	Anthropometry and bio-impedance	Fat-free mass did not differ significantly from controls	30% of patients malnourished, all receiving 5-ASA maintenance treatment
Geerling et al.[33]	18 F, 14 M with CD (long-standing disease but in remission (Van Hees Index 146). 32 healthy controls	Dual energy X-ray absorptiometry	No difference of lean tissue mass	Hamstring strength less than in controls, quadriceps strength preserved
Jahnsen et al.[34]	60 cases CD, 60 healthy controls; small bowel resection in 27 cases with CD	Dual energy X-ray absorptiometry	Lean body mass lower in CD than in UC or controls	Bone mineral content also reduced in CD; loss of LBM only in 43 cases treated with steroids
Sylvester et al.[35]	42 children with CD (exclusions – prior corticosteroid treatment or presence of other inflammatory conditions)	Dual energy X-ray absorptiometry	Low fat-free mass persisted over 2-yr follow-up when 27/42 received steroid treatment	Improvements of bone mineral composition associated with gains in fat-free mass.

Reference	Sample	Method	Measure	Findings
Tjellesen et al.[36]	13 M, 18F adults with long-standing CD compared to population norms; all in remission and none had received corticosteroids for 2 years	Dual energy X-ray absorptiometry	Z score for muscle mass −1.74. Muscle mass not significantly correlated with energy intake or small intestinal resection	Fat mass increased as % of body mass
Valentini et al.[37]	94 adult cases CD, 50 cases UC, all in remission (12/94, 8/50 on corticosteroids); 61 healthy controls	Anthropometry, bio-impedance	Low body cell mass in M and F; decrease of LBM in males only. In women, prolonged corticosteroids associated with low LBM	Associated decrease of grip strength
van Langenberg et al.[38]	27 adult cases of CD (2/27 on corticosteroids, 9/27 bowel resection), 22 controls	Quantitative computed tomography	Quadriceps cross-section reduced 14% in CD	Muscle loss associated with lower physical activity and reduced capacity to activate protein synthesis
Werkstetter et al.[39]	82 children with CD, 20 with UC	Quantitative computed tomography	Initial z score for muscle cross-sectional area −1.0	Treatment with 5-ASA, glucocorticoids and TNF-α antibodies increased muscle cross-sectional area
Werkstetter et al.[23]	27 children with CD, 12 with UC, in remission for >4 weeks	Bio-impedance	Reduced z-score for muscle mass even during remission	Associated low habitual physical activity scores
Wiroth et al.[24]	41 adult cases of CD in remission for >3 months, 25 controls	Bio-impedance	No difference in fat-free mass with CD	Lower limb endurance improved by recent use of steroids
Wiskin et al.[40]	55 adolescent children with IBD (37 CD, 18 UC; 22 had active disease)	Anthropometric estimate of fat-free mass	Fat-free mass inversely related to disease activity in CD; numbers insufficient to analyse in UC	Children had significant growth deficits; unclear whether active disease or growth deficit contributed to deficit of FFM
Zaltman et al.[25]	23 women with UC (15/23 active disease), 23 matched controls. Corticoid treatment in 9/23	Anthropometry and bio-impedance	No significant difference of lean tissue mass in UC	Associated low levels of habitual physical activity

continued

Table 7.2 Continued

Author	Subjects	Measurement techniques	Findings	Comments
Muscle function				
Bryant et al.[29]	137 20–50-year-old patients with CIBD (95 CD), 57% with active disease	Handgrip dynamometer	59% of patients with low lean body mass had grip strength >1SD below population norms	Odds ratio of sarcopaenia 2.03 if >12 months steroids
Geerling et al.[33,41]	18 F, 14 M with CD (long-standing disease but in remission)	Upper leg circumference, isokinetic dynamometer	Quadriceps strength normal, reduced hamstring strength	Hamstring strength correlated with fat-free mass only in controls
Valentini et al.[37]	94 adult cases CD, 50 cases UC, all in remission (12/94, 8/50 on corticosteroids), 61 healthy controls	Handgrip dynamometer	Handgrip decreased 9% in CD, 14% in UC (no sex difference)	Associated with loss of lean tissue mass, but decrease of LBM in males only
van Langenberg et al.[22]	27 adult cases of CD (2/27 on corticosteroids, 9/27 bowel resection), 22 controls	Isokinetic dynamometer	CD show greater fatigue over 30 successive isokinetic contractions of quadriceps	Findings correlated with self-reported fatigue; associated with low Mg, low Vit. D3, low IGF-1 and high IL-6
Werkstetter et al.[23]	27 children with CD, 12 with UC, in remission for >4 weeks, 39 age and sex-matched controls	Handgrip dynamometer	Z score for grip strength –1.02	Related to lower habitual physical activity and reduced LBM; LBM reduced even during remission
Wiroth et al.[24]	41 adult cases of CD in remission for >3 months, 25 controls	Lower limb extensor strength, leg endurance and sit-up tests	Scores 24–26% lower in CD	Strength not related to measures of habitual physical activity, LBM also had normalized
Zaltman et al.[25]	23 women with UC (15/23 active disease), 23 matched controls. Corticoid treatment in 9/23	Quadriceps and grip strength, timed sit-up	Quadriceps strength –6%, sit-up speed –32%, handgrip force normal	Strength loss associated with reduced habitual physical activity

Abbreviations: ASA = acetylsalicylic acid; CD = Crohn's disease; CIBD = chronic inflammatory bowel disease; FFM = fat-free mass; IBD = inflammatory bowel disease; IGF = insulin-like growth factor; IL–6 = interleukin 6; LBM = lean body mass; n.s. = non-significant; TNF-α = tumour necrosis factor alpha; UC = ulcerative colitis.

Although the adverse effects of CD can persist for several years,[23,35,36] four of the five studies reporting a normal lean tissue mass were of patients in remission,[24,30,32,33] and one concerned only women with UC.[25] In two of the five trials, despite a normal lean tissue mass, leg-muscle strength was nevertheless lower than that of controls.[24,33] Correlates of the low lean tissue have included disease activity,[40] a low serum albumin,[28] and prolonged steroid treatment.[34,37] Although no differences of muscle cross-sectional area were seen with the steroid treatment of adolescents,[28] and others saw an actual improvement of muscle dimensions during treatment that included the administration of glucocorticoids,[24,31] Bryant et al.[29] found a 2.03 odds ratio for finding a diagnosis of sarcopaenia in older patients who had received more than 12 months of steroid treatment.

Seven groups of investigators who looked at various aspects of muscle function in patients with CD (see Table 7.2) all found some decrease of muscular strength that persisted during periods of disease remission.[33,41] The strength impairment correlated with self-reported fatigue,[22] and in some[23,37] but not all reports[24] was correlated with a low lean tissue mass. Associated changes included a low thickness of cortical bone and a reduced trabecular bone density.[31,39] As many as 60% of patients with Crohn's disease were sarcopaenic, 30–40% developed osteopaenia, and 15% showed osteoporosis, with a doubling in the risk of fractures.[11,42–44] In 143 cases studied by Bechtold et al.,[28] the bone disease was thought secondary to muscle wasting, but other possible factors weakening bone structure are the inflammatory process itself, poor nutrient absorption, the sustained use of corticosteroids, and a low level of habitual physical activity. One study of 120 patients found no significant relationship between a self-reported 7-level classification of habitual physical activity and bone density,[45] but critics of this report have commented that this investigation did not classify physical activity in terms of the impact stimulus that it delivered to the bones.

Physical activity in the prevention of CIBD

The muscle and bone parameters of patients with CIBD are generally enhanced by an increase of habitual physical activity, although it is less clear whether physical activity is directly strengthening muscle and bone or whether benefits stem from associated improvements in nutrition, reduced levels of pro-inflammatory cytokines, and decreases in corticosteroid treatment. Regular physical activity might prevent the development of CIBD by increasing the production of the muscle-derived anti-inflammatory myokine interleukin (IL)-6[46,47] and heat-shock proteins,[48] while inhibiting the release of pro-inflammatory mediators from visceral fat.

Three of four published studies[12,15,19,20] have shown an association between regular physical activity and a reduced risk of developing CIBD, although leaving unanswered which was cause and which effect. Klein et al.[15] found a low-level of prior physical activity in recent onset cases (53 UC and 33 CD). The Nurses Health Study[61] identified 284 cases of CD and 363 cases of UC. The risk of developing CD was 0.64 among the most active quintile relative to those who were the least active, and this difference of disease prevalence persisted after adjusting for differences in smoking habits and body mass index. However, in this study the risk of developing UC was unrelated to habitual physical activity. In a sample of 12,014 Germans, Sonnenberg[20] noted a low prevalence of CIBD among those who worked vigorously in the open air (although conceivably the onset of CIBD could already have caused some of the sample to change to physically less demanding indoor work). Persson and colleagues[19] compared 145 cases of UC with 305 controls; in this study, the risk of UC was inversely related to reported physical activity (risk ratios of 0.6 and 0.5 for those reporting weekly and daily exercise), although again the onset of UC could have modified subsequent patterns of physical activity. Finally, a study of 177 incident cases of UC and 67 cases of CD saw no associations with a 5-level questionnaire assessment of habitual physical activity, even after adjusting data for inter-individual differences of BMI, total energy intake and smoking habits.[12]

Acute response to physical activity in CIBD

Perhaps because of low habitual physical activity levels, adolescents with CD metabolize less fat than healthy individuals when exercising at any given fraction of their maximal oxygen intake,[62] but they show few other adverse responses to moderate aerobic exercise.

D'Incà et al.[27] had six cases of CD who were currently in remission undertake one hour of treadmill exercise at 60% of their maximal oxygen intake. This caused no passing of faecal blood, no increase in stool frequency, no change in intestinal permeability and no evidence of lipid peroxidation. Moreover, any increase in oro-caecal transit time matched that seen in age-matched control subjects performing a similar amount of physical activity. In an uncontrolled study, Ploeger et al.[63] required 15 youth with CD to perform 30 minutes of cycling at a loading that demanded 50% of their peak aerobic power, and four 15-second bouts of maximal exercise. Both types of activity increased the numbers of immune cells, IL-6 and Il-17 and growth hormone (GH) concentrations and decreased levels of insulin-like growth factor (IGF)-1. The IL-6 was considered as muscle-derived and anti-inflammatory. IL-17 is not normally detectable in healthy individuals, but is possibly critical to the inflammation seen in Crohn's disease.[64]

Chronic responses to increased physical activity in CIBD

There are many potential areas where an increase of habitual physical activity might help a person with Crohn's disease,[48] including gains of nutrition, mood state, and body composition, with a reduction of disease activity, fatigue, poor performance and bone mineral loss.

Nutrition. Adolescent patients with CD often show growth retardation, with an increased resting energy expenditure and a low body mass index.[65] Potential causes of abnormal growth include a favouring of catabolism by chronic cortico-steroid administration, an inhibition of appetite by the accumulation of inflammatory cytokines, an impaired absorption of nutrients and protein loss in the diseased gut, and a diversion of food energy from normal growth to support the disease activity. Plainly, well-designed physical activity programmes could have a favourable effect upon many of these issues.

Disease activity. All of 11 human studies[49–59] (see Table 7.3) have reported reduced activity of the disease process following the introduction of exercise programmes (usually aerobic, but in one instance resistance training[49]). However, only five of these studies were controlled, and the exercise intervention was often poorly defined, sometimes including other significant modifications of life-style. Moreover, the subjects in the largest trial were patients with irritable bowel syndrome rather than CD or UC.[54] Focussing upon the four controlled trials of CIBD, it is clear that the exercise programme did not worsen the patients' condition, but on the other hand positive changes were relatively limited. There was a lessening of constipation, but not of pain or diarrhoea,[51] a reduction of disease activity on the IBDQ scale, but no decrease in plasma levels of tumour necrosis factor (TNF)- α,[52] and no change in indices of the severity of Crohn's disease despite an improved reported quality of life,[56] but improved scores on the IBDQ and Harvey Bradshaw index of disease activity.[59]

A study in a mouse model of colitis compared the effects of voluntary wheel exercise with a physical activity programme that was much more vigorous than in most human studies (the animals ran on a treadmill at speeds of 8–12 m/min for 40 minutes per day, 5 days a week for 6 weeks).[66] The moderate voluntary running alleviated the induced diarrhoea, and almost completely abolished the expression of inflammatory genes in the colonic mucosa, but in contrast the vigorous and enforced treadmill running worsened diarrhoea, led to expression of inflammatory genes (IL-6, IL-1-β and IL-17) in the colon and increased mortality. It was suggested that vigorous exercise increased bacterial penetration of the gut wall, and thus the tendency to inflammation and death.

Quality of life. Patients with IBD commonly,[23] but not always,[24] show an initial impairment in their quality of life relative to controls. Six studies of varying quality[50,52,56–59] (see Table 7.3) have all reported an increase in the quality of life following interventions that increased habitual physical activity, with changes commonly linked to the magnitude of functional gains.

Endocrine and immune function. Many have argued that physical activity benefits patients with IBD because it suppresses pro-inflammatory factors and augments anti-inflammatory mechanisms. Although moderate physical activity could have such an effect, very vigorous activity seems likely to increase inflammation, particularly if eccentric exercise is involved.[67] Regular moderate physical activity certainly reduces levels of the pro-inflammatory agent prostaglandin E2 in the intestinal mucosa.[68] Other possible sources of benefit from regular exercise are an increased production of heat shock proteins,[69] and an autophagy of the cells responsible for inflammation.[70]

Table 7.3 Beneficial effects of regular physical activity upon activity of the disease process, quality of life and endocrine and immune responses in CIBD

Author	Subjects	Methodology	Findings	Comment
Activity of disease process				
Candow et al.[49]	12 adult cases of CD, no controls	12 wks resistance training, 3/wk, 3 sets of 8–10 reps at 60–70% 1RM, 12 exercises	Disease activity as assessed by Harley and Bradshaw scale unchanged	Increased leg press (26%) and chest press (21%)
Crumbock et al.[50]	17 adult cases of CD, no controls	Physical activity questionnaire, IBDQ scale of disease activity	No relationship of disease activity to PA, stress or QOL	Uncontrolled correlational study
Daley et al.[51]	56 cases of CIBD randomized to experimental and usual care groups	Two 40-min exercise consultations that focussed on walking over 12-week programme increased physical activity (36.7 vs 15.0 on Godin scale)	Exercise reduced constipation, but not pain or diarrhoea over 12 weeks	18.3% recruitment of patients from hospital records; effects for >12 weeks not tested
Elsenbruch et al.[52]	30 cases of UC in remission or low activity randomized to exercise and control	IBDQ scale, Moderate exercise, 1/wk for 10 wks and lifestyle intervention	Disease activity reduced on IBDQ scale, but no change in TNF-α levels	Intervention included Mediterranean diet and stress management
Fraser and Niv[53]	6 cases of CIBD, no controls	3 weeks at Dead Sea spa, IBDQ, Harvey-Bradshaw Index of disease activity	Harvey-Bradshaw Index decreased from 9.0 to 3.5 over 1 week	Hyperbaric environment, Dead Sea immersion, controlled life of spa as well as advice on greater physical activity
Johannesen et al.[54]	102 cases of IBS randomized (51 experimental, 51 control)	Physiotherapist, set target of 20–60 min of moderate to vigorous exercise 3–5 days/week, contacted patients 1–2 times/month for 12 weeks	Exercised group showed fewer symptoms on overall IBS disease severity scale (−51 vs −5)	37/51 completed exercise programme; increase in peak oxygen intake of 0.11 min
Jones et al.[55]	Prospective 6-month study, 1308 cases of CD and 540 cases of UC initially in remission	CD activity vs average reported physical activity on Godin index	Activity score > median associated with a lower risk ratio for reactivation of CD and UC (respective unadjusted RRs 0.72 and 0.78).	Benefit significant for CD, n.s. for UC

Study	Subjects	Protocol	Outcome	Comments
Klare et al.[56]	30 cases of mild to moderate CD randomized to exercise or control	Indices of CD activity (Crohn's disease Activity Index and Rachmilewitz index), 10 wks moderate supervised outdoor running 3 times/wk	No significant change of Crohn's indices relative to controls, although improved health-related quality of life	Exercisers completed 24/30 sessions
Loudon et al.[57]	12 cases of CD, no controls	HBI; 12-wk walking programme, 20–35 min sessions, 3/wk, covering average of 3.5 km per session	Lessening of disease activity (Harvey-Bradshaw Index) 5.9 vs 3.6 ($p<0.02$)	Increase of aerobic capacity as predicted by Canadian aerobic fitness stepping test
Nathan et al.[58]	10 cases of CD, 1 case UC who had self-selected exercise, no controls	Walking, 3 of 11 subjects working up a sweat	Subjective benefit, no worsening of CIBD	3 reported severe fatigue day following excessive exercise
Ng et al.[59]	32 cases of CIBD, mild disease or in remission, randomized to walking and controls	Moderate walking (30 min, 3 times/wk, for 3 months, average distance 3.1 km/session)	Exercisers improved scores on IBDQ; and index of stress. Harvey-Bradshaw Index showed significant gain in exercisers, worsening in controls	No detrimental effects of exercise noted; gains seen after 1 month of exercise
Quality of life				
Crumbock et al.[50]	17 cases of CD, no controls	Physical activity questionnaire	More active individuals showed reduced stress and enhanced quality of life	Uncontrolled correlational study
Elsenbruch et al.[52]	30 cases of UC in remission or low activity randomized to exercise and control	Moderate exercise, 1/wk for 10 wks and lifestyle intervention	Gains on mental health and psychological health axes of SF-36 questionnaire	Intervention included Mediterranean diet and stress management
Klare et al.[56]	30 cases of mild to moderate CD randomized to exercise or control	10 wks moderate supervised outdoor running 3 times/wk	Significant gain on health-related quality of life scale	No changes of body composition; exercisers completed 24/30 sessions
Loudon et al.[57]	12 cases of CD, no controls	12-wk walking programme, 20–35 min sessions, 3/wk, covering average of 3.5 km per session	Increase of physical health, well-being and quality of life on CIBD stress index and CIBD quality of life score	7 of 12 patients reported gains on stress index

continued

Table 7.3 Continued

Author	Subjects	Methodology	Findings	Comment
Nathan et al.[58]	10 cases of CD, 1 case UC who had self-selected exercise, no controls	Walking, 3 of 11 subjects working up a sweat	Various subjective benefits reported from exercise – "feeling good, fatigued but energized, helped with lethargy and tiredness"	All 11 patients believed exercise was beneficial
Ng et al.[59]	32 cases of CIBD, mild disease or in remission, randomized to walking and controls	Moderate walking (30 min, 3 times/wk, for 3 months, average distance 3.1 km/session)	Enhanced quality of life as measured by CIBD stress index and CIBD questionnaire	No detrimental effects of exercise noted; gains seen after 1 month of exercise
Endocrine and immune responses				
D'Incà et al.[2,27]	6 cases of CD, 6 controls	Treadmill exercise at 60% of maximal oxygen intake	No differences in the post-exercise polymorphonuclear respiratory burst, lipo-peroxidation or oxidant stress	
Elsenbruch et al.[52]	30 cases of UC in remission or low activity randomized to exercise and control	Moderate exercise, 1/wk for 10 wks and lifestyle intervention	No significant changes in lymphocyte sub-set numbers or production of TNF-α relative to controls	Intervention included Mediterranean diet and stress management
Koek et al.[60]	31 cases of CD, 24 cases of UC, moderate activity levels, no controls	Measurement of expired NO	NO increased in active CIBD, both CD and UC, correlated with disease activity scores	Suggests CIBD is systemic disease
van Langenberg et al.[22]	27 adult cases of CD (2/27 on corticosteroids, 9/27 bowel resection), 22 controls	Measurements made prior to exercise tests	Increased levels of TBARS and decreased levels of IGF-1	Patients show low IGF-1 and high IL-6

Abbreviations: CD = Crohn's disease; HBI = Harvey-Bradshaw Index; CIBD = chronic inflammatory bowel disease; IBDQ = inflammatory bowel disease questionnaire; IBS = irritable bowel syndrome; IGF-1 = insulin-like growth factor 1; IL-6 = interleukin 6; 1RM = 1 repetition maximum; PA = physical activity; QOL = quality of life; RR = risk ratio; TNF-α = tumour necrosis factor alpha; UC = ulcerative colitis.

In practice, most human studies[2,22,27,52,60] have shown little change of endocrine or immune function in response to exercise programmes (see Table 7.3). On the other hand, benefit has generally been demonstrated in animal models. In mice, Hoffman-Goetz *et al.*[71] found that relative to control animals, three bouts of sustained and vigorous treadmill running increased levels of the anti-inflammatory cytokine IL-10 and decreased levels of TNF-α in intestinal lymphocytes. Likewise, in rats with chemically induced colitis, wheel running decreased pro-inflammatory genes, induced anti-inflammatory mediators, and modulated activity of the enzymes peroxidase and nitric oxide synthase.[72] In rats with an acetic acid-induced colitis, 6 weeks of moderate wheel running (0.4 km/h, for 30 minutes, 3 days/wk) reduced markers of oxidative stress and histological damage to the colon; stress as assessed by scores on psychological hole-board tests was also decreased.[73] Finally, in mice where colitis had been induced by dextran sodium sulphate treatment, some benefit was seen from vigorous physical activity (treadmill running for 55 min/day on a 5% slope at 18 km/h), with decreased levels of pro-inflammatory cytokines.[74]

Experience of exercise-centred rehabilitation in CIBD

Although an increase of physical activity seems to bring a variety of practical gains under laboratory conditions, poor adherence to exercise interventions can limit the realization of these benefits in clinical practice. The health professional must thus maximize the interest of affected individuals by tactics that include a discussion of goals and objectives, development of group camaraderie, and a regular feedback of information about improvements in physical condition.[48] Initial acceptance of the illness also seems important to compliance with a rehabilitation programme.[75]

Thirteen studies have provided data on acceptance of a rehabilitation programme[12,27,45,49,51–54,56–59,63] (see Table 7.4). In general, the patient response compares quite favourably with that seen in rehabilitation programmes for other clinical conditions. Typically, three-quarters of patients complete a moderate intensity aerobic programme of three months' duration. Resistance exercise at 60% of one repetition maximum force was also well tolerated in one study.[49] The single report where many patients reported difficulty in completing the required regimen involved low impact exercises designed to enhance bone strength.[45]

Physical activity and coeliac disease

Coeliac disease is basically an autoimmune disorder with a hypersensitivity of the intestines to dietary gluten, and in general there is little reason to expect that physical activity would alter the course of this condition. Nevertheless, by encouraging a greater intake of food, physical activity may counter some of the nutritional problems that are encountered in coeliac disease, particularly anaemia[76] and a loss of bone density.[77,78]

Table 7.4 Compliance with exercise rehabilitation programmes for patients with CIBD

Author	Subjects	Programme	Compliance	Comments
Candow et al.[49]	12 cases of CD, no controls	12 wks resistance training, 3/wk, 3 sets of 8–10 reps at 60–70% of 1RM, circuit of 12 exercises	Programme "well tolerated"	Increased leg press (26%) and chest press (21%)
Chan et al.[12]	918 cases of IBD (54% CD, 46% UC)	Online survey of exercise habits	80% of patients had to stop exercising at some point because of severity of symptoms	Exercise generally made them feel better
Daley et al.[51]	56 cases of IBD randomized to experimental and usual care groups	2 exercise consultations that focussed on walking over 12 weeks	Significant increase of activity reported on leisure index scale	
D'Incà et al.[27]	6 patients in remission	Cycle ergometer exercise at 60% of maximal oxygen intake	Exercise did not elicit symptoms	
Elsenbruch et al.[52]	30 cases of UC randomized to exercise and control	Moderate exercise, 1/wk for 10 wks	1 of 15 subjects dropped out due to miscarriage	
Fraser and Niv[53]	6 cases of IBD, no controls	3 weeks at Dead Sea spa	Full compliance	
Johannesen et al.[54]	102 cases of IBS (51 experimental, 51 control)	Physiotherapist, set target of 20–60 min of moderate to vigorous exercise 3–5 days/week	37/51 completed exercise programme	Motivation encouraged by training diary and cycle ergometer testing

Klare et al.[56]	30 cases of CD randomized to exercise or control	10 wks moderate outdoor running 3 times/wk	3 drop-outs from intervention (2 poor motivation, 1 injury)	Attendance averaged 24/30 sessions, 14/15 willing to repeat programme
Loudon et al.[57]	12 cases of CD, no controls	HBI; 12-wk walking programme, 20–35 min, 3/wk, covering average of 3.5 km per session	12/16 completed programme	
Nathan et al.[58]	10 cases of CD, 1 case UC, no controls	Walking, 3 of 11 subjects working up a sweat	Patients determined their own level of exercise, no drop-outs	3 subjects reported severe fatigue day following excessive exercise
Ng et al.[59]	32 cases of IBD, mild or in remission, no controls	Moderate walking (30 min, 3 times/wk, for 3/12)	All completed trial	
Ploeger et al.[63]	15 paediatric cases of CD in remission	30 min cycling at 50% peak power or 6 bouts of 4×15 sec cycling at 100% peak power	16 of 20 subjects completed exercise protocols	
Robinson et al.[45]	117 cases of CD randomized to low impact exercise or control group	12 low impact floor exercises, 2/wk for 12 months	85% completed programme, only 25% followed prescribed regimen	

Abbreviations: CD = Crohn's disease; CIBD = chronic inflammatory bowel disease; IBS = irritable bowel syndrome; 1RM = one repetition maximum; UC = ulcerative colitis.

Further, there is a small group of individuals who show an anaphylactic reaction to vigorous physical activity, and in some cases this is precipitated by eating some form of wheat before exercising.[79,80]

Areas for further research

Given that some studies have found a low level of physical activity before the onset of CIBD, there is a need to examine whether a low level of habitual physical activity contributes to development of CIBD, and if so, to explore underlying mechanisms. Apparent differences in the response of animals and humans to vigorous exercise also merit examination. Does the greater response in some animal models indicate that chemically induced colitis does not provide an effective way to evaluate the treatment of CIBD, or could humans show benefits similar to those seen in animals if they were to undertake an appropriately designed exercise programme? Finally, there is scope to explore practical tactics that could facilitate exercise participation for patients with exercise-induced diarrhoea. Possibilities include the use of bowel stabilizing medications such as loperamide ("Imodium"), the wearing of protective underwear that could relieve the anxiety that sometimes precipitates involuntary emptying of the bowels during physical activity, and choosing exercise locations that are close to public toilet facilities.

Practical implications for the management of CIBD

Most reports show that patients with CIBD have a low level of habitual physical activity relative to age and sex matched control groups. It needs to be clarified how far this is a consequence of such factors as a diarrhoea exacerbated by exercise, difficulties in managing an ileostomy, or a poor overall state of nutrition. Nevertheless, the disease process was in remission in some studies where activity levels were low, and the lack of adequate physical activity sometimes antedated clinical manifestations of CIBD. A lack of physical activity may then have contributed to disease development. Reasons remain to be explored, but one possible factor may have been that a favourable modulation of pro-inflammatory cytokines was lost because of low levels of physical activity.

Whatever the cause, the limitation of physical activity in CIBD has immediate negative consequences for the affected individual, including a low level of aerobic and muscular function, an increased fragility of bone structure, and a poor quality of life. There is also an adverse impact upon other aspects of overall health, with an increased risk of developing various chronic diseases. On the other hand, commitment to a programme of moderate aerobic and/or resistance exercise can improve functional capacity and the quality of life for a person with CIBD. Moreover, such treatment can be undertaken safely, without increasing activity of the disease process. There are thus strong arguments for making exercise rehabilitation an integral component in the management and treatment of CIBD.

Conclusions

Habitual physical activity is low in CIBD, with a resulting loss of functional capacity, muscle weakness and deterioration of bone structure. Lack of adequate physical activity may indeed contribute to the development of CIBD. Appropriately designed programmes of moderate aerobic or resistance activity can restore function to more satisfactory levels without exacerbating the disease process. As in many clinical conditions, a rehabilitation programme must be carefully designed and monitored in order to sustain patient compliance.

In a few patients with coeliac disease, a combination of exercise and eating gluten can cause a dangerous anaphylactic reaction. However, an increase of daily exercise may improve appetite, helping to counter anaemia and loss of bone mass.

References

1 Rocchi A, Benchimol EI, Bernstein CN *et al.* Inflammatory bowel disease: a Canadian burden of illness review. *Can J Gastroenterol* 2012; 26(11): 811–817.

2 D'Incà R, Varnuer M, D'Odorico A *et al.* Exercise and inflammatory bowel disease: Immunological aspects. *Exerc Immunol Rev* 2000; 6: 43–53.

3 Baumgart D, Sandborn WJ. Inflammatory bowel disease: clinical aspects and established and evolving therapies. *Lancet* 2007; 369(9573): 1641–1657.

4 Lees CW, Barrett JC, Parkes M *et al.* New IBD genetics: common pathways with other diseases. *Gut* 2011; 60: 1739–1753.

5 Winther KV, Jess T, Langholz E *et al.* Survival and cause-specific mortality in ulcerative colitis: follow-up of a population-based cohort in Copenhagen County. *Gastroenterology* 2003; 125: 1576–1582.

6 GBD 2013 Mortality and Causes of Death Collaborators. Global, regional, and national age–sex specific all-cause and cause-specific mortality for 240 causes of death, 1990–2013: a systematic analysis for the Global Burden of Disease Study 2013. *Lancet* 2015; 385(9963): 117–171.

7 Lakatos PL, Lakatos L. Risks for colorectal cancer in ulcerative colitis: Changes, causes and management strategies. *World J Gastroeneterol* 2008; 14(25): 3937–3947.

8 Terzić J, Grivennikov S, Karin E *et al.* Inflammation and colon cancer. *Gastroenterology* 2010; 138: 2101–2104.

9 Mayer R, Wong WD, Rothenberger DA *et al.* Colorectal cancer in inflammatory bowel disease: a continuing problem. *Dis Col Rectum* 1999; 42(3): 343–347.

10 Bøggild H, Tüchsen F, Ørhede E. Occupation, employment status, and chronic inflammatory bowel disease in Denmark. *Int J Epidemiol* 1996; 25(3): 630–637.

11 Boot AM, Bouquet J, Krenning EP *et al.* Bone mineral density and nutritional status in children with chronic inflammatory bowel disease. *Gut* 1998; 42: 188–194.

12 Chan SM, Luben R, Olsen A *et al.* Body mass index and the risk for Crohn's disease and ulcerative colitis: Data from a European prospective cohort study (The IBD in EPIC study). *Am J Gastroenterol* 2013; 108: 575–582.

13 Cucino C, Sonnenberg A. Occupational mortality from inflammatory bowel disease in the United States, 1991–1996. *Am J Gastroenterol* 2001; 96(4): 1101–1105.

14 Hlavaty T, Toth J, Koller T *et al.* Smoking, breastfeeding, physical inactivity, contact with animals, and size of the family influence the risk of inflammatory bowel disease: A Slovak case–control study. *United Eur Gastroenterol J* 2013; 1(2): 109–119.

15 Klein I, Reif S, Farbstein H *et al.* Preillness non-dietary factors and habits in inflammatory bowel disease. *Ital J Gastroenterol Hepatol* 1998; 30(3): 247–251.

16 Lustyk KB, Jarrett ME, Bennett JC *et al.* Does a physically active lifestyle improve symptoms in women with irritable bowel syndrome? *Gastroenterol Nurs* 2001; 24(3): 129–137.

17 Mack DE, Wilson PM, Gilmore JC *et al.* Leisure-time physical activity in Canadians living with Crohn's disease and ulcerative colitis. Population-based estimates. *Gastroenterol Nurs* 2011; 34(4): 288–294.

18 Ojerskog B, Hallstrom T, Kock NG *et al.* Quality of life in ileostomy patients before and after conversion to the continent ileostomy. *Int J Colorectal Dis* 1988; 3: 166–170.

19 Persson PG, Leijonmarck CE, Bernell O *et al.* Risk indicators for inflammatory bowel disease. *Int J Epidemiol* 1993; 22: 268–272.

20 Sonnenberg A. Occupational distribution of inflammatory bowel disease among German employees. *Gut* 1990; 31: 1037–1040.

21 Sørensen VZ, Olsen BG, Binder V. Life prospects and quality of life in patients with Crohn's disease. *Gut* 1987; 28: 382–385.

22 van Langenberg DR, Della Gatta P, Warmington SA *et al.* Objectively measured muscle fatigue in Crohn's disease: Correlation with self-reported fatigue and associated factors for clinical application. *J Crohn's Dis Colitis* 2014; 8(2): 137–146.

23 Werkstetter KJ, Ullrich J, Schatz SB *et al.* Lean body mass, physical activity and quality of life in paediatric patients with inflammatory bowel disease and in healthy controls. *J Crohn's Colitis* 2012; 6: 665–673.

24 Wiroth J-B, Filippi J, Schneider SM *et al.* Muscle performance in patients with Crohn's disease in clinical remission. *Inflamm Bowel Dis* 2005; 11: 296–303.

25 Zaltman C, Braulio VB, Outerail R *et al.* Lower extremity mobility limitation and impaired muscle function in women with ulcerative colitis. *J Crohn's Colitis* 2014; 8: 529–535.

26 Brevinge H, Berglund B, Bosaeus I *et al.* Exercise capacity in patients undergoing proctocolectomy and small bowel resection for Crohn's disease. *Br J Surg* 1995; 82: 1040–1045.

27 D'Incà R, Varnier M, Mestriner C *et al.* Effect of moderate exercise on Crohn's disease patients in remission. *Ital J Gastroenterol Hepatol* 1999; 31(3): 205–210.

28 Bechtold S, Alberer M, Arenz T *et al.* Reduced muscle mass and bone size in pediatric patients with inflammatory bowel disease. *Inflamm Bowel Dis* 2010; 16: 216–225.

29 Bryant R, Ooi S, Schultz C *et al.* Low muscle mass in inflammatory bowel disease (IBD): common and predictive of functional sarcopenia and osteopenia. *European Crohn's and Colitis Organisation Poster Presentation P* 190, 2014.

30 Capristo E, Mingrone G, Addolorato G *et al.* Metabolic features of inflammatory bowel disease in a remission phase of the disease activity. *J Intern Med* 1996; 2 43: 339–347.

31 Dubner SE, Shults J, Baldassano RN *et al.* Longitudinal assessment of bone density and structure in an incident cohort of children with Crohn's disease. *Gastroenterology* 2009; 136(1): 123–130.

32 Filippi J, Al Jaouni R, Wiroth JB *et al.* Nutritional deficiencies in patients with Crohn's disease in remission. *Inflamm Bowel Dis* 2006; 12: 185–191.

33 Geerling BJ, Badart-Smook A, Stockbrugger RW *et al.* Comprehensive nutritional status in recently diagnosed patients with inflammatory bowel disease compared with population controls. *Eur J Clin Nutr* 2000; 54: 514–521.

34 Jahnsen J, Falch JA, Mowinckel P *et al.* Body composition in patients with inflammatory bowel disease: a population-based study. *Am J Gastroenterol* 2003; 98: 1556–1562.

35 Sylvester FA, Leopold S, Lincoln M *et al.* A two-year study of persistent lean tissue deficits in children with Crohn's disease. *Clin Gastroenterol Hepatol* 2009; 7: 452–455.

36 Tjellesen L, Nielsen PK, Staun M. Body composition by dual-energy X-ray absorptiometry in patients with Crohn's disease. *Scand J Gastroenterol* 1998; 33: 356–360.

37 Valentini L, Schaper L, Buning C *et al.* Malnutrition and impaired muscle strength in patients with Crohn's disease and ulcerative colitis in remission. *Nutrition* 2008; 24: 694–702.

38 van Langenberg DR, Della Gatta P, Hill B *et al.* Delving into disability in Crohn's disease: Dysregulation of molecular pathways may explain skeletal muscle loss in Crohn's disease. *J Crohn's Colitis* 2014; 8(7): 626–634.

39 Werkstetter KJ, Pozza SB-D, Filipiak-Pittrof B *et al.* Long-term development of bone geometry and muscle in pediatric inflammatory bowel disease. *Am J Gastroenterol* 2011; 106: 988–998.

40 Wiskin AE, Wooton SA, Hunt TM *et al.* Body composition in childhood inflammatory bowel disease. *Clin Nutr* 2011; 30: 112–115.

41 Geerling BJ, Badart-Smook A, Stockbrügger RW *et al.* Comprehensive nutritional status in patients with long-standing Crohn's disease currently in remission. *Am J Clin Nutr* 1998; 67: 919–926.

42 Lee N, Radford-Smith G, Taaffe D. Bone loss in Crohn's disease: exercise as a potential countermeasure. *Inflamm Bowel Dis* 2005; 11: 1108–1118.

43 Abitol V, Roux C, Chaussade S *et al.* Metabolic bone assessment in patients with inflammatory bowel disease. *Gastroenterology* 1995; 108: 417–422.

44 Klaus J, Armbrecht G, Steinkamp M *et al.* High prevalence of osteoporotic vertebral fractures in patients with Crohn's disease. *Gut* 2002; 51: 654–658.

45 Robinson RJ, al-Azzawi F, Iqbal SJ *et al.* Osteoporosis and determinants of bone density in patients with CD. *Dig Dis Sci* 1998; 43: 2500–2506.

46 Bilski J, Brzozowski B, Mazur-Bialy A *et al.* The role of physical exercise in inflammatory bowel disease. *Biomed Res Internat* 2014; 2014: 429031.

47 Pedersen BK, Febbraio M. Muscle as an endocrine organ; focus on muscle-derived IL-6. *Physiol Rev* 2008; 88: 1379–1406.

48 Pérez CA. Prescription of physical exercise in Crohn's disease. *J Crohn's Colitis* 2009; 3: 225–231.

49 Candow D, Rizzi A, Chillibeck PD *et al.* Effect of resistance training on Crohn's disease. *Can J Appl Physiol* 2002; 27: S7–S8.

50 Crumbock SC, Loeb SJ, Fick DM. Physical activity, stress, disease activity and quality of life in adults with Crohn's disease. *Gastroenterol Nurs* 2009; 32(3): 188–195.

51 Daley AJ, Grimmett C, Roberts L *et al.* The effects of exercise upon symptoms and quality of life in patients diagnosed with irritable bowel syndrome: A randomized controlled trial. *Int J Sports Med* 2008; 29: 778–782.

52 Elsenbruch S, Langhorst J, Popkirowa K *et al.* Effects of mind-body therapy on quality of life and neuroendocrine and cellular immune functions in patients with ulcerative colitis. *Psychother Psychosom* 2005; 74: 277–287.

53 Fraser GM, Niv Y. Six patients whose perianal and ileocolic Crohn's disease improved in the Dead Sea environment. *J Clin Gastroenterol* 1995; 21: 217–219.

54 Johannesen E, Simrén E, Strid H *et al.* Physical activity improves symptoms in irritable bowel syndrome: A randomized controlled trial. *Am J Gastroeneterol* 2011; 106: 915–922.

55 Jones PD, Kappelman MD, Martin CF *et al.* Exercise decreases risk of future active disease in patients with inflammatory bowel disease in remission. *Inflamm Bowel Dis* 2015; 21: 1063–1071.

56 Klare P, Nigg J, Nold J *et al.* The impact of a ten-week physical exercise program on health-related quality of life in patients with inflammatory bowel disease: A prospective randomized controlled trial. *Digestion* 2015; 91: 219–247.
57 Loudon C, Coroll V, Butcher J *et al.* The effects of physical exercise on patients with Crohn's disease. *Am J Gastroenterol* 1999; 94: 697–703.
58 Nathan I, Norton C, Czuber-Dochan W *et al.* Exercise in individuals with inflammatory bowel disease. *Gastroenterol Nurs* 2013; 36(1): 437–442.
59 Ng V, Millard W, Lebrun C, Howard J. Low-intensity exercise improves quality of life in patients with Crohn's disease. *Clin J Sports Med* 2007; 17: 384–388.
60 Koek GH, Verleden GM, Evenpoel P *et al.* Activity related increase of exhaled nitric oxide in Crohn's disease and ulcerative colitis: a manifestation of systemic involvement? *Respiratory Med* 2002; 96: 530–535.
61 Khalili H, Ananthakrishnan AN, Konijeti GG *et al.* Physical activity and risk of inflammatory bowel disease: prospective study from the Nurses' Health Study cohorts. *Br Med J* 2013; 347: f.6633.
62 Nguyen T, Ploeger HE, Obeid J *et al.* Reduced fat oxidation rates during submaximal exercise in adolescents with Crohn's disease. *Inflamm Bowel Dis* 2013; 19: 2659–2665.
63 Ploeger H, Obeid J, Nguyen T *et al.* Exercise and inflammation in pediatric Crohn's disease. *Int J Sports Med* 2012; 33: 673–679.
64 Miossec P. IL-17 and Th17 cells in human inflammatory diseases. *Microbes Infect* 2009; 11: 625–630.
65 Zoli G, Katelaris PH, Garrow J *et al.* Increased energy expenditure in growing adolescents with Crohn's disease. *Dig Dis Sci* 1996; 41(9): 1754–1759.
66 Cook MD, Martin SA, Williams C *et al.* Forced treadmill exercise training exacerbates inflammation and causes mortality while voluntary wheel training is protective in a mouse model of colitis. *Brain Behav Immun* 2013; 33: 46–56.
67 Shephard RJ. *Physical activity, training and the immune response.* Carmel, IN: Benchmark Publicatiuons, 1997
68 Martinez ME, Heddens D, Earnest DL *et al.* Physical activity, body mass index, and prostaglandin E2 levels in rectal mucosa. *J Natl Cancer Inst* 1999; 91: 950–953.
69 Chen Y, Noble E. Is exercise beneficial to the inflammatory bowel diseases? An implication of heat shock proteins. *Med Hypoth* 2009; 72: 84–86.
70 He C, Bassik MC, Moresi V *et al.* Exercise-induced BCL2-regulated autophagy is required for muscle glucose homeostasis. *Nature* 2012; 481: 511–515.
71 Hoffman-Goetz L, Spagnuolo PA, Guan J. Repeated exercise in mice alters expression of IL-10 and TNF–a in intestinal lymphocytes. *Brain Behav Immun* 2008; 22: 195–199.
72 Szalai Z, Svász A, Nagy I *et al.* Anti-inflammatory effect of recreational exercise in TNBS-induced colitis in rats: Role of NOS/HO/MPO system. *Oxidat Med Cell Longev* 2014; 2014: ID 925981.
73 Kasimay O, Guzel E, Gemici A *et al.* Colitis-induced oxidative damage of the colon and skeletal muscle is ameliorated by regular exercise in rats: the anxiolytic role of exercise. *Exp Physiol* 2006; 91(5): 897–906.
74 Saxena A, Fletcher E, Larsen B *et al.* Effect of exercise on chemically-induced colitis in adiponectin deficient mice. *J Inflamm* 2012; 9: 30.
75 Watters C, Wright SJ, Robinson RJ *et al.* Positive and negative wellbeing as predictors of exercise uptake in Crohn's disease: An exploratory study. *Psychol Health Med* 2001; 6: 293–299.
76 Corazza GR, Valentin RA, Andreani ML *et al.* Subclinical coeliac disease is a frequent cause of iron-deficiency anaemia. *Scand J Gastroenterol* 1995; 30(2): 153–156.

77 Bodé S, Hassager C, Gudmand-Høyer E *et al.* Body composition and calcium metabolism in adult treated coeliac disease. *Gut* 1991; 32: 1342–1345.
78 McFarlane XA, Bhalla AK, Reeves DE *et al.* Osteoporosis in treated adult coeliac disease. *Gut* 1995; 36: 710–714.
79 Kidd JM, Cohen SH, Sosman AJ *et al.* Food-dependent exercise-induced anaphylaxis. *J Allergy Clin Immunol* 1983; 71(4): 407–411.
80 Palosuo K, Alenius H, Varjonen E *et al.* A novel wheat gliadin as a cause of exercise-induced anaphylaxis. *J Allergy Clin Immunol* 1999; 103(5): 912–917.

8 Physical activity and colo-rectal adenomas

Introduction

Fleshy growths of the colon and rectal endothelium (polyps) are usually found in the distal part of the colon and rectum. Often, these polyps develop into benign colo-rectal adenomas. The growths can be removed surgically, but unfortunately there is a high recurrence rate (around 20%/year). Moreover, the hyperplastic tissue can lose its normal cell characteristics and progress to a colonic or rectal cancer. Indeed, most colo-rectal carcinomas arise from adenomas, although only 1–10% of adenomas progress to cancers. The risk of progression to a malignant tumour is increased if the adenoma is large, if the histology is villous rather than tubular, and if the lesion contains many abnormal cells. A meta-analysis based on 18 studies suggested that in individuals of average risk, the prevalence of colo-rectal adenomas was 30.2%, but that of colo-rectal cancer was only 0.3%.[1] However, critics of this analysis have suggested that the apparently very high prevalence of colo-rectal adenomas may reflect in part the fact that data have often been collected on elderly people.

The effectiveness of ongoing surveillance of adenomas is limited by the relatively high costs of detection and low recurrence rates.[2] The screening costs associated with the detection of an advanced adenocarcinoma and a stage 1 colo-rectal cancer have been estimated at US$27,962 and US$922,762, respectively.[3] Given these high costs and the adverse prognosis following carcinogenic change, there is considerable interest in prevention by various lifestyle measures. This chapter looks specifically at the value of physical activity in preventing the development of colo-rectal adenomas.

There is now widespread agreement that an increase of habitual physical activity is helpful in reducing the likelihood of developing various types of benign and malignant tumours. Evidence on this point seems particularly strong for adenomas and carcinomas of the colon, where risks seem to be at least 20–40% lower among those individuals who are taking regular and adequate volumes of physical activity. Nevertheless, detailed analysis of the benefits of an active lifestyle has been hampered by a long disease latency. This has made it necessary to explore the physical activity patterns and overall lifestyle of large populations for periods of 20 years and more. Occupational comparisons have been helpful in that the physical demands of work have remained consistent for many people over long periods. On the other hand, mechanization and automation have progressively reduced energy expenditures in many previously "heavy" occupational categories, and it is now increasingly difficult for epidemiologists to find people who are employed in jobs that still require hard physical work.

Physical activity and the risk of developing colo-rectal adenomas

Given the high prevalence of adenomas, the appreciable risk of their progression to colo-rectal cancer and the strong likelihood of a recurrence after surgical removal, there is considerable interest in the potential of regular physical activity to reduce the risk of developing colo-rectal adenomas. This question has been examined in at least 25 human studies, 6 based upon inter-individual differences in the physical demands of occupation (see Table 8.1), and 19 on assessments of leisure or total activity (see Table 8.2). In general, there has been a trend towards a lower risk of adenoma formation in the more active individuals.

Occupational activity and colo-rectal adenomas

Only two of the six studies found no beneficial effect from occupational activity[7,9]; one of these investigations nevertheless found substantial benefit from a high level of leisure activity, and the other showed some positive trends from leisure activity and participation in sport. Most of the other studies showed positive but individually statistically non-significant trends. Pooling data from the occupational studies, the weighted risk of adenomas for sedentary individuals was a substantial 2.14 relative to those who were active. However, this high estimate of benefit was due in part to a risk ratio of 0.2 in one pair of active men[8]; ignoring this aberrant finding, the risk ratio for a sedentary occupation dropped to a weighted average of 1.74.

Leisure activity and colo-rectal adenomas

Often, the methods used to study leisure activity in these investigations have been relatively crude, and findings of a positive trend have not always reached statistical significance. The benefit reported in published articles is probably attenuated by this imprecision in the measurement of habitual physical activity, although in studies that have not included appropriate covariates such as age, sex and body mass index, it could also be exaggerated by linkages between such risk-influencing factors and the amount of regular physical activity undertaken.

Several of the 19 studies of leisure behaviour found no significant protection against colo-rectal adenomas in the more active members of their sample, although there was generally a reduced risk of colo-rectal cancers in the same samples.[6,10–12] The weighted average risk ratio of adenomata in those with sedentary leisure behaviour was 1.21 in the 18 reports with numerical values,

Table 8.1 Occupational activity and the risk of developing colo-rectal adenomas

Author	Sample	Physical activity	Risk ratios	Covariates and comments
*Boutron-Rualt et al. (2001)[4]	154 small, 208 large adenomas vs 426 controls	High vs low occupational activity	OR small adenomas 0.8 (0.5–1.3) large adenomas 0.6 (0.4–1.0) weighted effect 1.47 n.s.	Age, sex
Kato et al. (1990)[5]	525 adenomas, 578 controls	High vs low occupational activity	RR proximal colon 0.32 (0.19–0.53) distal colon 0.59 (0.43–0.82)	Age, marital status, alcohol smoking, family history
Klaus (1993)[6]	170 colo-rectal adenomas, 245 controls	Work activity (none vs >4.2 MJ/wk)	RR if sedentary work 1.19	Smoking, alcohol, use of NSAIDs
*Little et al. (1993)[7]	147 cases, 153 controls	Work activity above median vs none	No association with time spent sitting standing, walking or engaged in heavy work	Age, sex, social class
*Neugut et al. (1996)[8]	Colonoscopies: 506 normal, 298 adenomas, 345 past adenomas, 197 metachronous adenomas	Questionnaire and occupational title; high vs low activity	OR Incident adenomas M 0.2 (0.0–0.9) F 0.9 (0.6–1.6) Metachronous adenomas M 1.2 (0.2–5.9) F 3.6 (0.3–53.9)	Age, education, BMI, total energy intake, fibre, fat intake, smoking
*Sandler et al. (1995)[9]	86 M, 114 F Colo-rectal adenomas, 384 controls	Job activity questionnaire. Most vs least active quartile	No effect of job activity: OR M 1.1 (0.45–2.68) F 0.96 (0.49–1.88)	Benefit seen with leisure activity

Note
* Data presented for both occupational and leisure activity.
Abbreviations: BMI = body mass index; F = female; M = male; n.s. = nor significant; NSAIDs = non-specific anti-inflammatory drugs; OR = odds ratio; RR = relative risk.

Table 8.2 Leisure-time physical activity and risk of colo-rectal adenomas

Author	Sample	Physical activity	Risk ratios	Covariates and comments
*Boutron-Rualt et al. (2001)[4]	151 small, 204 large adenomas vs 426 controls	High vs low leisure activity	OR small adenomas 1.8 (1.0–2.3) large adenomas 0.9 (0.5–1.6) ns	Age, sex
Colbert et al. (2002)[17]	1905 adults in 3-yr prospective study of recurrences, 530 M, 203 F	Estimated time spent on vigorous activity vs least active	OR vigorous vs least active M 0.9 (0.6–1.2) F 0.7 (0.4–1.2)	Age
Enger et al. (1997)[16]	488 colo-rectal adenomas and matched pairs, aged 50–74 yrs	Questionnaire on recent physical activity (>6 METs vs >4 METs vs none)	OR >6 METs 0.7 (0.4–1.1) >4 METS 0.8 (0.6–1.2)	BMI, smoking, alcohol, diet
Giovannucci et al. (1995)[14]	586 adenomas in 47,223 health professionals over 6 yrs	Active vs inactive	RR if active 0.79 (0.57–1.09)	Age, parental history, endoscopy
Giovannucci et al. (1996)[15]	439 adenomas in 13,057 nurses over 6 yrs	High vs low quintiles of leisure activity	RR if active 0.58 (0.4–0.86)	Age, parental history, endoscopy
Guilera et al. (2005)[18]	226 adenomas, 494 controls	High vs low activity	OR of adenoma if obese: low activity 1.6 (0.7–3.4) high activity 0.8 (0.4–1.6)	Age, sex
Hauret et al. (2004)[19]	177 cases, 228 controls	MET-hr/day of moderate to vigorous activity (quartiles)	Highest vs lowest quartile OR 0.63 (0.34–1.17)	Age, sex, use of NSAIDs
Hermann et al. (2009)[10]	536 colo-rectal adenomas in 4-yr follow-up of 25,540 subjects	4-level classification of habitual activity	OR 1.02 (0.74–1.42), not a significant relationship	Age, sex, energy intake, diet, smoking, alcohol
Kahn et al.(1998)[20]	10-yr follow-up of 72,868 men, 81,356 women; cases 7504 M, 5111 F	3-level classification of physical activity (high vs low)	OR if high, M 0.83 (0.76–0.91) F 0.91 (0.78–1.03)	Age, diet, smoking, alcohol, aspirin use, family history and other factors

continued

Table 8.2 Continued

Author	Sample	Physical activity	Risk ratios	Covariates and comments
*Kato et al. (1990)[5]	525 adenomas, 578 controls	Sport >1–2 h/week	RR if active in sport proximal colon 0.67 (0.44–1.03), distal colon 0.57 (0.41–0.79)	Age, residence, smoking, alcohol, family history
*Klaus (1993)[6]	170 colo-rectal adenomas, 245 controls	Questionnaire	No effect of physical activity	Smoking, alcohol, use of NSAIDs
Kono et al. (1991)[21]	80 adenomatous polyps, 1148 normal subjects	Interview, 2–3 h/wk vs 0–1, 1–2 or 0–1 h/week	OR 2–3 h/wk 0.44 (0.22–0.87) 1–2 h/wk 0.70 (0.37–1.34) 0–1 h/wk 0.88 (0.49–1.58) p for trend=0.015	Smoking, alcohol, BMI, military rank
Larsen et al. (2006)[11]	443 adenomas, 3447 controls	4-quartile exercise scale	Most active: Low risk adenoma OR 1.19 (0.89–1.60)	
Lieberman et al. (2003)[22]	391 hyperplastic polyps vs 1441 controls	Framingham activity index 24–28 vs >36	RR 0.82 (0.60–1.10) if high activity	
*Little et al. (1993)[7]	147 colo-rectal adenomas, 153 controls	None vs run or cycle >30 min 1/wk	RR if active 0.46 (0.2–1.3)*	Age, sex, social class
Lubin et al. (1997)[23]	196 patients, matched controls	Highest vs lowest tertile physical activity	OR for most active 0.6 (0.3–0.9) (p for trend=0.03)	Age, smoking, fibre intake
*Neugut et al. (1996)[8]	Colonoscopies: 506 normal, 298 adenomas, 345 past adenomas, 197 metachronous adenomas	Very active vs inactive	OR if very active 0.4 (0.2–1.0) Incident adenomas M 0.7 (0.4–1.2) F 1.1 (0.6–1.7) Metachronous adenomas M 0.6 (0.3–1.0) F 1.0 (0.4–2.6)	Age, education, BMI, total energy intake, fibre, fat intake, smoking
Rosenberg et al. (2006)[24]	45,500 Black women, 6-yr follow-up; 1390 developed polyps	Walking and vigorous exercise >40 MET-hr/wk vs <5 MET-hr/wk	IR 0.72 vs 0.94 (p for trend=0.01)	Age, BMI, family history, smoking, education

Rozen et al. (1994)[25] (see also Lubin et al. (1997)[23])	243 colo-rectal adenomas, matched controls	Weekly activity report	OR leisure M 0.92 (0.36–2.31) F 0.64 (0.35–1.19) Sports M 0.76 (0.29–1.98) F 0.96 (0.52–1.77)	Diet, weight gain, BMI, smoking, alcohol
*Sandler et al. (1995)[9]	200 adenomas, 384 controls	Most leisure activity and most sports vs lowest quartiles; activity quartiles 2–4		
Shinchi et al.[26] (see also Kono et al. (1991)[21])	228 adenomas, 1484 controls	No exercise vs daily exercise	OR for daily exercise, all adenomas 1.2 (0.8–2.0) large adenomas 0.7 (0.3–1.3)	Smoking, alcohol, waist-hip ratio, military rank
Stemmerman et al. (1988)[27]	79 adenomas, 84 controls	Average number of polyps vs physical activity index	Lowest 1.37 Highest 1.19 (n.s.)	Diet, cholesterol, smoking, alcohol
Terry et al. (2002)[28]	441 non-advanced adenomas, 1866 controls	Activity >2h/wk vs <2h/wk	OR if active: non-advanced polyps M 0.8 (0.5–1.2) F 1.1 (0.6–1.7) advanced polyps M 0.4 (0.2–0.9) F 0.7 (0.4–1.0)	Age, sex, BMI, diet, hormone replacement therapy in women
Wallace et al. (2005)[12]	4-yr follow-up of 930 patients with previously resected colo-rectal adenoma	Weekday and weekend MET-hr of activity (>335 vs <2763)	No association with tubular adenomas (active RR 0.97 (0.73 = 1.28) or hyperplastic polyps 1.04 (0.73–1.49)	Age, sex, BMI treatment time
Wolin et al.[13]	Meta-analysis of 20 studies	Risk if active	RR if no activity M 0.81 (0.67–0.98) F 0.87 (0.74–1.02) Large adenomas M&F 0.70 (0.56–0.88)	

Note

* Data presented for both occupational and leisure activity.

Abbreviations: BMI = body mass index; F = female; IR = incidence ratio; M = male; n.s. = nor significant; NSAIDs = non-specific anti-inflammatory drugs; OR = odds ratio; RR = relative risk.

although this estimate was heavily weighted by one large study with 12,615 cases. The average risk ratio for the remaining 17 studies was 1.29. Five studies provided sex comparisons, with the increased risk of sedentary leisure pursuits being somewhat greater for men (1.25) than for women (1.14).

A meta-analysis based upon 20 investigations[13] largely confirmed the impression gained from the above analyses. The meta-analysis found a risk that was 23% greater among inactive men, and 15% higher in inactive women. The estimated protection against the development of adenomas was typically somewhat greater in men than in women (possibly because more men engage in vigorous physical activity, or because physically demanding domestic tasks undertaken by women are sometimes overlooked).

One report found the risk of sedentary work was greater for large adenomas (risk ratio 1.67) than for small ones (risk ratio 1.20).[4] In some[14,15] but not all[16] leisure studies, also, the beneficial effect of regular physical activity was greater for large than for small adenomas.

Animal experiments

Human biopsy specimens and in-vitro cell cultures have proven useful tools in studying factors favouring the genesis of colo-rectal adenomas. There has also been interest in developing animal models where lesions are limited to the large intestine, and cell characteristics mimic those seen in human adenomas and carcinomas. Experimental options include the study of spontaneous intestinal cancers in various species, chemically or environmentally induced cancers in small mammals, and tumours induced by genetic manipulation of mice.[29]

Data from controlled animal experiments have partially confirmed the findings from human epidemiological investigations. For example, a study of mice found 29% fewer polyps and 38% fewer larger polyps in male animals that undertook treadmill running for 60 minutes per day over a period of 9 weeks, although no change of risk was seen in female animals assigned to treadmill running, and no benefit was found from voluntary wheel-running in mice of either sex.[30]

Potential mechanisms

Likely mechanisms underlying the association between habitual physical activity and a reduced risk of colo-rectal adenomas include a better regulation of energy balance and a modulation of inflammatory responses.[19,31] Various studies including observations in experimental animals have consistently demonstrated the involvement in adenoma formation of an increased energy intake and obesity (as assessed by the body mass index or the waist hip ratio).[14,26] Moreover, the beneficial effects of a high level of physical activity upon the risk of adenomas are seen only in those who are not taking anti-inflammatory drugs, and prostaglandin E_2 apparently has an anti-apoptotic effect on colonic endothelial cells.[32]

Areas for further research

The vast majority of colonic cancers appear to have their origin in asymptomatic polyps.[33] It is thus important to identify and correct the multiple risk factors (possibly including physical inactivity) that influence the conversion of these initially benign growths into malignant tumours.[34] Analysis is hampered by the long disease latency. In particular, it has been necessary to explore the physical activity patterns and lifestyle of subjects over periods of 20 years and longer, and there remains scope to find a reliable objective method of summarizing a person's lifetime experience of an active lifestyle. Possibly, an emphasis needs to be placed on objective monitoring devices such as accelerometers, or on measuring the outcomes of regular physical activity, such as attained levels of aerobic fitness and muscular development.

Many investigators have reported a stronger protective effect of physical activity in men than in women. Data from controlled animal experiments have partially confirmed human epidemiological investigations in showing a larger response in male animals,[30] and the underlying reasons for this sex differential should be clarified.

There also remains opportunity to discover why the benefits of physical activity differ between proximal and distal adenomas, and between early and advanced adenomatous lesions.

Practical implications

Although most studies show substantial differences in the risks of colon and rectal cancer between those who are sedentary and those who have a very high level of physical activity either at work or in their leisure time, this does not necessarily imply that the enrolment of sedentary individuals in an exercise programme would yield an equivalent gain of health. There are two main reasons for caution. First, the risk of carcinogenesis was likely accumulated over 10 or 20 years of inadequate physical activity, and reversal of this process will probably require compliance with a vigorous exercise regimen for an equally long period. Second, the risk ratios presented in this chapter have been calculated by comparing the experience of sedentary individuals with the most active members of each sample, and in many instances the optimal level of weekly physical activity was much higher than would likely be attained if a sedentary person were encouraged to enter an exercise programme.

Nevertheless, the association between a physically active lifestyle and a reduced risk of colo-rectal cancer has now been amply demonstrated, and this is yet one more important reason for health professionals to encourage a greater level of habitual physical activity among the general population. The development of a colo-rectal cancer often provokes an evaluation of personal lifestyle, and some investigators have suggested that a discussion of the link between low levels of physical activity and colon cancer may be a useful means of persuading not only the patients but also their relatives[35-37] to exercise on a regular basis.

Conclusions

Life-long physical activity reduced the risk of developing adenomatous polyps in the colon and rectum, whether the source of activity is a physically demanding occupation, or an active lifestyle during leisure time. Possible mechanisms include a better modulation of energy balance and a reduction of local inflammation, with diminished concentrations of prostaglandin E_2, which reduces apoptosis in the endothelium of the colon and rectum.

References

1 Hellman SJ, Ronksley PE, Hilsden RJ *et al.* Prevalence of adenomas and colorectal cancer in average risk individuals: a systematic review and meta-analysis. *Clin Gastroenterol Hepatol* 2009; 7(12): 1272–1278.

2 Lund JN, Scholefield JH, Grainge MJ *et al.* Risks, costs, and compliance limit of colorectal adenoma surveillance: lessons from a randomised trial. *Gut* 2001; 49(1): 91–96.

3 Wong CS, Ching JYL, Chan VCW *et al.* The comparative cost-effectiveness of colorectal cancer screening using faecal immunochemical test vs colonoscopy. *Sci Rep* 2015; 5: 13,568.

4 Boutron-Rualt MC, Senesse P, Méance S *et al.* Energy intake, body mass index, physical activity, and the colorectal adenoma-carcinoma sequence. *Nutr Cancer* 2001; 39(1) 50–57.

5 Kato I, Tominga S, Matsuura A *et al.* A comparative case-control study of colorectal cancer and adenoma. *Jpn J Cancer Res* 1990; 81: 1101–1108.

6 Klaus DH. *Case-control study of colorectal adenomas and four potential risk factors: use of non-steroidal anti-inflammatory drugs and acetaminophen, physical activity, cigarette smoking, and alcohol consumption.* New Haven, CN; Yale University, 1993.

7 Little J, Logan RF, Hawtin PG *et al.* Colorectal adenomas and energy intake, body size and physical activity: a case-control study of subjects participating in the Nottingham faecal occult blood screening programme. *Br J Cancer* 1993; 67: 172–176.

8 Neugut AJ, Terry MB, Hocking G *et al.* Leisure and occupational activity and risk of colorectal adenomatous polyps. *Int J Cancer* 1996; 68: 744–748.

9 Sandler RS, Pritchard ML, Bangdiwala SI. Physical activity and the risk of colorectal adenomas. Epidemiology 1995; 6: 602–606.

10 Hermann S, Rohrmann S, Lineisen J. Lifestyle factors, obesity and the risk of colorectal adenomas in EPIC-Heidelberg. *Cancer Causes Control* 2009; 20: 1397–1408.

11 Larsen IK, Grotmol T, Almendingen K *et al.* Lifestyle as a predictor for colonic neoplasia in asymptomatic individuals. *BMC Gasstroenterol* 2006; 6: 5.

12 Wallace K, Baron JA, Karagas MR *et al.* The association of physical activity and body mass index with the risk of large bowel polyps. *Cancer Epidemiol Biomarkers Prev* 2005; 14(9): 2082–2086.

13 Wolin KY, Yan Y, Colditz GA. Physical activity and risk of colon adenoma: a meta-analysis. *Br J Cancer* 2011; 104: 882–885.

14 Giovannucci E, Ascherio A, Rimm EB *et al.* Physical activity, obesity, and risk for colon cancer and adenoma in men. *Ann Intern Med* 1995; 122: 327–334.

15 Giovannucci E, Coldlitz GA, Stampfer MJ *et al.* Physical activity, obesity, and risk of colorectal adenoma in women (United States). *Cancer Causes Control* 1996; 7: 253–263.

16 Enger SM, Longnecker MP, Lee ER *et al.* Recent and past physical activity and prevalence of colorectal adenomas. *Br J Cancer* 1997; 75: 740–745.

17 Colbert LH, Lanza E, Ballard-Barbash R *et al.* Adenomatous polyp recurrence and physical activity in the Polyp Prevention Trial (United States). *Cancer Causes Control* 2002; 13: 445–453.

18 Guilera M, Connelly-Frost A, Keku TO *et al.* Does physical activity modify the association between body mass index and colorectal adenomas? *Nutr Cancer* 2005; 51(2): 140–145.

19 Hauret KG, Bostick RM, Matthews CE *et al.* Physical activity and reduced risk of incident sporadic colorectal adenomas: observational support for mechanisms involving energy balance and inflammation modulation. *Am J Epidemiol* 2004; 159(10): 983–992.

20 Kahn HS, Tatham LM, Thun MJ *et al.* Risk factors for self-reported colon polyps. *J Gen Intern Med* 1998; 13: 303–310.

21 Kono S, Shinchi K, Ikeda N *et al.* Physical activity, dietary habits and adenomatous polyps of the sigmoid colon: a study of self-defense officials in Japan. *J Clin Epidemiol* 1991; 44: 1255–1261.

22 Lieberman DA, Prindiville S, Weiss DG *et al.* Risk factors for advanced colonic neoplasia and hyperplastic polyps in asymptomatic individuals. *JAMA* 2003; 290(22): 2959–2967.

23 Lubin F, Rozen P, Arieli B *et al.* Nutritional and lifestyle habits and water-fiber interaction in colorectal adenoma etiology. *Cancer Epidemiol Biomark Prev* 1997; 6: 79–85.

24 Rosenberg L, Boggs D, Wise LA *et al.* A follow-up study of physical activity and incidence of colorectal polyps in African-American women. *Cancer Epidemiol Biomark Prev* 2006; 15(8): 1438–1442.

25 Rozen PF, Lubin P, Arieli H *et al.* Nutritional and other life habits in colorectal adenoma etiology. *Cancer Res* 1994; 35: 295.

26 Shinchi K, Kono S, Honjo S *et al.* Obesity and adenomatous polyps of the sigmoid colon. *Jpn J Cancer Res* 1994; 85: 479–484.

27 Stemmemann GN, Heilbrun LK, Nomura AM. Association of diet and other factors with adenomatous polyps of the large bowel: A prospective autopsy study. *Am J Clin Nutr* 1988; 47: 312–317.

28 Terry MB, Neugut AI, Bostick RM *et al.* Risk factors for advanced colorectal adenomas: a pooled analysis. *Cancer Epidemiol Biuomark Prev* 2002; 11(7): 622–629.

29 Johnson TL, Fleet JC. Animal models of colorectal cancer. *Cancer Metastasis Rev* 2013; 32: 39–61.

30 Mehl KA, Davis JM, Clements JM *et al.* Decreased intestinal polyp multiplicity is related to exercise mode and gender in Apc $^{Min/+}$ mice. *J Appl Physiol* 1988; 98(6): 2219–2225.

31 Wolin KY, Tuchman H. Physical activity and gastrointestinal cancer prevention. *Recent Results Cancer Res* 2011; 186: 73–100.

32 Inaba A, Uchiyama T, Oka M. Role of prostaglandin E_2 in rat colon carcinoma. *Hepatogastroenterology* 1999; 46: 2347–2351.

33 Emmons KM, McBride CM, Puleo E *et al.* Project PREVENT: A randomized trial to reduce multiple behavioral risk factors for colon cancer. *Cancer Epidemiol Biomarkers Prev* 2005; 14(6): 1453–1459.

34 Emmons KM, McBride CM, Puleo E *et al.* Prevalence and predictors of multiple behavioral risk factors for colon cancer. *Prev Med* 2005; 40: 527–534.

35 Coups EJ, Hay J, Ford JS. Awareness of the role of physical activity in colon cancer prevention. *Patient Educ Counsel* 2008; 72(2): 246–251.
36 McGowan EL, Prapavessis H. Colon cancer information as a source of exercise motivation for relatives of patients with colon cancer. *Psychol Health Med* 2010; 15(6): 729–741.
37 McGowan EL, Prapavessis H, Campbell N *et al.* The effect of a multifaceted efficacy intervention on exercise behavior in relatives of colon cancer patients. *Int J Behav Med* 2012; 19: 550–562.

9 Physical activity and the risk of colo-rectal carcinomas

Introduction

Evidence of rectal cancer has been found in an Egyptian mummy from the era of Ptolemy. Almost all colo-rectal tumours are adenocarcinomas, and they are usually preceded by adenomas. They express the cyclooxygenase-2 (COX-2) enzyme, which is not present in healthy colonic tissue.

The current incidence of colo-rectal tumours varies some 20-fold between different countries, with rates being highest in developed societies. Migrants to developed societies quickly develop the higher rates, suggesting the importance of "Western" lifestyle factors in the origin of colo-rectal neoplasms – probably including not only low levels of physical activity, but also smoking habits, alcohol consumption, and a change of diet. Colo-rectal cancer is now the third most frequent type of cancer in North America, with 150,000 new cases diagnosed annually in the United States alone.[1]

The impact of these tumours upon health economics is substantial, particularly if the population has a sedentary lifestyle. There have been a number of analyses of the direct costs of colo-rectal cancer; in the U.S., the aggregate costs for all forms of medical care over a five-year period were $3.1 billion, measured in 2004 dollars.[2] Few investigators have examined the indirect costs, particularly the considerable amount of the patient's time that is occupied by prolonged treatment, but one report set the annual total of direct and indirect costs in the range $5.5–6.5 billion in 2003.[3] Based on a 2-fold increase in the risk of colon cancer among those who are totally inactive and a 40% increase of risk among those who are irregularly active, the added direct annual cost of tumours related to physical inactivity for 1.5 million Blue Shield/Blue Cross subscribers in Minnesota was estimated at US$2.9 million.[4] Katzmarzyk et al.[5] assumed a more modest (and probably a more realistic) increase in the risk of colo-rectal cancers (1.39) for those who were sedentary relative to their active peers; they attributed a total direct annual cost (hospital and physician care, drugs and research) of Cdn$66 million to the colo-rectal consequences of physical inactivity in a Canadian population of 30.5 million. Janssen[6] estimated that by the year 2009, the cost to 33.6 million Canadians had risen to a direct expenditure of Cdn$61 million and an indirect expenditure of Cdn$283 million for a total of Cdn$344 million. Another analysis for the Province of Ontario, with a population of almost 13 million, set the direct costs at Cdn$31.7 million, and the indirect costs at Cdn$151 million, a total of Cdn$183 million for a population of some 13 million.[7]

In Europe, the 5-year survival rate following the diagnosis of a colo-rectal cancer averages about 60%. However, much depends on the stage of development of the tumour. For Stage I tumours, the 5-year survival is around 90%, for Stage III it is 60–85%, and for tumours that have spread to other parts of the body survival drops to around 12%; hence, the importance not only of prevention, but also of early detection.

Physical activity and prevention of colo-rectal cancers

Observations on physical activity and the prevention of colo-rectal cancer have been based on cross-sectional and case-control studies of populations differing in both the physical demands of occupation and the extent of reported leisure activities. Several authors have measured both of these variables, and in general they have found a closer association of cancer risk with occupational coding than with reported leisure activity.[8–11] Most heavy occupational work is characterized by its duration rather than its intensity, and it may be that in terms of countering the development of bowel cancer, prolonged moderate physical activity is more effective than shorter periods of intensive leisure activity. Also, inter-individual differences of occupational activity may be more stable and easier to ascertain than differences in leisure activity.

Regular physical activity seems to reduce the risk of colon cancer, but many investigators have found it has less influence upon cancer rates for the rectum (see Tables 9.1 to 9.4). Occupational hazards also seem to affect the risk of colonic and rectal tumours differently.[12,13] Probably for this reason, the benefits of physical activity have been less clearly apparent and findings have been more widely divergent when risk ratios for colon and rectal tumours have been considered jointly.[8,9,14–18] We will examine in turn associations between physical activity and the risk of cancer in occupational studies for the colon and the rectum and then of leisure studies for the colon and the rectum.

Occupational studies

Occupational studies have typically attempted to categorize energy expenditures based upon job titles, or have asked study participants about the hours of sitting, standing and involvement in more active work at their place of employment. Occupational classifications have the advantage that a given activity pattern is typically sustained over many years, including the period when carcinogenic change is likely to have begun, but findings may also be confounded by other factors that can modify cancer risk, particularly exposure to industrial carcinogens and differences of socio-economic status, with the latter also influencing the individual's area of residence, smoking, consumption of alcohol, diet and opportunities to participate in various leisure activities.

Table 9.1 Low levels of occupational activity and the risk of colonic cancer

Author	Subjects	Physical activity	Risk ratio	Covariates
Arbman et al. (1993)[12]	98 cancer, 370 hospital and 430 population controls	Years of sedentary work, >20 vs 0	OR 1.5 (0.9–2.5)	Age, sex
Brownson et al. (1991)[23,24]	1830 colon cancer vs 15,309 cancers at other sites	Low vs high occupational activity	OR 1.2 (1.0–1.5)	Age, smoking
Chow et al. (1993)[25,26]	13,940 women, 4892 men; cases 1293 M, 936 F	Sedentary vs active job, low vs high energy expenditure (based on SIRs)	Sedentary: M 1.29, F 0.99, Low energy M 1.48, F 1.36	Age, occupation, area of residence
Dosemeci et al. (1993)[27]	93 cases (M), 5613 controls	<8 vs >12 kJ/min; >6 vs <2 hours sitting	OR 1.8 (0.9–3.8) 1.4 (0.5–4.1)	Age, smoking, socio-economic status
Fraser and Pearce (1993)[28]	1651 male cases	Low energy expenditure based on occupational registry	RR 1.2 (1.0–1.4)	Age
Fredriksson et al. (1989)[22]	329 cases, 658 controls	Self-reported high vs low activity*	OR M 0.82 F 0.68	Age, sex
Garabrant et al. (1984)[29]	2950 cases	Sedentary vs high activity on job classification	RR 1.6 (1.3–1.8) (2.7 descending, 2.0 transverse colon, 1.5 sigmoid colon)	Age, race, socio-economic status
Gerhardsson et al. (1986)[30]	19-yr incidence in 1.1 million Swedish men 352 cases	Sedentary vs active job classification	RR 1.3 (1.1–1.6)	Age, marital and socio-economic status, population density, area of residence

continued

Table 9.1 Continued

Author	Subjects	Physical activity	Risk ratio	Covariates
Gerhardsson et al. (1988)[31]	14-yr incidence in Swedish twins, 102 cases	Self-reported moderate vs highly active job	RR 1.6 (0.8–2.9)	Age, sex, meat and coffee intake, area of residence
Isomura et al. (2006)[21]	778 cases, 767 controls	Hard vs sedentary	OR Colon 0.7 (0.4–1.0) Proximal 0.7 (0.4–1.4) Distal 0.6 (0.4–1.0)	Age, smoking, alcohol, area of residence, BMI, leisure activities
Jarebinski et al. (1989)[32] and Vlajinac et al. (1987)[33]	186 cases, 372 controls	Sedentary vs active job	1.22 (n.s.)	Smoking, alcohol, education, profession
Kato et al. (1990)[34]	756 cases, 16,600 controls	Moderate vs high activity	Moderate 0.58 (0.37–0.90) High 0.51 (0.30–0.87)	Age, marital status, smoking, alcohol, family history
Le Marchand et al. (1997)[35]	Cases 467 M, 358 F, 1192 controls	Years in sedentary work (most vs least)	OR all colon and rectum M 1.3 (0.9–1.9), F 1.5 (0.9–2.3) R colon M 1.8 (p=0.06) F 2.1 (p=0.05) L colon M 1.3 (p=0.26), F 1.0 (p=0.88)	Age, alcohol, smoking, diet, family history
Longnecker et al. (1995)[19]	163 cases R. colon, 703 controls	Lifetime sedentary vs > light occupation	OR 0.68 (0.31–1.52)	Smoking, diet, BMI, family history, income race
Lynge and Thygesen (1988)[36]	10-year incidence in 2 million+ people, 39 M, 20 F	Sedentary vs non-sedentary	RR M 1.38 (1.01–1.89) F 1.73 (1.06–2.68)	Age, sex
Markowitz et al. (1992)[9]	307 men vs 1164 controls	High vs low occupational activity	OR 0.5 (0.3–0.8)	Age, race, area of residence, recreational activity

Study	Sample	Comparison	Result	Adjusted for
Marti and Minder (1989)[37]	1995 cases	Low vs high activity	SMR Low 115 (106–135) High 89 (82–96)	Age
Moradi et al. (2008)[20]	18-year follow-up of 2 million Swedes, activity classified for 10 years; 5900 M, 2000 F	Sedentary vs high or very high for 1960, 1970	RR M 1.3 (1.2–1.4), 1.2 (1.1–1.3) F 1.1 (1.1–1.3) 1.2 (1.1–1.4) Proximal (M/F) 1.25/1.2 Transverse 1.15/1.3 Distal 1.25/1.15 Descending 1.5/1.0	
Paffenbarger et al. (1987, 1992)[15,38]	6351 longshoremen, 22-year mortality, 21 colo-rectal cases	Light vs heavy activity	RR 0.85	Age, "heavy" smoking, blood pressure
Persky et al. (1981)[39]	3132 cases, 5784 controls	Resting heart rate vs colon cancer deaths	No relation to cancer in one population, significantly higher in second sample	
Peters et al. (1989)[40]	147 cases, 147 controls	Low activity in longest held job	Transverse and descending colon 3.0 (1.2–7.2) All colon 1.7 (0.9–3.4)	Age, diet, BMI, area of residence, occupational exposures
Pukkala et al. (1993)[41]	9/1499 phys. ed. teachers, 26/8619 language teachers	Job type	SIR PE teachers 1.61 (0.74–3.05) Lang. teachers 1.25 (0.81–1.81)	Age
Severson et al. (1989)[42]	172 cases in 7925 Hawaiian-Japanese	Moderate or heavy vs sitting	RR 0.72 (0.52–1.00)	Age, smoking, BMI
Steindorf et al. (2005)[43]	98 incident cases, 193 controls	>147 vs 0 MET-hr/wk lifetime activity	OR 0.32 (0.15–0.71) p=0.003 to active jobs	BMI, smoking, alcohol, fibre intake, calcium intake

continued

Table 9.1 Continued

Author	Subjects	Physical activity	Risk ratio	Covariates
Tavani et al. (1999)[11]	451 M, 356 F cases, 4154 controls	*High to low occupational activity for M and F at age 30–39 yrs*	OR M 0.64 (0.44–0.93), F 0.49 (0.33–0.72) Ascending 0.79/0.43 trans, descend 0.46/0.29 sigmoid 0.54/0.58	Age, smoking, diet, BMI, height, marital status
Thune and Lund (1996)[44]	16-yr follow-up of 53,242 M, 28,274 F Cases 228 M, 98 F	*Heavy manual vs sedentary work*	RR M 0.82 (0.59–13), F 0.69 (0.34–1.42)	
Vena et al. (1985)[45]	210 male cases, 431 controls	>20 years of sedentary work vs none	OR M 1.97	Age
Vena et al. (1987)[46]	Analysis of 455,000 deaths, 6459 M, 604 F	Low vs highly active	PMR* M Low 120–124 High 89–93 High 80	Age
Vetter et al. (1987)[47]	87 M, 13 F cases, 371 controls	High vs low sitting time, low vs high energy expenditure	OR 1.5, 1.6 (effect largest in men, OR=1.9)	Age, smoking
Vineis et al. (1993)[48]	131 cases, 463 controls	Intensity <8kJ/min vs >12 kJ/min	OR M 1.40 F 1.10	Age, social class, area of residence
Whittemore et al. (1990)[49]	Chinese, 466 cases, 2448 matched controls	Self-reported sedentary vs active job	OR M =2.5 (1.1–5.9) F =1.2 (0.43–3.2)	Age, sex, diet, body size, time since migration to Canada

Note
* Studies where effect is calculated for high rather than for low activity are italicized.
Abbreviations: BMI = body mass index; F = female; M = male; OR = odds ratio; PMR = proportionate mortality ratio; RR = relative risk; SIR = standardized incidence ratio; SMR = standardized mortality ratio.

Some studies have simply made ratings of current work-place activity, but other investigators[10,19,20] have attempted to capture data on occupational energy demands over periods of 10 or 20 years or longer. Multivariate assessments of risk or odds ratios have typically included quite a wide range of covariates, including age, sex, smoking and alcohol consumption, diet, BMI and family history. A few studies[9,21] have also covaried for the extent of recreational activity.

Colon cancer. In terms of colon cancer (see Table 9.1), at least 31 studies have examined the risks associated with sedentary employment relative to that for physically more demanding types of work. Some reports have shown risk ratios of $2^{20,22}$ and even $3^{11,40}$ when sedentary individuals were compared with the most active employees. In many instances, confidence limits for the association were quite broad, but 13 studies found a significantly higher risk in those with sedentary work, and in a further 14 there was a positive trend, whereas a trend to greater risk in the active individuals was seen in only 4 reports.

Among the negative reports, the analysis of Paffenbarger *et al.*[15] was based upon a limited number of colon cancer deaths in longshoremen. And Persky *et al.*[39] found no relationship between resting heart rate (a rather indirect surrogate of habitual physical activity) and the risk of death from colon cancer in one sample, but in a second population the heart rate was significantly higher in those dying from colon cancer. In their comparison, Pukkala *et al.*[41] made the documented assumption that language teachers were less active than physical education teachers in terms of the frequency, duration and intensity of leisure exercise throughout the lifespan, but they included no covariates other than age in their analysis; the standardized incidence ratio of colon cancer was higher for the physical education teachers than the language teachers, but on the other hand the physical education teachers had a much lower risk of rectal cancers. One other small study[32,33] found no protection from a high level of occupational activity.

Individual studies include differing proportions of men and women, differing criteria for grading levels of physical activity, and differing covariates; moreover, some investigators have provided varying assessments of effect, depending on the subject's age and the tumour site, making any meta-analysis difficult. However, the approximate weighted risk ratio for a sedentary lifestyle across all of the 31 cited reports is 1.35.

As discussed further below, benefit has commonly been thought larger in men than in women,[47] perhaps because the physical demands and frequency of active employment were greater for men. However, formal comparison in 11 studies found respective risk ratios of 1.32 for men and 1.39 for women. Whittemore *et al.*[49] found that benefit was larger in North Americans residents than in Chinese, possibly in part because of dietary differences or lower levels of non-occupational physical activity in North America. Gerhardsson *et al.*[31] eliminated the effect of genetic susceptibility by comparing responses in twin pairs; using this model, they still showed a substantial risk ratio of 1.6 for those in sedentary employment.

Table 9.2 Low levels of occupational activity and the risk of rectal cancer

Author	Subjects	Physical activity	Risk ratio	Covariates
Arbman et al. (1993)[12]	79 cases, 801 controls	>20 yr vs 0 yr sedentary occupation	OR 1.7 (1.0–3.0)	Age, sex
Brownson et al. (1991)[23,24]	812 cases, 15,309 cancers at other sites	Low vs high occupational activity	OR 1.2 (0.8–1.7)	Age, smoking
Dosemeci et al. (1993)[27]	120 male cases, 5613 controls	<8 vs >12 kJ/min; >6 vs <2 hours sitting	OR 1.5 (0.7–2.9) 1.1 (0.4–2.6)	Age, smoking, socio-economic status
Fraser and Pearce (1993)[28]	1046 cases	Low vs high occupational activity	RR 1.3 (effect greatest at ages 45–54 yrs)	Age
Garabrant et al. (1984)[29]	1213 cases aged 20–64 yrs	Low vs high occupational activity	RR 0.9 (0.7–1.1)	Age, race, socio-economic status
Gerhardsson et al. (1986)[30]	19-year incidence, 1.1 million Swedish men, 217 cases	Sedentary vs active job	RR 1.1 (1.0–1.2)	Age, marital and socio-economic status, population density, area of residence
Husemann et al. (1980)[50]	105 recto-sigmoid cases vs 99 gall stones	Sedentary time	1.40 (higher for rectal carcinoma than for gallstones)	
Isomura et al. (2006)[21]	208 M, 120 F cases, 470 controls	Hard vs sedentary (MET-h/wk)*	OR 0.6 (0.4–0.9)	Age, smoking, alcohol, area of residence, BMI, leisure activities
Jarebinski et al. (1989)[32] and Vlajinac et al. (1987)[33]	98 cases, 196 controls	Sedentary vs active job	OR 1.0 No effect	Smoking, alcohol, education, profession
Kato et al. (1990)[34]	753 cases, 16600 controls	Moderate vs high.	RR Moderate 1.24 (0.72–2.15) High 0.70 (0.36–1.38)	Age, marital status, smoking, alcohol, family history
Le Marchand et al. (1997)[35]	221 M, 129 F cases, 1192 controls	Years in sedentary work (most vs least)	OR M 1.2 (p=0.51) F 0.6 (p=0.19)	Age, alcohol, smoking, diet, family history
Longnecker et al. (1995)[19]	242 cases, 703 controls	Lifetime sedentary vs > light occupation	OR 0.99 (0.44–2.21)	Smoking, diet, BMI, family history, income race

Study	Cases	Comparison	Effect (95% CI)	Adjustments
Lynge and Thygesen (1988)[36]	25 M, 4 F cases relative to general population	Sedentary vs non-sedentary	RR M 0.96 (0.62–1.42) F 0.61 (0.17–1.57)	Age, sex
Markowitz et al. (1992)[9]	123 men vs 1164 controls	*High vs low occupational activity*	OR 0.6 (0.3–1.1)	Age, race, area of residence, recreational activity
Marti and Minder (1989)[37]	1066 cases	Low vs high activity	SMR Low 102 High 105	Age
Moradi et al. (2008)[20]	18-year follow-up of 2 million Swedes, activity classified for 10 years, 4206 M, 1122 F	Sedentary vs very high 1960 and 1970	RR M 1.1 F 1.05	
Pukkala et al. (1993)[41]	1/1499 phys ed. teachers, 15/8619 language teachers	Job type vs SIR	PE teachers 0.27 (0.01–0.52), lang. teachers 1.10 (0.62–1.81)	Age
Severson et al. (1989)[42]	172 cases in 7925 Hawaiian-Japanese	*Moderate or vigorous vs sitting*	RR 1.23 (0.71–2.15)	Age, smoking, BMI
Tavani et al. (1999)[11]	350 M, 214 F cases, 4154 controls	*High to low occupational activity for M and F at age 30–39 yrs*	M 1.32 (0.86–2.03) F 0.88 (0.48–1.60)	
Thune and Lund (1996)[44]	16-yr follow-up of 53,242 M, 28,274 F (168M, 55F cases)	*Heavy manual vs sedentary work*	RR M 1.00 (0.69–1.45) F 9.88 (0.33–2.36)	Age, smoking, diet, BMI, height, marital status
Vena et al. (1985)[45]	276 male cases, 431 controls	>20 years of sedentary work vs none	OR 1.13	Age
Vena et al. (1987)[46]	Analysis of 455,000 deaths cases 2617 M, 118 F	Low vs highly active	PMR M Low 100–138 High 83–95 F Low 113 High 113	Age
Whittemore et al. (1990)[49]	Chinese, 439 cases, 2448 matched controls	Self-reported inactive vs active job	OR M 1.60 (0.55–4.7) F 0.84 (0.32–2.2)	Age, sex, diet, body size, time since migration to Canada

Note

* Studies where effect is calculated for high rather than for low activity are italicized.

Abbreviations: BMI = body mass index; F = female; M = male; OR = odds ratio; PMR = proportionate mortality ratio; RR = relative risk. SIR = standardized incidence ratio.

Table 9.3 Leisure activity or combined leisure+occupational activity and the risk of colon cancer

Author	Subjects	Physical activity	Risk ratio	Covariates
Ballard-Barbash et al. (1990)[54]	73 M, 79 F with large bowel cancer from 1906 M and 2308 F	Least active vs most active tertile	RR M 1.8 (1.0–3.2) F 1.1 (0.6–1.8)	Age, BMI
Bostik et al. (1994)[55]	210 cases, prospective study of 35,215 women	3-level classification of physical activity, vigorous vs low*	RR 0.95 (0.68–1.39)	Multiple covariates
Calton et al. (2006)[56]	243 cases, prospective study of 31,783 women	Self-administered questionnaire, quintiles of activity over past 12 months	RR 1.15 (0.75–1.75) if active	Age, BMI, education, family history, smoking, alcohol, calcium, red meat, use of HRT and aspirin
Chao et al. (2004)[57]	536 M, 404 F cases in 70,403 M, 80,771 F	Self-reported: >8 hrs/wk vs 0 and >30 vs 0 MET-hrs/wk leisure activity	RR M 0.58 (0.39–0.87), 0.60 (0.41–0.87) F 0.65 (0.39–1.11), 0.77 (0.48–1.24) M 1.67 F 1.30	Age, education, prior exercise level, smoking, alcohol, red meat, folate, fibre, multivitamins and hormone replacement in women
Gerhardsson et al. (1986)[30]	19-yr incidence in 1.1 million Swedish men, 102 cases	Least vs most active	RR 1.6 (1.0–2.7) (combined)	Age, marital and socio-economic status, population density, area of residence
Gerhardsson et al. (1990)[58]	352 cases, 512 controls	Sedentary vs very active	RR 1.8 (1.0–2.7) (combined); L. colon 3.2, R. colon 1.1	Age, sex, BMI, diet, energy intake
Giovannucci et al. (1995)[59]	201 cases in 47,723 male health professionals over 6 yrs	46.8 vs 0 MET-h/wk	RR 0.53 (0.32–0.88)	
Isomura et al. (2006)[21]	248 cases, 468 controls	>16 vs 0 MET-h/wk leisure	OR Colon 0.8 (0.5–1.2) Proximal 1.3 (0.6–2.7) Distal 0.5 (0.3–1.1)	Age, smoking, alcohol, area of residence, BMI, leisure activities
Kato et al. (1990)[34]	221 cases, 578 controls	Sport <1 h/wk vs >1–2/wk	RR <1/wk 0.72 (0.44–1.19) >1–2/wk 0.55 (0.33–0.89)	Age, marital status, smoking, alcohol, family history

Study	Population	Activity measure	Result	Adjustments
Le Marchand et al. (1997)[35]	8467 M, 358 F cases, 1192 controls	Greatest vs least tertile of lifetime leisure activity	OR R colon M 0.7 (p=0.1), F 0.6 (p=0.08); L colon M 0.7 (p=0.34), F 0.6 (p=0.22)	Age, alcohol, smoking, diet, family history
Lee et al. (1991)[52]	17,148 Harvard alumni, 225 cases over 23 yrs	Leisure activity >10 vs <4 MJ/wk	RR 0.50 (0.27–0.93)	Age
Lee and Paffenbarger (1994)[53]	17,607 Harvard alumni, 280 cases	Leisure activity >10 vs <4 MJ/wk	RR 1.08 (0.81–1.46), 0.94 (0.54–1.64)	Age, BMI, parental history. Note: positive effect if BMI >26 units
Lee et al. (1997)[60]	21,807 physicians, 217 cases	Vigorous exercise vs >5/wk vs none	RR 1.1 (0.7–1.6)	Age, obesity, alcohol
Longnecker et al. (1995)[19]	163 cases R. colon, 703 controls	Vigorous activity >2h/wk vs none	OR 0.57 (0.33–0.97)	Smoking, diet, BMI, family history, income race
Marcus et al. (1994)[61]	536 F cases, 2315 controls	Active >7 vs 0–1 times/wk	OR 0.46 (0.19–1.10)	Benefit only seen with high frequency
Martinez et al. (1997)[62]	396 cases colon cancer in F	Self-reported >20 vs <2 MET-h/wk leisure activities	RR 0.54 (0.33–0.90); no difference by colonic site	Age, smoking, family history, BMI, HRT, red meat and alcohol
Polednak (1976)[51]	107 cases in 8393 men	Sedentary vs minor and major university athletes	Mortality rates: Major athletes 15.2 Minor athletes 13.3 Non-athletes 12.3	Body size
Schnohr et al. (2005)[63]	14-yr follow-up of 13,216 F and 18,718 M; colon cancer 180 (F), 215 (M)	Self-reported leisure activity, RR for moderate and vigorous activity	RR Moderate M 1.08 (0.74–1.57) F 1.02 (0.70–1.50) Vigorous M 0.72 (0.47–1.11) F 0.90 (0.56–1.46)	Age, smoking, alcohol, education, birth cohort, BMI

continued

Table 9.3 Continued

Author	Subjects	Physical activity	Risk ratio	Covariates
Severson et al. (1989)[42]	172 cases in 7925 Hawaiian-Japanese	*Physical activity index high vs low*	RR 0.71 (0.51–0.99)	Age, smoking, BMI
Slattery et al. (1988, 1990)[64,65]	229 cases, 384 controls	*High activity vs no activity 2 yrs before diagnosis*	0.70 (0.38–1.29) Intense 0.27 (0.11–0.65) Low 1.25 (0.68–2.29)	Age, sex, BMI, smoking, education, area of residence
Slattery (2002)[66]	1993 cases, 2410 matched controls	*Highest vs lowest lifetime leisure*	OR 0.6 (0.5–0.7)	Age, BMI, tumour site
Steindorf et al. (2005)[43]	98 incident cases, 193 controls	*>74 vs <23 MET-hr/wk*	OR 0.82 (0.36–1.90) for active	BMI, smoking, alcohol, fibre intake, calcium intake
Thun et al. (1992)[67]**	1150 cases in 764,343 patients over 6 yrs	*High vs low leisure activity*	RR 0.60 (0.27–1.27)	Ager, smoking, diet, BMI, height, marital status
Thune and Lund (1996)[44]	230 M, 99 F cases in 80,616 people over 16 yrs	*Regular training vs sedentary*	RR M 1.33 (0.90–1.98) F 0.84 (0.43–1.65)	Age, smoking, BMI, lipids, height, marital status
White et al. (1996)[68]	444 cases, 427 controls	*2/wk vs no leisure activity >4.5 METs*	RR 0.70 (0.49–1.00)	Age, sex, BMI, health behaviours
Whittemore et al. (1990)[49]	274 M, 192 F cases, 2448 matched controls	Sedentary vs active	OR M (N. Am) 1.6 (1.1–2.4) M (China) 0.85 (0.39–1.9) F (N. Am) 2.0 (1.2–3.3) F (China) 2.5 (1.0–6.3)	Diet, BMI, time in N. America
Yang et al. (1994)[69]	267 L, 247 r-sided colon cancer		Physical activity related more to L-sided cancer	

Notes

* Studies where effect if for high rather than for low activity are italicized.

** Thun[67] and Waterbor et al.[70] (Table 9.4) also focussed on the interaction between physical activity and fatalities rather than the incidence of colon cancer.

Abbreviations: BMI = body mass index; F = female; M = male; HRT = hormone replacement therapy; METs = metabolic equivalents; N. Am = North America; OR = odds ratio; RR = relative risk.

Rectal cancer. In contrast to colon cancer, the association between a high level of occupational activity and rectal cancer is inconsistent, with some reports suggesting a substantial benefit, and others either no effect or even an adverse response (see Table 9.2). Of 23 investigations, 5 showed a significant adverse association with sedentary work, and a further 9 a similar trend, but 9 studies showed no effect or even an adverse association with physically demanding employment. The weighted mean risk across the 23 studies approximated 1.18 for those with sedentary work. Eight studies allowed a sex comparison, and in these reports the weighted risk ratio for sedentary employment was 1.15 in men and 0.91 in women.

Studies of leisure activity

Studies of associations between reported patterns of leisure activity and the risks of colon and rectal cancer generally confirm the inferences drawn from occupational studies.

Colon cancer. A total of 25 studies have evaluated the effect of a low level of leisure activity upon the risk of colon cancer. The findings are somewhat similar to those for occupational activity, with 13 reports showing a significant association between a sedentary lifestyle and an increased risk, and 7 other investigations finding a similar trend, against only 5 studies finding an adverse association with an active lifestyle, one of these 5 being based on death rates rather than the incidence of colonic cancer.[51] The weighted risk ratio is 1.58 (see Table 9.3).

In a few instances, the findings reported by the same laboratory have been quite inconsistent; thus, Lee *et al.* reported a risk ratio of 0.50 for active Harvard alumni in 1991,[52] but 3 years later, an analysis for almost the same group of subjects but over a differing time period reported a risk of only 1.08.[53] Seven studies compared responses in men and women, with respective risk ratios of 1.55 and 1.40. Polednak[51] compared major and minor university athletes with non-athletes who had attended the same institutions; the death rates were higher and the ages of death from colon cancer lower for the athletes than for the non-athletes, even after controlling for differences of body build.

Rectal cancer. There have been at least 15 studies of leisure activity and rectal cancer; 8 of these have shown a favourable trend, but this was statistically significant in only one report (see Table 9.4); moreover 7 reports showed no effect or a trend to a negative association. Averaging across the 15 studies, the weighted risk ratio approximated 1.20 for those with a sedentary lifestyle (see Table 9.4). Five of these reports compared effects in men and women, finding weighted risk ratios of 1.46 for men and 1.16 for women.

Conclusions. The data presented in this chapter show that for colon cancer there have been at least 31 occupational studies, and 25 studies of leisure activity, a number of the latter described in the same reports. Of these, 26 found a significant advantage to the more active individuals, and a further 21 showed a similar trend, with neutral or negative findings in only 9 studies; the average benefit over the 56 studies was 40%.

Table 9.4 Leisure activity or combined leisure + occupational activity and the risk of rectal cancer

Author	Subjects	Physical activity	Risk ratio	Covariates
Chao et al. (2004)[57]	390 cases in 70,403 M, 80,771 F	Self-reported, >8 hrs/wk vs 0*	0.83 (0.59–1.16)	Age, education, prior exercise level, smoking, alcohol, red meat, folate, fibre, multivitamins and hormone replacement
Gerhardsson et al. (1988)[31]	14-yr incidence in 16,447 Swedes	Recreational activity	RR 1.2 (0.7–2.2)	Age, sex, diet
Gerhardsson et al. (1990)[58]	Cases 107 M, 110 F, 512 controls	Sedentary vs very active	RR M 0.90 (0.3–2.4) 1.40 F 1.4 (0.4–4.9)	Age, sex, BMI, diet, energy intake
Isomura et al. (2006)[21]	198 M, 132 F cases, 470 controls	>15 vs, 0 MET-h/wk leisure	OR 0.5 (0.3–0.8)	Age, smoking, alcohol, area of residence, BMI, leisure activities
Kato et al. (1990)[34]	221 cases, 578 controls	Sport <1 h/wk vs >1–2/wk	RR <1 h/wk 0.86 (0.50–1.50) >1–2/wk 0.54 (0.30–0.97)	Age, marital status, smoking, area of residence
Le Marchand et al. (1997)[35]	221 M, 129 F cases, 1192 controls	Greatest vs least tertile lifetime recreation	OR M 0.5 (p=0.07) F 0.8 (p=0.97)	Age, alcohol, smoking, diet, family history
Lee et al. (1991)[52]	17,148 Harvard alumni, 44 cases over 23 yrs	Leisure activity >10 vs <4 MJ/wk	RR 1.43 (0.78–2.60)	Age
Lee and Paffenbarger (1994)[53]	17,607 Harvard alumni, 53 cases	Leisure activity >10 vs <4 MJ/wk	RR 1.71 (0.88–3.31) 2.75 (0.50–15.12)	Age, BMI, parental history

Study	Sample	Activity measure	Result	Adjustments
Lee et al. (1997)[60]	21,807 physicians, 217 cases	*Vigorous exercise >5/wk vs none*	RR 1.1 (0.7–1.6)	Age, obesity, alcohol
Longnecker et al. (1995)[19]	242 cases, 703 controls	*Vigorous activity >2h/wk vs none*	OR 1.19 (0.70–2.04)	Smoking, diet, BMI, family history, income race
Schnohr et al. (2005)[63]	14-yr follow-up of 13,216 F and 18,718 M; colon cancer 180 (F), 215 (M)	*Self-reported leisure activity, RR for moderate and vigorous activity*	RR Moderate M 0.87 (0.53–1.41) Vigorous M 0.89 (0.53–1.49)	Age, smoking, alcohol, education, birth cohort, BMI
Severson et al. (1989)[42]	172 cases in 7925 Hawaiian-Japanese	*High vs low activity index*	RR 1.41 (0.84–2.36)	Age, smoking, BMI
Thune and Lund (1996)[44]	228 cases in 80,616 people over 16 yr	*Regular training vs sedentary*	RR M 0.98 (0.60–1.61) F 1.49 (0.53–4.22)	Age, smoking, BMI, lipids, height, marital status
Waterbor et al. (1988)[70]	985 baseball players	Mortality, sedentary vs players	0.95	Playing position, waist/height ratio
Whittemore et al. (1990)[49]	236 M, 203 F cases	Sedentary	OR M (N. Am) 1.5 (0.93–2.5) M (China) 0.71 (0.32–1.6) (0.32–1.6) F (N Am) 1.9 F (China) 0.69 (0.34–1.4)	Diet, BMI, time in N. America

Note
* Studies where effect if for high rather than for low activity are italicized.
Abbreviations: BMI = body mass index; F = female; M = male.

There have now been more than 40 reports looking at the relationship between physical activity and colon cancer, mostly showing a graded inverse relationship.[71-73] A review of 48 leisure and occupational studies published in 2001 reached similar conclusions to those stated above. It found 35 of 48 investigations showing a 10–70% reduction of colon cancer risk, with benefit most apparent in those practising at least moderate activity (>4.5 METs, >10 MJ/wk).[73] A meta-analysis to 2008 accessed 52 articles.[74] It estimated a relative risk of 0.76 (0.72–0.81) in the more active individuals, and little difference between men and women. However, this report underlined that benefit was more clearly shown in case-control studies (RR 0.69 (0.65–0.74)) than in cohort studies (RR 0.83 (0.78–0.88)). Another recent review article and meta-analysis found a fairly consistent association between habitual physical activity and a 25–30% protection against colon cancer.[75]

Not all of the studies in women have demonstrated statistically significant effects of leisure or total activity. However, this may reflect the small proportion of women who engage in physically demanding employment and imprecision in the ascertainment of other forms of vigorous physical activity such as housekeeping responsibilities over the life span.[56]

The findings are a little less conclusive for rectal than for colonic tumours. Of 23 occupational and 15 leisure studies analysed in this chapter, only 6 have found a significant advantage to the more active individuals, with 16 showing a positive trend, and 16 neutral or negative conclusions. The average benefit associated with an active lifestyle was about 19%.

Moderating factors

Pattern of exercise. The preventive value of physical activity is modulated not only by its intensity and duration, but also by its timing relative to a carcinogenic process that can continue for 20 years or more. Fraser and Pearce noted that occupational activity seemed particularly effective in reducing the risk of colon cancer if practised between 35 and 54 years of age, while for rectal cancer the critical age range was 45–54 years.[28] Likewise, Tavani et al.[11] found the greatest effect with activity at 15–19 years. Vetter et al. also saw the largest response in those less than 45 years old,[47] and Markowitz et al. found the largest effect from activity in the age range 22–44 years.[9] However, Steindorf et al.[43] noted substantial benefit from activity at all ages from 20 to 50 years.

Chao et al.[57] showed a clear dose–response relationship to the reported volume of leisure activity for colon cancer, whether measured in hours per week or MET-hours per week. However, no benefit was associated with physical activity that had occurred ten years prior to the analysis. Interestingly, in this study a similar benefit was associated with slight or moderate/heavy recreational activity, provided that the weekly time allocation was similar. Marcus et al.[61] also looked at the influence of the frequency of exercise, and in their sample little difference of risk was observed between 0 and 7 times per week, but in the serious exercisers (>7 times per week), there was a substantial trend to a reduction of risk (0.46 (0.19–1.10)). Schnohr *et al.*[63] also found that the trend to benefit was much greater for vigorous than for moderate physical activity, and in the study of Slattery *et al.*[64] highly significant benefit was associated with intense activity (OR 0.27 (0.11–0.66)) but light activity had no effect (OR 1.25 (0.68–2.29)).

Most studies have focussed upon the benefits of aerobic exercise. However, a study of resistance exercise, based on 870 cases and 996 controls[75] found non-significant trends to a possible benefit from resistance training of a similar order to that seen in many of the aerobic studies (OR 0.70 (95% confidence interval 0.45–1.11)).

Region of benefit. Several investigations have compared the effects of physical activity upon the risk of cancer for various parts of the colon, but perhaps because of relatively small sample sizes the findings have not agreed. The greatest benefit has been reported variously in the caecal region,[23,28] the ascending colon,[20,28,29,34,42,44] the transverse colon[30,40] or the distal colon.[20–22,40,76] A recent review and meta-analysis of 21 studies concluded that the benefit of increased physical activity was distributed equally across the various colonic sites,[75] a finding also noted in several individual studies.[62]

Sex differences in exercise response. Many investigators have reported a stronger protective effect of physical activity in men than in women.[8,14,41,44,54,55,63,77–80] Although there could be a hormonal explanation for this apparent difference, this could also reflect greater difficulty in assessing all of the habitual physical activity of women with current questionnaires, a lower overall level of physical activity, or in some studies a smaller number of cases of colonic cancer in the women.

Mechanisms of protection

One plausible explanation of the reduced susceptibility of physically active individuals to colon cancer would be that exercise increases colonic motility, and thus reduces mucosal exposure to carcinogenic toxins within the bowels. The effect of both single bouts of exercise and habitual training upon colonic motility give some support to this concept. An increase of prostaglandin secretion may also be involved. Prostaglandins can stimulate colonic motility and thus reduce colonic exposure to toxins. Demers *et al.*[81] noted that completion of a marathon run led to significant increases in plasma levels of several prostaglandins (PGE2, PGF2α and 6-keto PGF1α).

Exercise may also influence the process of colonic segmentation. Thus, Holdstock *et al.*[82] used radio-opaque markers and pressure sensors to demonstrate a substantial increase of postprandial intra-luminal pressures, with physical activity (walking vs sitting or lying) converting activity into a forward, propulsive movement of the gut contents.

Many other possible mechanisms could be involved in protecting active individuals against colonic cancer, such as a change of diet or personal lifestyle, a reduction of body fat content and a modulation of hormone levels or immune function.[83] The person who exercises regularly is likely to be a non-smoker, is usually less obese than a sedentary individual, and may opt for a diet that is high in fibre and low in fat. The possible importance of obesity was underlined in the study of Lee and Paffenbarger,[53] where the overall response to an active lifestyle tended to be negative, but a large positive trend was seen in those with a body mass index $>26 \text{kg/m}^2$; by 2 methods of calculation, the relative risk in those spending >10 vs <4 MET-h/week were 0-.56 (0.29–1.09, p=0.09) and 0.19 (0.02–1.52, p=0.09).

The active individual is also protected against diabetes mellitus, and several studies have shown that those with diabetes are more likely to develop colo-rectal cancer over a 13-year follow-up (risk ratio for diabetics 1.30, in men; 1.16, not significant, in women[79]; male diabetics no significant effect, women risk ratio of 1.55[77]; risk ratio of 1.40 in male diabetics, 1.43 in women[17]). It could simply be that those with diabetes are under increased medical surveillance, and thus colonic tumours are detected more readily. Alternatively, the tumour could exacerbate a sub-clinical case of diabetes, leading to its diagnosis. Finally, the diabetes may have distorted hormonal balance, favouring tumour growth.

Physical activity and management of colo-rectal neoplasms

There is now some evidence that a substantial volume of physical activity (perhaps as much as 18 MET-hours per week of reported leisure pursuits) may decrease mortality in those who have previously been treated for colo-rectal cancers,[76,84] although further research is needed to be sure that a poor prognosis is not impeding an active lifestyle rather than regular physical activity having a positive effect upon prognosis. Benefit may reflect exercise-induced enhancement of immuno-surveillance, or a decrease in inflammation and oxidant stress.

For some who have undergone colonic resection, the challenge may be to continue exercising while controlling an ileostomy. However, this is not an impossible task, as shown by the example of the American football player Rolf Benirschke, who continues to ski, swim and play hockey after the creation of an ileostomy.[85] McGowan *et al.* have suggested that the encouragement of sport may be a useful tactic in increasing physical activity among survivors of a colo-rectal cancer.[86]

Areas for further research

The vast majority of colonic cancers appear to have their origin in asymptomatic polyps.[87] It is thus important to identify and correct the multiple risk factors (possibly including physical inactivity) that influence the conversion of these initially benign growths into malignant tumours.[88] Analysis is hampered by the long disease latency. In particular, it has been necessary to explore the physical activity patterns and lifestyle of subjects over periods of 20 years and longer, and there remains scope to find a reliable objective method of summarizing a person's lifetime experience of an active lifestyle. Possibly, greater emphasis needs to be placed on measuring the outcomes of regular physical activity, such as attained levels of aerobic fitness and muscular development.

Many investigators have reported a stronger protective effect of physical activity in men than in women. Data from controlled animal experiments have partially confirmed human epidemiological investigations in showing a larger response in male animals,[89] and the underlying reasons for this sex differential should be clarified.

Further work is also needed to determine optimal patterns of physical activity for the prevention of colo-rectal tumours. To date, almost all studies have been based on aerobic programmes, and there is scope to compare the benefits of aerobic and resistance exercise.

Finally, there is need for additional study to confirm the benefits of physical activity in those who have been treated for established cancers,[84] and to identify methods of encouraging an active lifestyle among cancer survivors. Moreover, research is required to ensure that the better prognosis of active individuals is due to their activity, rather than that a poor prognosis is impeding exercise participation.

Practical implications

Although most studies show substantial differences in the risks of colon and rectal cancer between those who are sedentary and those who have a very high level of physical activity either at work or in their leisure time, this does not necessarily imply that the enrolment of sedentary individuals in an exercise programme would yield an equivalent gain of health. There are two main reasons for caution. First, the risk of carcinogenesis was likely accumulated over 10 or 20 years of inadequate physical activity, and reversal of this process will probably require compliance with a vigorous exercise regimen for an equally long period. Second, the risk ratios presented in this chapter have been calculated by comparing the experience of sedentary individuals with the most active members of each sample, and in many instances the optimal level of weekly physical activity was much higher than would likely be attained if a sedentary person were encouraged to enter an exercise programme.

Nevertheless, the association between a physically active lifestyle and a reduced risk of colo-rectal cancer has now been amply demonstrated, and it seems of a clinically important magnitude. This is thus yet one more important reason for health professionals to encourage a greater level of habitual physical activity among the general population. The development of a colo-rectal cancer also provokes a careful evaluation of personal lifestyle, and some investigators have suggested that a discussion of the link between low levels of physical activity and colon cancer may be a useful means of persuading not only the patients but also their relatives[86,90,91] to begin exercising on a regular basis.

Conclusions

Life-long physical activity, whether due to a physically demanding occupation or vigorous leisure pursuits, is associated with a reduced risk of developing cancers of the large intestine, with protection being greater for the colon than for the rectum. The common assumption that physical activity has more effect in men than in women is probably due either to the fact that men more commonly engage in hard physical work, or that questionnaires fail to capture many of the physical activities performed by women. Benefit seems to occur equally in various regions of the colon, and is associated with aerobic exercise, but the benefits of resistance exercise have yet to be confirmed. Possible mechanisms that could be involved in protecting active individuals against colonic cancer include an increased intestinal motility and differences in colonic segmentation, possibly mediated by altered prostaglandin secretions, with a resulting reduced mucosal exposure to carcinogenic toxins. Other possibilities are a change of diet or personal lifestyle, a reduction of body fat content and a modulation of hormone levels or immune function.[83] Physical activity should be maintained as far as is possible following successful treatment of the cancer, as regular exercisers seem to have better survival prospects.

References

1 Haggar FA, Boushey RB. Colorectal cancer epidemiology: incidence, mortality, survival, and risk factors. *Clin Colon Rectal Surg* 2009; 22(4): 191–197.

2 Yabroff KR, Borowski LL, J. Economic studies in colorectal cancer: Challenges in measuring and comparing costs. *J Natl Cancer Inst Monogr* 2013; 2013(46): 62–78.

3 Redaelli A, Cranor CW, Okano GJ *et al.* Screening, prevention and socioeconomic costs associated with the treatment of colorectal cancer. *Pharmacoeconomics* 2003; 21(17): 1213–1238.

4 Garrett NA, Brasure M, Schmitz KH *et al.* Physical inactivity. Direct cost to a health plan. *Am J Prev Med* 2004; 27(4): 304–309.

5 Katzmarzyk PT, Gledhill N, Shephard RJ. The economic burden of physical inactivity in Canada. *Can Med Assoc J* 2000; 163(11): 1435–1440.

6 Janssen I. Health care costs of physical inactivity in Canadian adults. *Appl Physiol Nutr Metab* 2012; 37: 803–806.

7 Katzmarzyk PT. The economic costs associated with physical inactivity and obesity. *Health Fitness J Canada* 2011; 4(4): 31–40.

8 Albanes D, Blair A, Taylor PR. Physical activity and risk of cancer in the NHANES I population. *Am J Publ Health* 1989; 79: 744–750.

9 Markowitz S, Morabia A, Garibaldi K *et al.* Effect of occupational and recreational activity on the risk of colorectal cancer among males: a case-control study. *Int J Epidemiol* 1992; 21(6): 1057–1062.

10 Slattery ML, Edwards S, Curtin K *et al.* Physical activity and colorectal cancer. *Am J Epidemiol* 2003; 158(3): 214–224.

11 Tavani A, Braga C, La Vecchia C *et al.* Physical activity and risk of cancers of the colon and rectum: an Italian case-control study. *Br J Cancer* 1999; 79(11/12): 1912–1916.

12 Arbman G, Axelson O, Fredricksson M *et al.* Do occupational factors influence the risk of colon and rectal cancer in different ways? *Cancer* 1993; 72: 2543–2549.
13 Weisburger JH, Wynder EL. Etiology of colorectal cancer with emphasis on mechanism of action and prevention. *Important Adv Oncol* 1987: 197–220.
14 Levi F, Psche C, Lucchini F *et al.* Occupational and leisure-time physical activity and the risk of colorectal cancer. *Eur J Cancer Prevention* 1999; 8: 487–493.
15 Paffenbarger RS, Hyde RT, Wing AL. Physical activity and the incidence of cancer in diverse populations: A preliminary report. *Am J Clin Nutr* 1987; 45: 312–317.
16 Peters HP, Bos M, Seebregts L *et al.* Gastrointestinal symptoms in long-distance runners, cyclists and triathletes: prevalence, medication and etiology. *Am J Gastroenterol* 1999; 94: 1570–1581.
17 Steenland K, Nowlin S, Palu S. Cancer incidence in the National Health and Nutrition Survey 1. Follow-up data: diabetes, cholesterol, pulse and physical activity. *Cancer Epidemiol Biomarkers Prev* 1995; 4: 807–811.
18 Zhang C. A case-control study of colorectal cancer in Beijing. *Chung Hua Liu Hsing Ping Hsueh Tsa Chih* 1992; 13: 321–324.
19 Longnecker MP, Gerhardsson de Verdier M, Frumkin H *et al.* A case-control study of physical activity in relation to risk of cancer of the right colon and rectum in men. *Int J Epidemiol* 1995; 24: 42–50.
20 Moradi T, Gridley G, Björk J *et al.* Occupational physical activity and risk for cancer of the colon and rectum in Sweden among men and women by anatomic subsite. *Eur J Cancer Prev* 2008; 17(3): 201–208.
21 Isomura K, Kono S, Moore MA *et al.* Physical activity and colorectal cancer: The Fukuoka colorectal cancer study. *Cancer Sci* 2006; 97: 1099–1104.
22 Fredriksson M, Bengtsson N-O, Hardell L *et al.* Colon cancer, physical activity, and occupational exposure. *Cancer* 1989; 63: 1838–1842.
23 Brownson RC, Zahm SH, Chang JC *et al.* Occupational risk of colon cancer. An analysis by anatomical subsite. *Am J Epidemiol* 1989; 130(4): 675–687.
24 Brownson RC, Chang JC, Davis JR *et al.* Physical activity on the job and cancer in Missouri. *Am J Publ Health* 1991; 81: 639–642.
25 Chow WH, Dosemeci M, Zheng R *et al.* Physical activity and occupational risk of colon cancer in Shanghai, China. *Int J Epidemiol* 1993; 22: 23–29.
26 Chow WH, Malker HS, Hsing AW *et al.* Occupational risks for colon cancer in Sweden. *J Occup Med* 1994; 36: 647–651.
27 Dosemeci M, Hayes RB, Vetter R *et al.* Occupational physical activity, socioeconomic status, and risks of 15 cancer sites in Turkey. *Cancer Cause Control* 1993; 4: 313–321.
28 Fraser G, Pearce N. Occupational physical activity and risk of cancer of the colon and rectum in New Zealand males. *Cancer Causes Control* 1993; 4(1): 45–50.
29 Garabrant DH, Peters JM, Mack TM *et al.* Job activity and colon cancer risk. *Am J Epidemiol* 1984; 119: 1005–1114.
30 Gerhardsson M, Norell SE, Kiviranta H *et al.* Sedentary jobs and colon cancer. *Am J Epidemiol* 1986; 123: 775–780.
31 Gerhardsson M, Floderus B, Norell SE. Physical activity and colon cancer risk. *Int J Epidemiol* 1988; 17: 743–746.
32 Jarebinski M, Adanja B, Valjinac H. Case-control study of relationship of some biosocial correlates to rectal cancer patients in Belgrade, Yugoslavia. *Neoplasma* 1989; 36: 369–374.
33 Vlajinac H, Jarebinski M, Adanja B. Relationship of some biosocial factors to colon cancer in Belgrade (Yugoslavia). *Neoplasma* 1987; 34(4): 503–507.

34 Kato I, Tominga S, Matsuura A, Yoshii Y *et al.* A comparative case-control study of colorectal cancer and adenoma. *Jpn J Cancer Res* 1990; 81: 1101–1108.

35 Le Marchand L, Wilkens LR, Kolonel L *et al.* Associations of sedentary lifestyle, obesity, smoking, alcohol use, and diabetes with the risk of colorectal cancer. *Cancer Res* 1997; 57: 4787–4794.

36 Lynge E, Thygesen L. Use of surveillance systems for occupational cancer: Data from the Danish national system. *Int J Epidemiol* 1988; 17: 493–500.

37 Marti B, Minder CE. Physische Berufsaktivität und Kolonkarzinommortalität bei Schweizer Männern 1979–1982 [Physical activity at work and colon carcinoma in Swiss men 1979–1982]. *Sozial Praeventivmed* 1989; 34: 30–37.

38 Paffenbarger RS, Lee I-M, Wing AL. The influence of physical activity on the incidence of site-specific cancers in college alumni. *Adv Exp Med Biol* 1992; 322: 7–15.

39 Persky V, Dyer AR, Leonas J *et al.* Heart rate: A risk factor for cancer? *Am J Epidemiol* 1981; 114: 477–487.

40 Peters RK, Garabrandt DH, Yu MC *et al.* A case-control study of occupational and dietary factors in colorectal cancer in young men by subsite. *Cancer Res* 1989; 49: 5459–5468.

41 Pukkala E, Poskiparta M, Apter D *et al.* Life-long physical activity and cancer risk among Finnish female teachers. *Eur J Cancer Prev* 1993; 2(5): 369–376.

42 Severson RK, Nomura AMY, Grove JS *et al.* Prospective analysis of physical activity and cancer. *Am J Epidemiol* 1989; 130(3): 522–529.

43 Steindorf K, Jedrychowski W, Schmidt M *et al.* Case-control study of lifetime occupational and recreational physical activity and risks of colon and rectal cancer. *Eur J Cancer Prev* 2005; 14: 363–371.

44 Thune I, Lund E. Physical activity and risk of colorectal cancer in men and women. *Br J Cancer* 1996; 73: 1134–1140.

45 Vena JE, Graham S, Zielezny M *et al.* Lifetime occupational exercise and colon cancer. *Am J Epidemiol* 1985; 122(3): 357–365.

46 Vena JE, Graham S, Zielezny M *et al.* Occupational exercise and risk of cancer. *Am J Clin Nutr* 1987; 45: 318–327.

47 Vetter R, Dosemeci M, Blair S *et al.* Occupational physical activity and colon cancer risk in Turkey. *Eur J Epidemiol* 1992; 8: 845–850.

48 Vineis P, Ciccone G, Magnino A. Asbestos exposure, physical activity and colon cancer: a case-control study. *Tumori* 1993; 79: 301–303.

49 Whittemore AS, Wu-Williams AH, Lee M *et al.* Diet, physical activity, and colorectal cancer among Chinese in North America and China. *J Natl Cancer Inst* 1990; 82(11): 915–926.

50 Husemann B, Neubauer MG, Duhme C. Sitzende Tätigkeit und Rektum-Sigma-Karzinoma [Sitting activity and recto-sigmoid carcinomna]. *Onkologie* 1980; 4: 168–171.

51 Polednak AP. College athletics, body size and cancer mortality. *Cancer* 1976; 38: 382–387.

52 Lee IM, Paffenbarger RS, Hsieh C. Physical activity and risk of developing colorectal cancer among college alumni. *J Natl Cancer Inst* 1991; 83: 1324–1329.

53 Lee I-M, Paffenbarger RS. Physical activity and its relation to cancer risk: a prospective study of college alumni. *Med Sci Sports Exerc* 1994; 26: 831–837.

54 Ballard-Barbash R, Schatzkin A, Albanes D *et al.* Physical activity and risk of large bowel cancer in the Framingham study. *Cancer Res* 1990; 50: 3610–3613.

55 Bostick RM, Potter JD, Kushi LH *et al.* Sugar, meat, and fat intake, and non-dietary risk factors for colon cancer incidence in Iowa women (United States). *Cancer Causes Control* 1994; 5(1): 38–52.

56 Calton BA, Lacey JV, Schatzin A *et al.* Physical activity and the risk of colon cancer among women: A prospective cohort study (United States). *Int J Cancer* 2006; 119: 385–391.

57 Chao AC, Connell CJ, Jacobs EJ *et al.* Amount and timing of recreational physical activity in relation to colon and rectal cancer in older adults: the Cancer Prevention Study II Nutrition Cohort. *Cancer Epidemiol Biomarkers Prev* 2004; 13: 2187–2195.

58 Gerhardsson de Verdier M, Steineck G, Hagman U *et al.* Physical activity and colon cancer: A case referent study in Stockholm. *Int J Cancer* 1990; 46: 985–989.

59 Giovannucci E, Ascherio A, Rimm EB *et al.* Physical activity, obesity, and risk for colon cancer and adenoma in men. *Ann Intern Med* 1995; 122: 327–334.

60 Lee I-M, Manson JE, Ajani U *et al.* Physical activity and risk of colon cancer: the Physicians' Health Study (United States). *Cancer Cause Control* 1997; 8: 568–574.

61 Marcus PM, Newcomb PA, Storer BE. Early adult physical activity and colon cancer risk among Wisconsin women. *Cancer Epidemiol Biomark Prev* 1994; 3: 641–644.

62 Martinez ME, Giovannucci E, Spiegelman D *et al.* Leisure-time physical activity, body size, and colon cancer in women. *J Natl Cancer Inst* 1997; 89: 948–955.

63 Schnohr P, Grønbaek M, Petersen L *et al.* Physical activity in leisure time and risk of cancer: 14-year follow-up of 28,000 Danish men and women. *Scand J Publ Health* 2005; 33: 244–249.

64 Slattery ML, Schumacher MC, Smith KR *et al.* Physical activity, diet and risk of colon cancer in Utah. *Am J Epidemiol* 1988; 128: 989–999.

65 Slattery ML, Abd-Elghany N, Kerber R *et al.* Physical activity and colon cancer: A comparison of various indicators of physical activity to evaluate the association. *Epidemiology* 1990; 1: 481–485.

66 Slattery ML, Potter J, Caan S *et al.* Energy balance and colon cancer – beyond physical activity. *Cancer Res* 1997; 57: 75–80.

67 Thun MJ, Calle E, Namboodiri MM *et al.* Risk factors for fatal cancer in a large prospective study. *J Natl Cancer Inst* 1992; 84: 1491–1500.

68 White E, Jacobs EJ, Daling JR. Physical activity in relation to colon cancer in middle-aged men and women. *Am J Epidemiol* 1996; 144: 42–50.

69 Yang G, Gao Y, Ji B. Comparison of risk factors between left- and right-sided colon cancer. *Chung Kuo I Hsueh Yuan Hsueh Pao* 1994; 16: 63–68.

70 Waterbor J, Colke P, Delzell E *et al.* The mortality experience of major league baseball players. *N Engl J Med* 1988; 318(19): 1278–1280.

71 Giovannucci E. Modifiable risk factors for colon cancer. *Gastroenterol Clin N Am* 2002; 31(4): 925–943.

72 Slattery ML. Physical activity and colorectal cancer. *Sports Med* 2004; 34(4): 239–252.

73 Thune I, Furberg A-S. Physical activity and cancer risk: dose-response and cancer risk: dose-response and cancer, all sites and site-specific. *Med Sci Sports Exerc* 2001; 33(6 Suppl.): S530–S550.

74 Wolin KY, Tuchman H. Physical activity and gastrointestinal cancer prevention. *Recent Results Cancer Res* 2011; 186: 73–100.

75 Boyle T, Keegel T, Bull F *et al.* Physical activity and risks of proximal and distal colon cancers: A systematic review and meta-analysis. *J Natl Cancer Inst* 2012; 104(20): 1548–1561.

76 Boyle T, Fritschi L, Platell C *et al.* Lifestyle factors associated with after colorectal cancer diagnosis. *Br J Cancer* 2013; 109: 814–822.
77 Lund Nilsen TI, Vatten LJ. Prospective study of colorectal cancer risk and physical activity, diabetes, blood glucose and BMI: exploring the hyperinsulinaemia hypothesis. *Br J Cancer* 2001; 84(3): 417–422.
78 Tang R, Wang JY, Lo SK *et al.* Physical activity, water intake and risk of colorectal cancer in Taiwan: A hospital-based case-control study. *Int J Cancer* 1999; 82: 484–489.
79 Will JC, Galuska DA, Vinicor F *et al.* Colorectal cancer: another complication of diabetes mellitus? *Am J Epidemiol* 1998; 147: 816–825.
80 Wu AH, Paganini-Hill A, Ross RK *et al.* Alcohol, physical activity and other risk factors for colorectal cancer: A prospective study. *Br J Cancer* 1987; 55: 687–694.
81 Demers LM, Harrison TS, Halbert DR *et al.* Effect of prolonged exercise on plasma prostaglandin levels. *Prostaglandins Med* 1981; 6(4): 413–418.
82 Holdstock DJ, Misiewicz JJ, Smith T *et al.* Propulsion (mass movements) in the human colon and its relationship to meals and somatic activity. *Gut* 1970; 11: 91–99.
83 Shephard RJ, Shek PN. Associations between physical activity and susceptibility to cancer: Possible mechanisms. *Sports Med* 1998; 26: 293–315.
84 Meyerhardt JA, Heseltine D, Niedzwiecki D *et al.* Impact of physical activity on cancer recurrence and survival in patients with stage III colon cancer: Findings from CALGB 89803. *J Clin Oncol* 2006; 24(22): 3535–3541.
85 Pressel P. Interview with Rolf Benirschke: Ileeostomate and second leading 1980 NFL scorer. *Jet* 1981; 8: 22–56.
86 McGowan EL, Speed-Andrews AE, Rhodes RE *et al.* Sport participation in colorectal cancer survivors: an unexplored approach to promoting physical activity. *Support Care Cancer* 2013; 21: 139–147.
87 Emmons KM, McBride CM, Puleo E *et al.* Project PREVENT: A randomized trial to reduce multiple behavioral risk factors for colon cancer. *Cancer Epidemiol Biomarkers Prev* 2005; 14(6): 1453–1459.
88 Emmons KM, McBride CM, Puleo E *et al.* Prevalence and predictors of multiple behavioral risk factors for colon cancer. *Prev Med* 2005; 40: 527–534.
89 Mehl KA, Davis JM, Clements JM *et al.* Decreased intestinal polyp multiplicity is related to exercise mode and gender in Apc [Min/+] mice. *J Appl Physiol* 2005; 98(6): 2219–2225.
90 Coups EJ, Hay J, Ford JS. Awareness of the role of physical activity in colon cancer prevention. *Patient Educ Couns* 2008; 72(2): 246–251.
91 McGowan EL, Prapavessis H. Colon cancer information as a source of exercise motivation for relatives of patients with colon cancer. *Psychol Health Med* 2010; 15(6): 729–741.

10 Exercise-related transient abdominal pain (ETAP)

Introduction

The "stitch in the side" induced by prolonged and vigorous exercise is well known to athletes, coaches and sports physicians, and it is an important topic with which to conclude our survey of issues relating to physical activity and function of the gastro-intestinal tract. Alternative names for this problem include side-cramp, side-ache, sub-costal pain, and ETAP (exercise-related transient abdominal pain); we will here use the acronym ETAP.

One group of investigators found that more than 60% of runners had experienced symptoms of ETAP during the past year, and that a fifth of participants were affected in any given long-distance running event.[1,2] The condition has a major negative impact upon an athlete's competitive performance, but nevertheless, it has received relatively little attention in the sports medicine literature. This chapter looks at early views, and summarizes more recent information on the prevalence and characteristics of ETAP. It considers differential diagnosis and likely causes, including relationships to the ingestion of food and fluids, before making practical recommendations for its prevention, mitigation and treatment.

Early views on ETAP

Sports physicians and kinesiologists have made repeated claims that the phenomenon of the athlete's "stitch" in the side was described by both Pliny the Elder and Shakespeare (for example[2-5]). However, such assertions have dubious merit. Pliny was suggesting a remedy of dubious efficacy for a condition where the body was arched violently backwards: "For the painful cramp, attended with inflexibility, to which people give the name of opisthotony, the urine of a she-goat is injected into the ears" (Pliny the Elder, Book 28, Chapter 52). Likewise, in *The Tempest* (l. 326–328), Shakespeare has Prospero speak of a night-time cramp, apparently unrelated to any form of physical activity: "tonight thou shalt have cramps, side-stitches, that shall pen thy breath up; urchins shall, for that vast of night that they may work, all exercise on thee".

The condition was briefly mentioned by Mossler in a nineteenth-century German medical text,[6] and was the subject of vigorous discussion during the

1920s and 1930s, with many rival explanations of physiopathology summarized by Kugelmass[7] and Capps.[3] More recently, interest in this problem was rekindled by the research of Koistinen *et al.* in Finland[8] and by Morton and his colleague in Australia.[1]

Prevalence of ETAP

Some reports have suggested that a third or more of endurance athletes are affected at least occasionally by problems of a "stitch" during distance running.[12,22] However, several factors complicate determination of the true prevalence of this condition. The symptoms of ETAP are rather varied and non-specific. Moreover, questionnaires on abdominal symptoms have often been distributed at the end of an athletic event, and with a response rate that has sometimes been less than 40% of race participants[10] (see Table 10.1), it is likely that the apparent prevalence of ETAP was boosted because individuals were more interested to return questionnaires if they were affected by abdominal pain than if they had remained symptom-free.[11,12] Some authors have focussed on the numbers affected during a given event, but others have looked at any occurrence of exercise-related abdominal pain during the entire previous year. In the latter type of survey, there has thus been some confusion as to whether a symptom occurring "rarely" during a year should be regarded as present or absent.[10,12,17] Furthermore, ETAP is by definition exercise-related and transient, but few investigators have enquired about whether those who were surveyed also experienced abdominal pain when they were not exercising. In fact, many of those who have reported abdominal symptoms during exercise also have such complaints when they are sitting at rest.[17] Finally, the upper abdominal pain typical of ETAP has not always been distinguished clearly from lower abdominal pain. Athletes more commonly complain of lower than of upper abdominal pain, and these seem to be two different entities.[23]

Despite these issues, the reported prevalence of ETAP during long-distance walking and running events seems relatively consistent across surveys. A questioning of 848 participants in the 14-km Sydney "City2Surf" event had 30% of runners and 16% of walkers reporting ETAP.[16] Symptoms were less severe and less frequent in the walkers than in the runners, suggesting that motivation to extreme effort may be a factor precipitating ETAP. In contrast, the prevalence of ETAP during a run in Northern Finland was 32% in those covering 10.5 km, 21% in those running 21 km, and 16% in those completing the full marathon course.[8] Here, a higher level of training may have accounted for the lower prevalence in those running the longer distances (the respective weekly training distances for the 3 groups were 26, 48 and 63 km). A third study found a "side-ache" in 19% of contestants during a 67-km ultramarathon involving substantial changes of altitude.[19]

Symptoms of ETAP are experienced relatively equally across a surprising number of sports. A survey of 965 regular participants in 6 different types of activity found that the prevalence of abdominal pain over the previous year was 69% in runners, 75% in swimmers, 52% in aerobics participants, 47% in basketball players and 62% in horse riders, although only 32% in cyclists.[1] Other investigators have also noted a lower prevalence of ETAP in cyclists,[24] and in the cycling segment of a triathlon event.[11,14,17] One factor differentiating cyclists from runners is a less marked oscillatory movement of the body, a point confirmed by accelerometer measurements of body motion made during the performance of both activities.[24] In triathlon participants, the cumulative duration of physical activity may also be a factor, since the running segment of the event typically follows the cycling portion.[11] Sinclair[25] maintained that abdominal symptoms were particularly likely to occur if a person was running downhill, although this view has not been supported by some later work.[16]

Some observers have found no sex differences in the prevalence of ETAP (see Table 10.2), but many have encountered ETAP more frequently in female than in male athletes.[9,10,12,17] The condition also seems more common in young than in older adults, a point noted in three studies[10,12,15] but not in a fourth report.[9] Possibly, the younger individuals exert themselves to a greater extent than those who are older. The severity of the pain was either uninfluenced[16] or moderated[10,26] by training status, and the frequency of occurrence was also less in those who were well trained.[27]

Pain characteristics

The pain was well localized in 88% of those affected, most commonly in the right (46%) or the left (23%) lumbar region, and it was described as an aching (25%), sharp (22%) or cramping (22%) sensation. It was of sufficient severity to cause a deterioration of performance in 20%[9,29] to 42%[16] of complainants, and abdominal symptoms of this type accounted for 23% of drop-outs from a 161-km ultramarathon.[30]

In the survey of 848 participants in the Sydney City2Surf run, ETAP was weakly correlated with reports of nausea, and bore some relationship to shoulder-tip pain, a site of reference for diaphragmatic sensations. However, in the Sydney study, ETAP was unrelated to other gastro-intestinal symptoms such as belching and flatulence.[16] A second report, based on a small sample of triathlon contestants, found a relationship between side-ache and belching, both of which were correlated with one measure of the intensity of effort, the peak serum lactate concentration.[11]

In general, if the problem is indeed ETAP, symptoms are relieved soon after a person stops exercising, but if the pain has been severe, some residual soreness may persist after completion of the event.[4]

Differential diagnosis of ETAP

Exercise-induced abdominal pain usually has a functional explanation, but it is important to exclude more serious chronic disorders, many of which can be distinguished from ETAP because they have a sudden onset in individuals who have previously exercised many times without experiencing a pain of this type. Pointers to a condition other than a functional stitch include difficulty in swallowing, recent weight loss, bloody stools, the presence of an abdominal mass

Table 10.1 Reported prevalence of exercise-related transient abdominal pain (ETAP) in endurance athletes

Authors	Activity	Population	Sample	Prevalence	Comment
Overall prevalence					
Halvorsen et al.[9]	Marathon running	Marathon participants	279/2800 runners = 10% of participants	53/279 = 19% reported ETAP	3% also reported abdominal pain post-race
Keeffe et al.[10]	Marathon running	Marathon participants, 85% men, median age 30–40 yrs	707/1700 runners (41.6% of runners), median running distance 41–50 miles/week	Hard runs 19.3%, average runs 13.9%, easy runs 10.9%	Runners classified as occasionally or frequently vs rarely or never
Morton and Callister[1]	6 different sports	54% male, mean age 28.5 yrs	965/1016 = 95% of participants	589/965 = 61% reported ETAP	ETAP experienced within past year, commonly on less than 10% of occasions
Peters et al.[11]	Running Cycling Triathlon	Marathoners Elite cyclists Elite triathletes	165/177 = 93% of participants 160/191 = 84% 143/201 = 71%	71% had ETAP 45% (cycling) 79% (running)	Lower abdominal symptoms in past year (never vs sometimes (<50%), often (>50%) or always. ETAP not distinguished from other lower abdominal problems
Riddoch and Trinick[12]	Marathon running	Marathon runners, 92% male, average age 34 yrs, running 36 miles/wk	471/1750 participants in Marathon	146/471 = 31% had ETAP	Symptoms more common after hard than after easy run, seen both during and after run
Sullivan[13]	Distance running	Recreational and competitive runners	57 of ?	14/57 = 25%	
Sullivan[13]	Triathlon	Triathletes	110 of ?	39/110 = 35%	

Study	Activity	Participants	Prevalence	Comments
Sullivan and Wong[14]	Distance running	Running club, men and women	31/109 = 28%	Often associated with diarrhoea
Worobetz and Gerrard[15]	Endurance event (swim/cycle/canoe/run)	"Enduro" participants	70 of 119 (59%) of participants	29/70 = 35% reported abdominal cramps
Prevalence in a single event				
Koistinen et al.[8]	Distance running (10.5, 21 or 42 km)	Joggers to national competitors,	230 of 426 (55% of participants)	Stitch in 32% of 10.5 km, 21% of 21 km, 16% of 42 km runners	Performance hindered in 19–16% of respondents
Morton et al[16]	14-km fun run (76% runners, 24% walkers)	Varied level of running experience	848/893 (95% of participants)	ETAP in 30% of runners, 16% of walkers	Performance hindered in 42% of participants who developed pain
Peters et al.[11]	3-h laboratory cycle ergometry and treadmill running	Male triathletes	32 of 32 participants	Cycling 3/32 (9%), running 9/32 27%	Symptoms in final 90 min, similar for those taking semi-solid, isotonic and placebo fluids
Peters et al.[17]	4-day walk, walking 40–50 km/day	79 men, 76 women aged 30–49 yrs	154/480 = 32% of participants	3/154 = 2% developed ETAP	No time loss vs delayed walk vs dropping out; 1 drop-out from "abdominal cramps"
Rehrer et al.[18]	25-km race and marathon	114 initially untrained subjects	44/114 = (39% of participants)	25 km 16% report ETAP Marathon 23%	Same subjects completed marathon at later stage in training
Rehrer et al.[19]	67-km ultramarathon with 1900 m change of altitude	158 men, 12 women distance runners	170/?	32/170 = 18.8% developed ETAP	
ter Steege et al.[20] and ter Steege and Kolkman[21]	Recreational running, 10, 21 or 42 km	Recreational runners, 70% male	1281/2076 = 62% of participants	17% developed ETAP	Internet response up to 1 month after event; most had hardly any vs moderate, severe or very severe complaints

Table 10.2 Possible age and sex differences in the prevalence of exercise-related transient abdominal pain (ETAP) among endurance athletes

Authors	Activity	Population	Sample	Effects of age and sex	Comment
Halvorsen et al.[9]	Marathon running	Marathon participants	279/2800 = 10% of participants	Gastro-intestinal problems more frequent in females. No effect of age	Unclear if sex difference is in ETAP or other GI problems. Mean age 39 yrs; 52/279 females
Keeffe et al.[10]	Marathon running	Marathon participants	707/1700 runners (41.6% of participants), median training distance 41–50 miles/week	Abdominal cramps greater if age <20 yr than if >40 yr; also twice as frequent in women as in men with all categories of run	ETAP occasionally or frequently vs rarely or never. Median age 30–40; 85% men
Koistinen et al.[8]	Distance running (10.5, 21 or 42 km)	Joggers to national competitors	230 of 426 (55% of participants)	No effect of age; symptoms more frequent in women	Average age 32 yrs (10.5 km), 35 yrs (21 km), 38 yrs (42 km); 45 of 230 were women
Morton and Callister[27]	6 different sports		965/1016 (95% of participants)	Prevalence and severity of ETAP decreased with age; no effect of sex	Mean age 28.5 yrs, 54% male

Study	Activity	Participants	Prevalence	Findings	Notes
Morton et al.[16]	14-km fun run (76% runners, 24% walkers)	Varied level of running experience	848/893 (95% of participants)	ETAP more common in women and in younger individuals	Sex differences in pre-event meal. Median age 21–30 yrs; Runners: 186/627 women Walkers: 132/198 women
Peters et al.[11]	Running Cycling Triathlon	Marathoners Elite cyclists Elite triathloners	165/177=93% of participants 160/191=84% of participants 143/201=71% of participants	Lower abdominal symptoms more frequent in young, and in women (with exception of triathlon)	(ETAP never vs sometimes (<50%), often (>50%) or always. Narrow age range, roughly equal numbers of men and women
Peters et al.[28]	4-day walk covering 40–50 km/day	79 men, 76 women aged 30–49 yrs	154/480 = 32% of participants	No effect of age (narrow age range). No mention of effect of sex	No time loss vs delayed walk vs dropping out. Aged 30–49 yrs, 243/480 women
Rehrer et al.[19]	67-km ultramarathon with 1900 m change of altitude	158 men, 12 women distance runners	170/?	Side-ache more common in women than in men	Mean age 40 yrs (men), 35 yrs (women), 12/170 women
Riddoch and Trinick[12]	Marathon running	Marathon runners, 92% males, average age 34 yrs, running 36 miles/wk	471/1750 (27% of participants)	Abdominal cramps more frequent in women and younger runners (<34 yrs)	Mean age 34 yrs; 38/471 women

Table 10.3 A partial listing of conditions that must be differentiated from exercise-related transient abdominal pain (ETAP)

- visceral ischaemia (see text)
- median arcuate ligament syndrome (see text)
- lesions of the abdominal muscles (see text)
- myocardial ischaemia
- pulmonary embolus[31]
- oesophagitis, gastritis and gastro-oesophageal reflux[32–34]
- gastro-intestinal motility disorders[35]
- gastro-duodenal ulcer or malignant tumour[34]
- colonic spasm[36]
- caecal volvulus[37]
- chronic constipation[38]
- ovarian cyst[39]
- splenic infarction
- diaphragmatic rupture[40]
- excessive mobility of the kidney[41]
- renal colic[42]
- acute renal failure &/or rhabdomyolysis[43,44]
- cholangitis[45,46]
- pancreatitis[46]
- stress fracture of the ribs
- chronic inflammatory bowel disease
- intra-abdominal and gall-bladder adhesions[45,47]
- various infections including appendicitis[4,48]

---

and the persistence or worsening of discomfort after physical activity has ceased. A long list of more serious pathologies can give rise to abdominal pain (see Table 10.3). We will comment specifically upon visceral ischaemia, median arcuate ligament syndrome, and a lesion of the abdominal muscles.

Visceral ischaemia

A reduction of blood flow through the vessels supplying the viscera is a normal component of the physiological response to a bout of vigorous and prolonged exercise,[49] and visceral ischaemia may be a factor contributing to ETAP in a healthy adult. Mensink *et al.*[50] found that 48% of 107 patients with chronic visceral ischaemia developed abdominal symptoms during exercise. Often, severe visceral ischaemia is associated with a bloody diarrhoea.[51]

In an elderly person, ischaemia-related symptoms may develop with less vigorous effort, particularly if there is an atherosclerotic narrowing of the coeliac arteries. Demetriou *et al.*[52] described an elderly man who developed severe epigastric pain after walking a short distance. Angiography demonstrated a severe narrowing of the coeliac artery, and the patient's symptoms were relieved by performing an angioplasty to relieve blockage of this vessel. A chronic insufficiency of blood flow to the viscera can be detected by making serial blood gas determinations during exercise.[53]

Median arcuate ligament syndrome

Severe, exercise-related abdominal pain and diarrhoea can arise if the median arcuate ligament compresses the coeliac artery, causing a reduction of visceral blood flow. This syndrome usually includes a history of weight loss and pain after eating, and sometimes compression of the blood vessel causes a distinct sound, an "epigastric bruit" that can be detected with a stethoscope. Symptoms are relieved by surgical division of the ligament that is constricting the coeliac artery.[54]

Lesions of the abdominal muscles

A mechanical strain of the rectus abdominis or oblique muscles of the abdomen, or a haematoma in the sheath of the rectus muscle can give rise to abdominal pain. Although symptoms are sometimes precipitated by a specific bout of vigorous exercise, the pain associated with each of these conditions usually persists and even becomes worse in the period following a bout of physical activity. Creatine kinase levels are elevated following muscle injury, and a rectal sheath haematoma is usually accompanied by scrotal swelling and pain.[55-58]

The gut can also be compressed by a hypertrophied psoas muscle, but this seems more likely to cause diarrhoea than ETAP.[59]

Possible causes of ETAP

Many possible causes of ETAP have been suggested. Disagreement reflects in part the reporting of spurious associations arising from reliance on univariate rather than multivariate analysis of the relationship to postulated causes.[11] Suggested origins include visceral ischaemia, visceral vibration, ischaemia and/or spasm of the respiratory muscles, postural disorders, peritoneal irritation, and psychological factors.

Visceral ischaemia

Visceral ischaemia is one of the older and more popular explanations of ETAP.[6,22,51] It is widely agreed that prolonged and vigorous exercise causes a major decrease in blood flow to the viscera. Moreover, as noted above, severe visceral ischaemia can be extremely painful, and in extreme cases it can damage the endothelium of the gut wall, allowing penetration of endotoxins into the circulation, sometimes with fatal consequences.[51,60] Against this hypothesis, the timing of ETAP seems poorly correlated with the decrease of visceral blood flow that is seen in young athletes during vigorous physical activity.[61]

Some early investigators linked the symptoms of ETAP to a congestion or contraction of the spleen and liver. Benjamin[62] maintained that faulty neural regulation of the blood vessels during exercise led to a swelling of the liver and spleen. However, in reaching this conclusion, he relied upon the very fallible technique of abdominal percussion to determine the extent of liver enlargement, and his hypothesis has now been rejected. Other early investigators argued for a painful contraction of the spleen,[63,64] or splenic tension.[65] There is indeed some evidence that the human splenic capsule contains contractile muscle fibres, and that splenic volume decreases during vigorous exercise,[66–68] but there is as yet no strong evidence that this is the cause of ETAP.

Visceral vibration

Because pain is typically sub-costal in location, and is seen more commonly during running than in cycling, many have espoused the hypothesis that the visceral vibration associated with locomotion places a mechanical stress on the visceral ligaments at their site of attachment to the diaphragm.[25,61,69,70] This tension could be exacerbated by a slowing of gastric emptying and the increase in oscillating mass associated with a fluid distended stomach.[1,61] In support of the vibration hypothesis, symptoms are eased by exercises to strengthen the abdominal muscles, raising abdominal pressure by breathing out through pursed lips, and/or the wearing a supportive abdominal belt.[4] On the other hand, there is a high prevalence of ETAP among distance swimmers, although one might anticipate support of the abdominal organs and relatively little movement of the viscera while a person was swimming. Moreover, the symptoms of the runner are not increased by running on a hard surface or by deliberate relaxing of the abdomen,[4] tactics that seem likely to increase visceral vibration, and fluoroscopy shows no defect of diaphragmatic movement when a person is running following the eating of a large meal.[25]

The abdominal muscles typically tighten as the runner's foot hits the ground, and there is a brief check in body momentum that tends to throw the caecum against the abdominal wall. This mechanical trauma, repeated many times during a run, can thus cause what has been termed the caecal slap syndrome,[71] as well as provoking an excessive movement of the kidneys,[41] with an associated release of prostaglandins[72] and/or vasoactive intestinal polypeptide,[73,74] with resulting pain or discomfort.

Respiratory muscle ischaemia or spasm

Another early explanation of ETAP was an ischaemia and/or spasm of the diaphragm[1,3,4,49] or the intercostal muscles.[7] The idea of respiratory muscle involvement was sparked by the periumbilical/sub-diaphragmatic localization of the pain and the referral of symptoms to the shoulder tip, although the latter feature (typical of diaphragmatic involvement) is seen in only about a quarter of cases of ETAP.[27]

Against any respiratory muscle hypothesis, subjects can engage in vigorous hyperventilation when they are running on a treadmill at near maximal effort.[75] Moreover, blood flow does not seem to be shunted away from the respiratory muscles during vigorous effort, as would be required to cause a local ischaemia,[76] the volumes recorded at spirometry are not reduced with the development of

ETAP,[77] and symptoms are commonly encountered in horse riders (where visceral vibration is considerable, but levels of ventilation are relatively low).[4]

Cramping of the respiratory muscles also seems an unlikely explanation, since electromyographic recordings show no change in the electrical activity of the respiratory muscles coincident with the development of ETAP.[78]

Postural disorders

A long-standing postural disorder might adversely affect respiration, thus causing ETAP. This hypothesis has quite a long history. Herxheimer[70] and Kugelmass[7] both suggested that the symptoms of ETAP could be reduced by teaching patients to adopt a better posture, with a resulting facilitation of breathing. Capps also noted that kyphosis was a factor predisposing to ETAP.[3] More recently, Morton and Callister[79] suggested that spinal problems had a role in causing ETAP. In support of this idea, it was noted that symptoms could be reproduced in many athletes by palpating facets T8 to T12 of the thoracic vertebrae, and that relief was obtained by body inversion.[80]

Nassau[81] developed a somewhat related explanation, arguing that symptoms were caused by a perversion of the normal respiratory pattern. In his view, shallow breathing and a relaxation of the abdomen during inspiration led to a stagnation of blood in the viscera, with a congestion and distension of the visceral organs.

Irritation of the parietal peritoneum

Irritation of the parietal peritoneum can give rise to a sharp and localized abdominal pain,[82] and one more suggestion is that exercise could cause ETAP through friction between the parietal and visceral layers of the peritoneum, causing an exertional peritonitis. Friction might possibly be exacerbated by the effects of ingesting hypertonic liquids upon the lubricant properties of the peritoneal fluid.[1,11]

Psychological factors

Finally, ETAP is most frequently seen in young and inexperienced athletes, and some manifestations of the condition are aggravated by anxiety and competitive stress, suggesting that psychological factors may play at least a secondary role in causation.[12,14,27,83]

Influence of food and fluid ingestion

Several authors have reported that the ingestion of a large volume of various types of fluid can increase the risk of developing ETAP.[11,61,84,85] This question was examined systematically in a study of 40 subjects who reported vulnerability to ETAP.[84] Each individual performed 4 23-minute bouts of treadmill exercise at a self-selected recreational running speed (average 10.3 km/h); 16 of 40 reported

ETAP if no fluid was ingested before or during exercise; 28 of 40 were affected if they drank flavoured water or Gatorade; and 32 of 38 were affected if they drank a fruit juice with a high carbohydrate content and osmolarity. Possibly, the hypertonic drink slowed gastric emptying, thus increasing tension on the gastric ligaments, or it could have altered the composition of the peritoneal fluid. However, the fact that a substantial proportion of the runners experienced symptoms when no fluid was ingested speaks against bloating of the stomach and other side-effects of sports drinks as a major cause of ETAP. Plainly, dehydration can itself cause symptoms,[18,86] and complaints may also be initiated by drinking after a period of dehydration.[29]

Information on the effects of eating a meal before an event remains conflicting. One precursor of ETAP identified in the questioning of participants in the City2Surf fun run was the consumption of a large meal relative to body mass in the period one to two hours prior to the event.[16] Sinclair also observed ETAP in 30 of 35 individuals when they ran in the postprandial state.[25] On the other hand, Stuempfle *et al.* found gastric cramp was less likely if subjects took fluids and a high fat meal prior to an event.[87]

Conclusions

Points can be cited for and against each of the various proposed explanations of ETAP, and further research is required before a definite role can be ascribed to any one or more of these potential causes.

Areas for further research

There are points in favour of and against each of the causes of ETAP that have yet been advanced, and further research is required before the condition can be definitively ascribed to one or more of these postulated factors. Such research is obviously an important preliminary to developing effective evidence-based prevention and treatment of the problem. As yet, most of the proposed antidotes are based simply upon clinical impressions.

In terms of prevention, mobilization and/or manipulation of the thoracic spine has been advocated by some chiropractors, apparently with success relative to placebo treatments.[42,90–92] Others have advocated a stretching of the psoas and quadratus lumborum musscles.[42] However, the efficacy of such remedies requires further verification on larger samples of athletes.

Finally, there is a need to clarify conflicting information on the potential roles of food and fluid ingestion in causing the symptoms of ETAP.

Practical implications for prevention, diagnosis and management

What are the practical implications of current research findings in terms of prevention, diagnosis and management of ETAP?

If what seems to be ETAP should develop, it is first important to exclude any of the more serious causes of abdominal pain listed in Table 10.3. For most of these conditions, a cessation of exercise and medical advice is urgently required. Given that the aetiology of ETAP itself still remains very much under debate, most of the proposed methods of preventing and treating the condition are based upon clinical impressions, and as yet they lack a solid evidence-base.

In terms of prevention, one potentially useful measure is to strengthen the diaphragm, postural and abdominal muscles. A recent study of 50 runners found that symptoms were less common in individuals with strong trunk muscles and a large transversus abdominis.[88] These muscles contribute to spinal stability,[89] and probably influence the extent of visceral vibration. Mobilization and/or manipulation of the thoracic spine has been advocated by some chiropractors, apparently with success relative to placebo treatments.[42,90–92] If confirmed, these findings would place some of the responsibility for ETAP upon spinal dysfunction. Others have advocated a stretching of the psoas and quadratus lumborum muscles,[42] but the efficacy of such techniques requires further verification.

It may be helpful to breathe with a full exhalation, coordinating breathing with foot strikes, and thus minimizing torso movement.[4] Symptoms generally tend to be less frequent in those who are well trained,[34] and thus physical conditioning for an event should be optimized. It also seems wise to limit consumption of food and drink in the two hours preceding an event, and in particular to avoid drinks with a high carbohydrate content,[84] although the findings from nutritional research remains conflicting.

Classical sources of immediate relief for ETAP have been to bend over, to apply local abdominal pressure or an abdominal binder, to breathe through pursed lips, to tighten the abdominal muscles, and to slow the pace until symptoms disappear.[70] If an athlete recognizes the symptoms of ETAP from previous experience, he or she should be advised that there do not seem any serious sequelae to this condition, and where possible they should be encouraged to run through their pain.

Conclusions

ETAP is a frequent occurrence in many classes of endurance event, affecting a fifth or more of participants, particularly younger, less experienced and female athletes during a distance run. It is important to rule out other more dangerous conditions, but ETAP in itself, although painful, does not appear to have any serious sequelae. Athletes who recognize from past experience that they are affected by ETAP can thus be encouraged to run through their pain. Many causes have been postulated, including visceral ischaemia, visceral vibration, ischaemia and/or spasm of the respiratory muscles, postural disorders, peritoneal irritation, and psychological factors, but further research is still needed to distinguish among these possibilities and to develop evidence-based prevention and treatment. The risks of ETAP seem to be reduced by optimizing physical condition, strengthening abdominal and spinal muscles, and avoiding food and hypertonic fluids immediately before an event. A slowing of pace, bending, local pressure and an abdominal binder may give immediate relief. The merits of spinal manipulation have yet to be confirmed.

References

1 Morton DP, Callister R. Characteristics and aetiology of exercise-related transient abdominal pain. *Med Sci Sports Exerc* 2000; 32(2): 432–438.
2 Morton DP, Callister R. Exercise-related transient abdominbal pain (ETAP). *Sports Med* 2015; 45: 23–35.
3 Capps RB. Causes of the so-called side-ache in normal persons. *Arch Intern Med* 1941; 68: 94–101.
4 Eichner ER. Stitch in the side: causes, workup, and solutions. *Curr Sports Med Rep* 2006; 5: 289–292.
5 Morton DP. Exercise related transient abdominal pain. *Br J Sports Med* 2003; 37: 287–288.
6 Mossler F. *Ziemssen's Handbuch*, Vol. 8. Leipzig, Germany F.C.W. Vogel, 1878.
7 Kugelmass IN. The respiratory basis of periodic subcostal pain in children. *Am J Med Sci* 1937; 194: 376–381.
8 Koistinen PO, Jauhonen P, Lehtola J *et al.* Gastrointestinal symptoms during endurance running. *Scand J Med Sci Sports* 1991; 1: 232–234.
9 Halvorsen FA, Lyng J, Glomsaker T *et al.* Gastrointestinal disturbances in marathon runners. *Br J Sports Med* 1990; 24: 266–268.
10 Keeffe EB, Lowe DK, Goss R *et al.* Gastrointestinal symptoms of marathon runners. *West J Med* 1984; 141(4): 481–484.
11 Peters HP, Van Schelven FW, Verstappen PA *et al.* Gastrointestinal problems as a function of carbohydrate supplements and mode of exercise. *Med Sci Sports Exerc* 1993; 25(11): 1211–1224.
12 Riddoch C, Trinick T. Gastrointestinal disturbances in marathon runners. *Br J Sports Med* 1988; 22: 71–74.
13 Sullivan SN. The gastrointestinal symptoms of running. *N Engl J Med* 1981; 304: 915.
14 Sullivan SN, Wong C. Runners' diarrhea. Different patterns and associated factors. *J Clin Gastroenterol* 1992; 14: 101–104.
15 Worobetz LJ, Gerrard DF. Gastrointestinal symptoms during exercise in enduro athletes: prevalence and speculation on the aetiology. *N Z Med J* 1985; 98(784): 644–666.
16 Morton DP, Richards D, Callister R. Epidemiology of exercise-related transient abdominal pain at the Sydney City-to-Surf community run. *J Sci Med Sport* 2005; 8(2): 152–162.
17 Peters AM, Bos M, Seebregts L *et al.* Gastrointestinal symptoms in long-distance runners, cyclists, and triathletes: prevalence, medication and etiology. *Am J Gastroenterol* 1999; 94: 1570–1581.
18 Rehrer NJ, Janssen GME, Brouns F *et al.* Fluid intake and gastrointestinal problems in runners competing in a 25-km race and marathon. *Int J Sports Med* 1989; 10(Suppl. 1): S22–S25.

19 Rehrer NJ, Brouns F, Beckers EJ *et al.* Physiological changes and gastro-intestinal symptoms as a result of ultra-endurance running. *Eur J Appl Physiol* 1992; 64: 1–8.

20 ter Steege RW, Van der Palen J, Kolkman JJ. Prevalence of gastrointestinal complaints in runners competing in a long-distance run: an internet-based observational study in 1281 subjects. *Scand J Gastroenterol* 2008; 43(12): 1477–1482.

21 ter Steege RW, Kolkman JJ. Review article: the pathophysiology and management of gastrointestinal symptoms during physical exercise, and the role of splanchnic blood flow. *Aliment Pharmacol Ther* 2012; 35(5): 516–528.

22 Gil SM, Yazaki E, Evans DF. Aetiology of running-related gastrointestinal dysfunction. *Sports Med* 1998; 26: 365–378.

23 Moses FM. The effect of exercise on the gastro-intestinal tract. *Sports Med* 1990; 9: 159–172.

24 Rehrer NJ, Meijer CA. Biomechanical vibration of of the abdominal region during running and bicycling. *J Sports Med Phys Fitness* 1991; 31: 231–234.

25 Sinclair JD. Stitch: the side pain of athletes. *N Z Med J* 1951; 50(280): 607–612.

26 Brouns F, Saris WHM, Rehrer NJ. Abdominal complaints and gastrointestinal function during long-lasting exercise. *Int J Sports Med* 1987; 8(3): 175–189.

27 Morton DP, Callister R. Factors influencing exercise-related transient abdominal pain. *Med Sci Sports Exerc* 2002; 34: 745–749.

28 Peters HP, Zweers M, Backx FJ *et al.* Gastrointestinal symptoms during long-distance walking. *Med Sci Sports Exerc* 1999; 31(6): 767–773.

29 Halvorsen FA, Ritland S. Gastrointestinal problems related to endurance event training. *Sports Med* 1992; 14(3): 157–163.

30 Hoffman MD, Fogard K. Factors related to successful completion of a 161-km ultramarathon. *Int J Sports Physiol Perf* 2011; 6: 25–37.

31 Ouyang DL, Chow AY, Daly TK, Garza D, Matheson GO. Bilateral pulmonary emboli in a competitive gymnast. *Clin J Sports Med* 2010; 20: 64–65.

32 Moustafellos P, Hadjianstasiou V, Gray D. Postural epigastric pain as a sign of CMV gastritis. *Transplant Proc* 2006; 38: 1357–1358.

33 Kraus BB, Sinclair JW, Castell DO. Gastroesophageal reflux in runners: characteristics and treatment. *Ann Intern Med* 1990; 112: 429–433.

34 Waterman JJ, Kapur R. Upper gastrointestinal issues in athletes. *Curr Sports Med Rep* 2012; 11(2): 99–104.

35 Green GA. Exercise-induced gastro-intestinal symptoms. A case-oriented approach. *Phys Sportsmed* 1993; 21(10): 60–70.

36 McMahon JM, Underwood ES, Kirby WE. Colonic spasm and pseudo-obstruction in an elongated colon secondary to exertion: Diagnosis by stress barium enema. *Am J Gastroenterol* 1999; 94(11): 3362–3364.

37 Pruett TL, Wilkins ME, Gamble WG. Cecal volvulus: a different twist for the serious runner. *N Engl J Med* 1985; 312: 1262–1263.

38 Anderson CR. A runner's recurrent abdominal pain. *Phys Sportmed* 1992; 20(3): 81–83.

39 Liu Y-P, Shih S-L, Yang F-S. Sudden onset of right lower quadrant pain after heavy exercise. *Am Fam Physician* 2008; 78(3): 379–384.

40 Yang YM, Yang HB, Park JS *et al.* Spontaneous diaphragmatic rupture complicated by perforation of the stomach during Pilates. *Am J Emerg Med* 2010; 28: 259.e1–e.3.

41 Leslie BR. Exercise-induced abdominal pain. *JAMA* 1983; 250: 3283 (letter).

42 Muir B. Execise related transient abdominal pain: a case report and review of the literature. *J Can Chirop Assoc* 2009; 53(4): 251–260.

43 Haas DC, Bohnkewr BK. Abdominal crunch induced rhabdomyolysis presenting as right upper quadrant pain. *Mil Med* 1999; 163(2): 160–161.

44 Martinez Lopez AB, Hidalgo Cebrián R, Rivas Garcia A. Otras causas de dolor abdominal: rabdomiólisis aguda en relación con el ejercicio físico. [Other causes of abdominal pain: acute rhabdomyolysis associated with physical exercise] *An Pediatr* (Barc) 2012; 77(6): 352–353.

45 Dimeo FC, Peters J, Guderian H. Abdominal pain in long distance runners: case report and analysis of the literature. *Br J Sports Med* 2004; 38(5): 324.

46 Touzios JG, Krzywda B, Nakeeb A *et al.* Exercise-induced cholangitis and pancreatitis. *HPB* (Oxford) 2005; 7: 124–128.

47 Lauder TD, Moses FM. Recurrent abdominal pain from abdominal adhesions in an endurance athlete. *Med Sci Sports Exerc* 1995; 27: 623–625.

48 Egloff BP, Dombrowsky J, McKinnon H *et al.* Abdominal pain in a marathon runner. *Curr Sports Med Rep* 2009; 8(2): 49–51.

49 Shephard RJ. *Physiology & Biochemistry of Exercise.* New York, NY: Praeger Publications, 1982.

50 Mensink PB, van Petersen AS, Geelkerken RH *et al.* Clinical significance of splanchnic artery stenosis. *Br J Surg* 2006; 93: 1377–1382.

51 Moses FM. Exercise-associated intestinal ischemia. *Curr Sports Med Rep* 2005; 4: 91–95.

52 Demetriou V, Liong WC, Warakaulle D. Exercise-induced abdominal pain: an unusual presentation of mesenteric ischaemia. *J R Soc Med* 2010; 103: 455–457.

53 Otte JA, Geelkerken RH, Oostveen E *et al.* Clinical impact of gastric exercise tonometry on diagnosis and management of chronic gastrointestinal ischemia. *Clin Gastroenterol Hepatol* 2005; 3: 660–666.

54 Desmond CP, Roberts SK. Exercise-related abdominal pain as a manifestation of the median arcuate ligament syndrome. *Scand J Gastroenterol* 2004; 19: 1310–1313.

55 Auten JD, Schofer JM, Banks SL *et al.* Exercise-induced bilateral rectus sheath hematomas presenting as acute abdominal pain with scrotal swelling and pressure: case report and review. *J Emerg Med* 2010; 38(3): e9–e12.

56 Costello J, Wright J. Rectus sheath haematoma: "a diagnostic dilemma"? *Emerg Med J* 2005; 22: 523–524.

57 Johnson R. Abdominal wall injuries: rectus abdominis strains, oblique strains, rectus sheath haematoma. *Curr Sports Med Rep* 2006; 5: 99–103.

58 Jones E, Ho G, Howard T. Abdominal pain in a female runner. *Curr Sports Med Rep* 2010; 9(2): 99–102.

59 Dawson M. Psoas muscle hypertrophy: mechanical cause for jogger's trots. *BMJ* 1985; 291: 787–788.

60 Jeukendrup AE, Vet-Joop K, Sturk A *et al.* Relationship between gastrointestinal complaints and endotoxaemia, cytokine release and the acute-phase reaction during and after a long-distance triathlon in highly trained men. *Clin Sci* 2000; 98: 47–55.

61 Plunkett BT, Hopkins WG. Investigation of the side pain "stitch" induced by running after fluid ingestion. *Med Sci Sports Exerc* 1999; 31(8): 1169–1175.

62 Benjamin K. Zur Pathogenese der Wachstumsblässe. Nervöse Kreisslauffreaktioinen bei Körperarbeit. [Pathogenesis of growth pallor. Nervous circulatory reaction to bodily work]. *Jahrbuch Kinderheilk* 1923; 102: 203 (cited by A Bethe *et al. Handbuch der normalen und pathologischen Physiologie. 7. Blutzykulation.* Berlin, Germany, Springer, 1926).

63 Barcroft J. Die stellung der milz im Kreislaufsystem. Ergebnisse der Physiologie. [The position of the spleen in the circulation. Physiological results]. *Ergebnisse Physiol* 1926; 25: 818–861.

64 Mosse M. Ertrinkungstod und Wiederbelebung. [Drowning and resuscitation]. *Med Welt* 1927; 1: 17 (cited by Kugelmass, 1937).

65 Rautmann HL. Ertrinkungstod und Wiederbelebung. [Drowning and resuscitation]. *Medizin Welt* 1927; 1, 1047 (cited by Kugelmass, 1937).

66 Stewart IB, McKenzie DC. The human spleen during physiological stress. *Sports Med* 2002; 32(6): 361–369.

67 Otto AC, Rona du Toit DJ, Pretorius PH *et al.* The effect of exercise on normal splenic volume measured with SPECT. *Clin Nucl Med* 1995; 20(10): 884–887.

68 Laub M, Hvid-Jacobsen K, Hovind P *et al.* Spleen emptying and venous hematocrit in humans during exercise. *J Appl Physiol* 1993; 74: 1024–1026.

69 Schmidt FA. *Unser Körper.* [Our Body]. Leipzig, Germany, Voigtländer, 1931.

70 Herxheimer H. Ueber das "Seitenstechen" [On the side-stitch]. *Dtsch Med Wochschr* 1927; 53: 1130–1131.

71 Porter AMW. Marathon running and the caecal slap syndrome. *Br J Sports Med* 1982; 16(3): 178.

72 Beubler E, Juan H. PGE release, blood flow and transmucosal water movement after mechanical stimulation of the rat jejunal mucosa. *Naunyn Schmiedeberg's Arch Pharmacol* 1978; 305: 91–95.

73 Opstad PK. The plasma vasoactive intestinal peptide (VIP) response to exercise is increased after prolonged strain, sleep and energy deficiency and extinguished by glucose infusion. *Peptides* 1987; 8: 175–178.

74 MacLaren DP, Raine NM, O'Connor AM *et al.* Human gastrin and vasoactive intestinal polypeptide responses to endurance running in relation to training status and fluid ingested. *Clin Sci* (Lond) 1995; 89: 137–143.

75 Shephard RJ. The maximum sustained voluntary ventilation in exercise. *Clin Sci* 1967; 32: 167–176.

76 Roussos C, Macklem PT. The respiratory muscles. *N Engl J Med* 1982; 307(13): 786–797.

77 Morton DP, Callister R. Spirometry measurements during an episode of exercise-related transient abdominal pain. *Int J Sports Physiol Perf* 2006; 1: 336–346.

78 Morton DP, Callister R. EMG activity is not elevated during exercise-related transient abdominal pain. *J Sci Med Sport* 2008; 11: 569–574.

79 Morton DP, Callister R. Influence of posture and body type on the experience of exercise-related transient abdominal pain. *J Sci Med Sport* 2010; 13: 485–488.

80 Morton DP. Runner's stitch and the thoracic spine. *Br J Sports Med* 2004; 38: 240 (letter).

81 Nassau E. Uber das sogenannate "Seitenstechen" der kinde. [On the so-called side-stitch of children]. *Klin Wschr* 1935; 14: 1252–1254.

82 Capps JA, Coleman GH. Experimental observations on the localization of the pain sense in the parietal and diaphragmatic peritoneum. *Ann Intern Med* 1922; 30: 778–789.

83 Priebe M, Priebe J. Runner's diarrhoea – prevalence and clinical symptomatology. *Am J Gastroenterol* 1988; 79: 827–828.

84 Morton DP, Aragón-VargaS LF, Callister R. Effect of ingested fluid composition on exercise-related transient abdominal pain. *Int J Sport Nutr Exerc Metab* 2004; 14: 197–208.

85 Pauwels N. Bet 1. Is exercise-related abdominal pain (stitch) while running prevent-able? *Emerg Med J* 2012; 29: 930–931.
86 de Oliveira EP, Burini RC. Food-dependent exercise-induced gastrointestinal distress. *Int Soc Sports Nutr* 2011; 8: 12.
87 Stuempfle KJ, Hoffman MD, Hew-Butler T. Association of gastrointestinal distress in ultramarathoners with race diet. *Int J Sport Nutr Exerc Metab* 2013; 23(2): 103–109.
88 Mole JL, Bird M-L, Fell JW. The effect of transversus abdominis activation on exercise-related transient abdominal pain. *J Sci Med Sport* 2014; 17: 261–265.
89 Hodges P. Is there a role for transversus abdominis in lumbo-pelvic stability? *Man Ther* 1999; 4(2): 74–86.
90 DeFranca GG, Levine LJ. The T4 syndrome. *J Manipulative Physiol Ther* 1995; 18(1): 34–37.
91 Morton DP, Aune T. Runner's stitch and the thoracic spine. *Br J Sports Med* 2004; 38(2): 240.
92 Schiller L. Effectiveness of spinal manipulative therapy in the treatment of thoracic spine pain: a pilot randomized clinical trial. *J Manipulative Physiol Ther* 2001; 24(6): 394–401.

Index

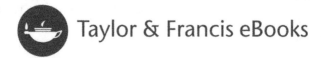

Taylor & Francis eBooks

Helping you to choose the right eBooks for your Library

Add Routledge titles to your library's digital collection today. Taylor and Francis ebooks contains over 50,000 titles in the Humanities, Social Sciences, Behavioural Sciences, Built Environment and Law.

Choose from a range of subject packages or create your own!

Benefits for you

- » Free MARC records
- » COUNTER-compliant usage statistics
- » Flexible purchase and pricing options
- » All titles DRM-free.

REQUEST YOUR **FREE** INSTITUTIONAL TRIAL TODAY

Free Trials Available
We offer free trials to qualifying academic, corporate and government customers.

Benefits for your user

- » Off-site, anytime access via Athens or referring URL
- » Print or copy pages or chapters
- » Full content search
- » Bookmark, highlight and annotate text
- » Access to thousands of pages of quality research at the click of a button.

eCollections – Choose from over 30 subject eCollections, including:

Archaeology	Language Learning
Architecture	Law
Asian Studies	Literature
Business & Management	Media & Communication
Classical Studies	Middle East Studies
Construction	Music
Creative & Media Arts	Philosophy
Criminology & Criminal Justice	Planning
Economics	Politics
Education	Psychology & Mental Health
Energy	Religion
Engineering	Security
English Language & Linguistics	Social Work
Environment & Sustainability	Sociology
Geography	Sport
Health Studies	Theatre & Performance
History	Tourism, Hospitality & Events

For more information, pricing enquiries or to order a free trial, please contact your local sales team: www.tandfebooks.com/page/sales

Routledge
Taylor & Francis Group

The home of
Routledge books

www.tandfebooks.com